The Good News

About Nutrition, Exercise & Weight Control

The Good News

About Nutrition, Exercise & Weight Control

By Dr. Fred W. Stransky

with R. Todd Haight

Momentum Books Ltd.
Troy, Michigan
and
Oakland University Press
Rochester, Michigan

Throughout *The Good News*, we have provided success stories of some of our patients. These are actual case histories, however we have changed their names to protect their privacy.

This book is a collaborative venture of Momentum Books, Ltd. and Oakland University Press.

Momentum Books, Ltd.
1174 E. Big Beaver Rd
Troy, Michigan 48083

Oakland University Press
119 North Foundation Hall
Rochester, Michigan 48309

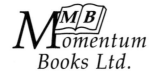

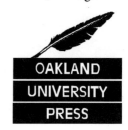

ISBN: 1-879094-35-5, Hardcover
ISBN: 1-879094-66-5, Paperback

Library of Congress Cataloging-in-Publication
Stransky, Fred W., 1947–
    The good news about nutrition, exercise & weight control / Fred W.
        Stransky; with R. Todd Haight
    p. cm.
    ISBN 1-879094-66-5
    1. Weight loss. 2. Nutrition. 3. Health. I. Title: Good news. II. Haight, R.
Todd, 1962– III. Title

RM222.2 .S8535 2001
613.7--dc2l

00-045211

To my inspiration and partner in life, Jeanne, and our children, Trew, Krista and Allison, who each, in their own way, have become my heroes.

Contents

Acknowledgments

Hopefully, as you read this book, it becomes obvious that I passionately believe that for the vast majority of Americans, their quality of life and life expectancy are primarily driven by the way they choose to live. I have been fortunate to be the Director of the Meadow Brook Health Enhancement Institute on the campus of Oakland University. Many of my clinical observations come from the health enhancement programs that emanate out of the Institute.

Our very active Institute Advisory Board has inspired much of the recent success that the Meadow Brook Health Enhancement Institute has had in influencing the health behavior of people in our region. The Advisory Board includes John Modetz, Chairman, Dick Derington, Jim Zboril, D.D.S., Alice Gustafson, John Melstrom, Ted Zellers, Ernie Kosch, Leonard Hendricks, William Potere, Gail Duncan and Andrew Madak, D.O. The Advisory Board, as part of a Strategic Planning Process, strongly recommended that this book be written. Their encouragement, particularly from John Modetz, William Potere, Gail Duncan and John Melstrom, was instrumental in completing the manuscript.

The staff of the Meadow Brook Health Enhancement Institute were extremely accommodating as this book was being prepared. Janet Peabody-Kratt and Ann Besaw adjusted my schedule and supported my efforts to complete this project above and beyond any reasonable expectation. Both Jan and Ann are two of the most dedicated and loyal coworkers I have ever had the pleasure to work with.

Thank you to Gary Kratt, who provided technological support, which made the manuscript preparation efficient and achievable.

Geoff Upward, Director of Communications and Marketing at Oakland University, was responsible for orchestrating the book project. By bringing together Momentum Books Ltd., Oakland University Press and my editor, the project became a reality. His ongoing support of the Meadow Brook Health Enhancement

Institute has expanded our role as a disseminator of preventive medicine education.

Bill Haney, President of Momentum Books Ltd., has a personal commitment to health enhancement. In production meetings, it became obvious that his experience in the publishing business was extensive and that he was highly respected in his field.

Also from Momentum Books, Managing Editor Kyle Scott has been a tremendous support and guide throughout the course of being published. Her expertise and encouragement have been most welcome.

Graduate students in Exercise Science also contributed to the overall project. Special thanks to Sue Hewitt and Toni Navarro for their support and interest in the project.

A special thanks to Todd Haight, my editor, who is clearly a rising star in his field. I look forward to working on many additional projects with Todd, who is one of the most understanding, accommodating and competent professionals I have had the pleasure to work with.

The illustrator for the book, Pam Hardin, is a nationally recognized portrait artist who has made a personal commitment to health enhancement herself. I was honored that she would consider contributing, through her illustrations, to the understanding and enjoyment of reading this book.

Finally thanks, to Yvonne Moses, R.D., the dietician to the Meadow Brook Health Enhancement Institute, for her major contributions to the support materials, which should make application more probable.

Todd gives special thanks as well to Colleen Christopher, R.N., for reading and critiquing drafts of the work, and for Eric Bishop's sharp eyes and fast fingers on the keyboard; to Debbie, Lauren and Rebecca for their sacrifice and patience these past four months; to Momentum Books for opening doors; and to Fred for sticking to his guns.

Introduction

Everyone loves good news. Good news about your job. Good news about your friends. Good news about your family.

Good news about your health.

It's about time you heard some good news about the potential that exists to improve your health. After more than 25 years of helping people lose body fat and achieve enhanced health, I'm ready to help you, too. Not with the same old tirades about what you've done wrong, nor with the empty promises of miracle cures for reducing body fat. No, I can only offer you nearly three decades of research, clinical experience and patient success stories in the areas of disease prevention and weight management.

In *The Good News*, I'll present a lifestyle program that is different in that you are encouraged to determine your own health outcomes. Along the way, I'll explain why the high-protein/low-carbohydrate diet fad may help you lose weight, but potentially at the expense of your health in the long run.

Before we start, though, let me tell you the stories of some people you may be able to identify with. These three individuals started out with high hopes for health enhancement, but ended up experiencing the familiar disappointments associated with dieting.

Meet Shannon, Helen and Brad.

Shannon's Story

At age 26, Shannon weighed 105 pounds, worked out each day at the gym, watched what she ate—and felt good about her physical appearance.

Six years later, her weight had increased to 140 pounds. Now with two children, she was unable to lose her pregnancy weight gain. With energetic toddlers underfoot, she had little time to work out, much less to count calories grams of fat. It was much easier to stop at McDonald's than to look for healthy alternatives.

Frustrated, she began to try the latest diet craze. First the grapefruit diet, then The Zone and Atkins. Life became an endless cycle of diets that worked—for a short time. Time after time, she regained the weight she had lost.

She gave up, then tried again, and then gave up again. And with each attempt, the depression associated with failure set in. She didn't eat right, feel good or look healthy.

And each time she tried and failed, the same question returned: "Why can't I find a diet that really works?"

Helen at 60

For Helen, middle age was a difficult reminder that her body seemed hopelessly out of control.

She had always struggled with dieting and was typically 20 percent above her ideal body weight. Since reaching age 50, however, she found herself more than 30 percent above her recommended weight. At 5'4", she was now 167 pounds. Her body fat measurement suggested she was at increased risk for heart disease, cancer and diabetes.

Helen took the diet counselor route. From Weight Watchers to Medical Weight Loss Clinics, she sampled them all. While some of the weight-reducing programs were clinically acceptable, she still couldn't seem to find the diet that worked for her.

Now nearing her sixtieth birthday, she began to question her approach to weight control.

Could other lifestyle factors, beyond her diet, be contributing to her weight control problem?

Brad, Looking for a Lifetime Plan

Brad was a strong, muscular man, standing nearly six feet tall. Since turning 30, however, he had begun to gain weight. Working nearly 60 hours a week, he no longer had time to exercise regularly.

So, to lose 25 pounds that had subtly appeared on his tall frame, he began the program everyone was talking about—the Atkins Diet. After all, it was being discussed on all the talk shows and written about in the print media. The diet sounded so easy to implement and promised incredible results. Just eat lots of protein and fat—which Brad loved—and lose weight! What could be easier?

But what were the long-term health consequences, he began to wonder. After all, Atkins advocated meals loaded with bacon, hamburger, steak, cheese, eggs—the same foods he always thought would cause high cholesterol, weight gain and cardiovascular problems later in life. How could these foods be good for him?

Even more important, would Atkins' approach help him keep the weight off after he stopped the diet?

Like Shannon and Helen, Brad decided it was time to find a permanent solution to weight control, rather than a temporary fix—a lifetime plan, not a short-term diet bandage.

Good News, Bad News

Our health in America is currently being ravaged by an epidemic of obesity. We're now being romanced by the latest fad approach to weight reduction—high-protein/low-carbohydrate diets.

Sadly, these diets are being promoted by some physicians, health care professionals and best-selling authors. Americans have been seduced by promises they can eat whatever they want while losing weight.

Americans traditionally have fallen for fads. We've made icons out of hula-hoops, yo-yos and pet rocks. Why not fad diets? Why not sell the idea that we can achieve weight loss quickly and effortlessly, all while eating the foods we love to eat?

French-fries? Ice cream? Steak? No counting calories, exercise isn't required and weight loss is "effortless."

What could be easier?

In the last few years, so-called health experts have deluged us with books and well-placed media articles, making these claims that weight control is easily achieved. Bookshelves are stocked with new secrets for losing weight, from taking a pill to reducing body fat while you sleep to products that "vibrate" away fat deposits.

These outrageous assertions are inconsistent with research observations. Many of the claims made by the high-protein/low-carbohydrate diet advocates on today's talk-show circuit are also based on flawed reason, poor research or—more likely—no research at all. In fact, science is more likely not to support their contentions.

Ah, but there is good news to report on the potential that exists to achieve weight control and health enhancement. That's what this book is all about. The time has come to expose the fallacies associated with high-protein/low-carbohydrate diets. Just as important, it's time to offer a healthy, research-supported alternative to weight control that can help you lose body fat safely and increase your life expectancy.

You will learn that your nutritional habits can profoundly influence your risk for developing coronary artery disease, strokes, cancer and diabetes. You may actually be able to reverse heart disease and recover from other health problems just by changing your diet and lifestyle. How's that for good news?

We'll talk about the role of exercise and nutrition in maintaining an optimal body fat content, with a simplified plan to make it practical for you to live a healthy lifestyle. And I'll share 10 steps for living to be a century old (and if you follow these steps, you'll likely be healthy enough to enjoy it!).

Also in *The Good News*, you'll find: an extensive food reference that will make it easy to keep track of your fiber and fat intake; gourmet recipes to support my dietary plan; *The Good News* Food Diary; and meal plans so you can prepare complete meals that not only taste great but also support health enhancement goals for you and your family.

It's time to share *The Good News*.

I

REALITY CHECK— THE TRUTH ABOUT HIGH-PROTEIN DIETS

1

Empty Promises from Modern-Day Sirens

In This Chapter:
- ✔ A brief history of high-protein/ low-carbohydrate diets
- ✔ Our fascination with fad diets
- ✔ Four reasons high-protein/ low-carbohydrate diets are popular

One of the most fascinating stories in Greek mythology remains that of the Sirens. These beautiful maidens, described in Homer's classic, *Odyssey*, would sit on an island's rocks overlooking the ocean and wait for ships to appear on the horizon. Then the creatures would begin their enchanting, seductive song.

The Sirens claimed to possess extraordinary knowledge, which they promised to share with any man who would come to them. This promise was irresistible, making sailors lose their reason and leading them to their deaths on the reefs surrounding the isle when they neglected to navigate.

Ship after beautiful ship, the legend says, was dashed on the shore, drawn to the glorious song of the Sirens.

Today, our nation is captivated by another kind of Siren, one that also promises remarkable knowledge. These Sirens offer something greatly desired by so many in our world today—the promise of effortless weight control. It's an astonishing guarantee that you'll lose weight and stay fit while enjoying any food you want, as much as you want.

Not surprisingly, this fast and easy solution to our obesity epidemic is as deceiving as those Sirens. Just look back at the diet craze of the last three decades, and you'll understand what I mean.

America's Health Roller Coaster

When I began my clinical work in disease prevention almost thirty years ago, the United States led the world in deaths caused by coronary artery disease (atherosclerosis or heart attacks). At that time, more than 40 percent of the calories we consumed were from fat. But a healthier nutritional trend was on the horizon, as research began to demonstrate a relationship between fat consumption and atherosclerosis.

Since then, we've experienced a significant decline in heart attack deaths in the United States. In fact, we've actually led the world in decline in deaths due to heart attacks. This drop is clearly linked to our success in lowering blood cholesterol levels. And we've done that primarily by reducing fat consumption—saturated fats in particular.

Even in the midst of this generation's fried food frenzy, our overall fat consumption has declined. As we entered the 1990s:

- Fat consumption in our nation dropped to 33 percent of our calorie intake. (That's down from 40 percent in 1970.)

- Blood cholesterol levels in the United States decreased from an average of 235mg% in the 1960s to 205mg% in the 1990s.

- Heart disease and stroke deaths both declined by more than 60 percent in the last 40 years.[1]

I have defined in this book some truly good news—a health and lifestyle profile that, if followed, could actually *lead to the end of coronary artery disease* (heart attacks) as a public health issue in our country. Imagine that! A plan to eliminate the number-one cause of death in America. No hocus-pocus—just straight research and clinical findings. One of the core elements of this health and lifestyle profile is a low blood cholesterol level, which most Americans can achieve by adopting a diet low in fat content.

Over the last three decades, fad diets have come and gone. As a disease prevention clinician, I assumed that high-protein diets popular in the 1990s would quickly fade away. I believed that we would resume our national attack on heart disease and related chronic degenerative diseases—strokes, cancer, hypertension and diabetes—by continuing to decrease fat consumption in the United States.

After all, the high-protein diet popularized by the *Dr. Atkins' Diet Revolution* and *The Complete Scarsdale Medical Diet* appeared on the American scene in the early 1970s, yet they seemed to have no impact on our new

Decline in Death Rate Due to Heart Attacks (in the U.S.)

Death Rate (per 100,000 population)

Death Rate

national trend toward consuming less fat. At the same time, it was reported that 98,000 Americans were consuming—as their sole source of food, for at least one month—liquid protein. Remember that fad? You may also recall that fifty-eight deaths were reported among people who undertook those liquid protein diets.

The liquid protein fad came to an abrupt end when such supplemental diets were banned in the United States. The high-protein diet promoted by Dr. Atkins and others also disappeared at about the same time.

So What Happened?

Fast forward to the year 2000. Best-selling books touting high-protein or low-carbohydrate diets resurfaced in the form of *Dr. Atkins' New Diet Revolution* by Robert C. Atkins, M.D.; *Enter the Zone* by Barry Sears; *Protein Power* by Michael and Mary Eades; and *Healthy for Life* by Richard and Rachael Heller.

The proliferation of diet books unsubstantiated by research once again began to get my attention. When I went to the bookstore, I was unable to find a best-selling book that contradicted the outrageous claims being made by many of these authors. Once again, I assumed that with all the weight of science on the side of low-fat, high complex-carbohydrate diets, the high-protein/low-carbohydrate diets would begin to disappear. Instead, it got worse.

Weight control programs that de-emphasize animal products and promote regular exercise require changes in lifestyle and discipline. It's no surprise then that some patients were quickly being seduced by claims that they can lose weight without long-term consequences while eating all the high-fat foods they want—the same foods that had *created* our epidemic of heart disease. The national impact was fascinating; published reports indicated that beef and pork consumption across the country was increasing.

Once again, our nation was being seduced by those charming Sirens.

Two final experiences led to my decision to take action and write this book. I host the weekly show, "The Secrets of Good Health," on Detroit's WJR-AM 760, one of the nation's oldest and farthest-reaching radio stations. Late in 1999, I interviewed Dr. Robert Atkins on the show and asked him specific clinical questions regarding his high-protein diet.

Imagine my disappointment in his responses to my questions and concerns about his diet. He was able to "spin" answers as effectively as any politician. Interestingly, the audience didn't seem to pick up on his lack of clinical and research substance.

Secondly, physicians throughout the country were adopting a high-protein/low-carbohydrate diet for themselves and their patients. They too were caught up in the hype. If physicians could be misled, I knew it was time to set the record straight.

It was time to silence the song of the Sirens.

Our Fascination with Fad Diets

As a nation, we certainly are taken with fad diets. Yet we have failed miserably in controlling weight. Americans, despite all of our technology and affluence, despite our extensive knowledge about health and fitness, are by far the fattest people on the globe. More than half our population is significantly overweight.

How can that be? Many of my research colleagues are convinced obesity is primarily a genetic problem. I often ask these same researchers if they believe all of the obesity genes have migrated to the United States. After all, we're a mixture of people from throughout the world.

Meanwhile, some health organizations actually define our obesity problem in epidemic terms. It has become a cause celebre, a disorder that requires a national program of medical doctors, psychologists, physiologists, and dieticians to resolve.

How easy it would be to blame our obesity on things out of our control, such as genetics, rather than to admit, that the true culprit is lifestyle, something based on personal choice.

The consequences of our poor lifestyle decisions go far deeper. Because of our inability, as a nation, to control body fat content, we idolize people who have the "perfect" body. That makes us easy targets for products or methods that promise to make us look like the celebrity on the weight-loss commercial, no matter how outrageous the claim.

In many cases, Americans are actually willing to sacrifice their long-term health to achieve short-term weight-loss success. We're ready to trade a healthy tomorrow for a phantom perfect body shape today. Except in most cases, we don't even get the payoff, because fad diets typically fail either to take the fat off or keep it off. Now how's *that* for a deal.

Just as concerning, high-protein, high-fat/low-carbohydrate diets promote the foods we learned to love when America led the world in heart disease. Imagine being able to eat cheeseburgers, bacon, eggs, Jell-O gelatin with artificially sweetened heavy cream and lobster bathed in rich butter—and then witness "amazing results in fourteen days." That's the claim by cardiologist Dr. Robert Atkins. Furthermore, Dr. Atkins says his diet will help prevent heart disease!

Suddenly animal fat, cream and butter are heart-attack fighters? This claim has even grabbed the attention of the American Medical Association (AMA), which has expressed grave concerns about the Atkins diet.

Here's what the AMA said:

> *The rationale advanced to justify the diet [Atkins] is, for the most part, without scientific merit.*

> *Council is deeply concerned about any diet that advocates an "unlimited" intake of saturated fats and cholesterol-rich foods.*

> *Physicians should counsel their patients as to the potentially harmful results that might occur because of adherence to a "ketogenic diet."*[2]

Dr. Atkins is not alone, though. Other fad diets have made similar claims over the last thirty years. So how do I explain their increasing popularity and acceptance?

Faulty Reasoning

For the most part, the popularity of these diets is based on a fabricated notion that high-carbohydrate diets promote an *excessive production of insulin*. Later in this book, we'll address this fallacy in more detail.

A Fancy Name, a Slogan and a Celebrity Endorsement

Let's face it, fad diets become popular because of a gimmick. People love to hear that their inability to control weight is not their fault. By correcting a physiological problem or adding more protein to the diet, suddenly they can achieve their weight-loss goals with little effort or health consequences. Not a bad idea—if only it were *true*.

Amazingly, the authors of these high-protein, high-fat diets even get away with denouncing the medical establishment. These diet advocates have even suggested that traditional medicine is *conspiring to keep Americans fat* so that health-care revenues will continue to flow. Dr. Atkins and others, both directly and indirectly, have criticized recommendations by The Senate Select Committee on Nutrition, The American Heart Association, The American Cancer Society, The Diabetic Association and The American Dietetic

Like looking through a different set of glasses

Bill Mountain's health status was never of particular concern. Trouble is, he wasn't close to having optimal health either.

He didn't smoke, drank only an occasional beer and ate meals of the meat-and-potatoes variety. He enjoyed volleyball and racquetball from time to time, but had no regular aerobic activity. Cola soft drinks and coffee were staples.

Bill never strayed far from the path of a healthy lifestyle. Standing 6'3" and just reaching his 50th birthday in 1989, he was 18 pounds overweight—less than 10 percent above his ideal body weight. But he knew the added weight and prevailing stress from his business were a potentially high-risk combination.

Before a health problem developed, he came to Oakland University's Meadow Brook Health Enhancement Institute for a comprehensive physical exam.

"I had heard the Institute was highly into research, studies and statistics of health data," he recalls. "They were not just into the medical side but more into helping you create a healthy way of life. A doctor just tells you what's wrong with you. I hoped the Institute would teach me how to relieve stress and get myself into good condition."

But he didn't take it seriously—until several years later when he found himself 32 pounds overweight. His 34-inch waist had grown to 38 inches.

"I was sick of having to get pants in a 37 or 38," he says. "My blood pressure was up, my cholesterol was in the 280 range and I wasn't doing anything physical. I was a perfect candidate for a stroke or heart attack."

In 1997, at age 58, he returned to the institute. This time he meant business. He was ready to make some simple changes that would leave him, well, uncommonly healthy.

"After my exam, I went in for a consultation with Fred Stransky, the director. He gave me

Association that suggest Americans should eat fewer animal products
and more complex carbohydrates. Some of Dr. Atkins' assertions:

> *The AMA's ad hoc nutrition panel had to phrase it that
> way, because they knew, of course, that they could not
> find any evidence that would have allowed them to
> make a stronger indictment.* [3]

> *We allow them to eat bacon and eggs and butter and
> cheese and meat. And we end up with a better lipid pro-
> file without the medication than they had when they
> were taking it and trying to follow a low-fat diet, albeit
> one as foolish as the American Heart Association
> version.* [4]

several options. I could continue what I was doing and see few results, or cut out the meats and fats a few times a week. Or, at the other end of the scale, I could become a complete vegetarian. He left the choice up to me. It depended on how healthy I wanted to be."

Like most Americans, Bill was raised on a steady menu of steaks, burgers, pork chops, gravy and other fat-laden foods. Vegetarianism had never crossed his mind.

"I had never considered it, never even thought about it. It just wasn't for me. I like my meats and heavy foods. I like butter and desserts, and I love my beer. But I was beginning to see how they were affecting my health. I was tired of putting on weight."

He and his wife decided on the spot to become vegetarians. As they walked out of the Institute, it began to sink in.

"We looked at each other and said, 'What did we tell Dr. Stransky we would do?' But we made a commitment and we stuck with it. We haven't had meat since."

It didn't take long to see results. By summer 1998, he was back to a 34-inch waist—and he's stayed there since.

"I'm 182 pounds again. I've lost almost 30 pounds," he boasts. "I walk four or five times a week, up to four miles each time, at a brisk pace. I was a heavy Coke and Pepsi drinker; now I only drink diet sodas. My diet now includes a lot of water, fruits and vegetables—things I didn't really eat before. And I've cut out all alcohol."

Best of all, he feels great.

"I have the energy to walk and exercise. I feel better about myself and I haven't found the diet to be that different. That surprised me. I don't really miss the foods I used to eat. This lifestyle is interesting, achievable and beneficial.

"Now when I start my day, I've already decided where I'm going to fit in my exercise. It's part of my daily planning. It's like looking through a different set of glasses."

They Work... for a Time

There's another important reason for the popularity of these diets, one that may surprise you: They work. But there's a catch ... they may compromise your health and long-term weight control.

You can lose weight on nearly every diet. By restricting carbohydrate intake, for example, you can lose a significant amount of weight initially, but it's almost all water. Carbohydrate stored in the body is associated with large amounts of water, so a low-carbohydrate diet lowers the amount, and thus the weight, of water in the body.

Surprised? The large rapid weight change you experience with these low-carbohydrate diets, at least initially, is almost all water. Because it's not primarily body fat loss, your efforts—and weight—mislead you. After a period of time, many people regain most of the weight they lost from this initial dehydration. While it is possible to achieve long-term weight loss on these diets, you also have the substantial potential to compromise your health.

They Claim Fast Results

Life today involves microwaves, cell phones and fast food; instant coffee, instant soup and instant tea. Even our children wear beepers! Americans are impatient and want immediate gratification. We know that responsible physicians recommend losing only one or two pounds of weight per week, but we frequently reject a methodical fat reduction plan as being unacceptably slow.

Despite substantial evidence that successful weight loss usually occurs over a period of many months, we want instant gratification.

If America can send a man to the moon, we should be able to create a weight loss plan that produces rapid weight loss with little effort, right?

Enter the high-protein, low-carbohydrate diets of the 1990s.

Time For a Little Pep Talk

The *Journal of the American Medical Association* has concluded that physicians should counsel their patients on the potentially harmful results of a diet such as the one by Dr. Atkins.

With concerns being expressed about cancer and animal fat and protein consumption, what's left to eat? Complex carbohydrates. Isn't it interesting to see so much data that links fat consumption with death and disease—yet there is not *one* study that I am aware of that links complex carbohydrates to the major causes of death, either in this country or anywhere in the world?

So ask yourself one question. Why would you want to potentially sacrifice your long-term health by adopting a dietary plan that's denounced by science and research-oriented medicine? Especially when there is a way to lose weight and get the results you want—lower body fat, better overall health and a better opportunity to prevent the major causes of death in America.

Some people have suggested to me that Americans aren't going to listen to my message. They say you don't want to hear that discipline and effort are required to achieve your health goals. You want a health "silver bullet." On the other hand, millions of people have chosen reasonable dietary plans like the McDougal Plan, Dr. Mirkin's 20/30 Plan or the Ornish Plan—all of whom recommend a plant-based diet.

As I review with you the research linking nutrition to optimal health, I'm confident that you will reject the high-protein/low-carbohydrate diets as just another fad.

I want to get you fired up to make the health and lifestyle choices most likely to enhance your health and feeling of well-being.

Forget the silver bullet—it's a blank.

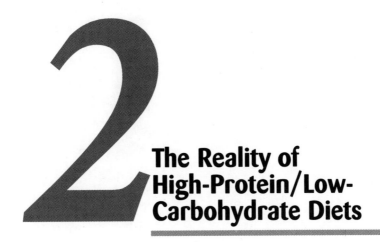

2
The Reality of High-Protein/Low-Carbohydrate Diets

In This Chapter:
- ✔ Lessons from the Pima Indians
- ✔ Weight loss on a high-protein/low-carbohydrate diet
- ✔ High-protein/low-carbohydrate diet health concerns
- ✔ The true key to weight loss

One reason high-protein/low-carbohydrate diets such as the one advocated by Dr. Atkins are popular is they promote the fallacy that eating more carbohydrates will cause obesity and high blood insulin levels.

Tell that to the Pima Indians.

Sometime during the Middle Ages, the Pima Indians split into two groups.[1] One group ultimately found its way to southern Arizona; the other ended up in the Sierra Madres in Mexico. We know both groups share the same genetic roots. You might assume then, that the health status of both groups would be comparable.

Remarkably, there are distinct differences. And why their health profiles are so different offers tremendous insight into the influence of diet and lifestyle on health and disease.

What The Pima Indians Teach Us

The Mexican Pimas, to this day, live a life of physical labor and subsistence farming.[2] Farm machinery is virtually nonexistent and the Indians prepare fields with a plow and ox. It's estimated that a Mexican Pima spends twenty-nine hours every week in physical labor. Also, they eat beans and corn tortillas at most meals, so their diet is high in carbohydrates. They rarely eat meat.

The Arizona Pimas, by contrast, ended most of their farming activities in the 1970s and now average only two hours of physical labor per week. Their diet is consistent with the average American—higher in fat and protein; lower in carbohydrate—than their Mexican counterparts.

Now, the remarkable part. Arizona adult Pimas are, on average, about 60 pounds heavier than Mexican Pimas; in fact, they now have the *highest incidence of obesity in the world*. Nearly half of the Arizona Pimas develop diabetes by age 35, also one of the highest rates in the world. On the other hand, few Mexican Pimas ever develop diabetes.[3] Remember, these two groups have the same genetic roots.

Note the key difference between these groups—lifestyle. Physical activity and dietary differences have combined to create dramatic variances in health status. Americans simply don't appreciate the powerful potential to prevent chronic degenerative diseases, including diabetes, by optimizing their lifestyles.

If a high-carbohydrate diet causes obesity and high insulin levels, as suggested by Dr. Atkins and others, how do they explain this apparent discrepancy? How would you?

Genetically, Pima Indians are more susceptible to obesity and high blood insulin levels (diabetes) than other populations. But while the Arizona Pimas struggle with these health problems, the *Mexican* Pimas have rendered them clinically insignificant—in spite of genetics—simply by maintaining a high-carbohydrate (plant-based) diet accompanied by habitual physical activity.

By studying the Mexican Pimas, we can see that even people who are genetically predisposed to obesity and diabetes can prevent the weight gain that often causes diabetes—if they follow a diet low in fat and high in complex carbohydrates, coupled with regular physical activity.

If you have ever doubted that your diet can make a health difference, the Pima Indians provide very dramatic evidence that it can.

The Japanese provide even further insight into the claim that carbohydrates cause obesity. The Japanese people who live in Japan eat rice, and other complex carbohydrates, as a dietary staple. But those who relocate to the United States and adopt an American diet, which is higher in fat and protein and lower in carbohydrate, tend to gain weight and become more susceptible to numerous chronic degenerative diseases including diabetes.[4]

Again, how would high-protein/low-carbohydrate advocates explain these observations?

But Can I Lose Weight on High-Protein or Low-Carb Diets?

Yes, but you may be compromising your long-term health. For this concern to make sense, let me first explain how you lose weight on high-protein/low-carbohydrate diets.

Initial weight loss, which can be rapid, is unequivocally related to water loss. As I'll discuss later, your body stores glucose (carbohydrate) in the form of glycogen. Remember that carbohydrates require water to be stored in the body, and about three grams of water are stored with every gram of glycogen. When you begin a low-carbohydrate diet, your body's store of glycogen is not replenished and so you lose large amounts of water. This rapid, initial "success" can seem encouraging at first, especially when so many of us have failed so many times in our attempts to lose weight.

Unfortunately, most people assume they're losing *body fat*. It's simply too bad the authors of these diets have been allowed to deceive those who are desperately trying to lose weight.

After this initial water reduction, you may still lose weight due to two factors:

1. High-Protein/Low-Carb Diets Generally Restrict Your Caloric Intake

Caloric restriction, not the nutrient composition of the diet, creates weight loss. In one study that demonstrates this principle, obese subjects were given a diet made up of 32 percent protein, 15 percent carbohydrate and 53 percent fat. A diet given to a similar group consisted of 29 percent protein, 45 percent carbohydrate and 26 percent fat. Each diet contained 1,200 calories per day. The researchers were unable to find a difference in weight loss between the two diets.[5] Other studies have provided similar results.

It's important to remember that the authors of high-protein/low-carbohydrate diets have failed to provide adequate research to support their theories. Yet the authors of these dietary programs sell millions of books without presenting research evidence to support their claims.

2. Appetite Suppression

Dr. Atkins claims his dietary plan creates *ketosis*, a metabolic condition that occurs during starvation and in individuals who have uncontrolled diabetes. During ketosis, carbohydrate is not metabolized (broken down by your body and used for energy). This means your body must take most of its fuel from your fat stores.

Ketone bodies are produced from the breakdown of fat. As ketone bodies accumulate in your blood, acidosis develops. And acidosis, while suppressing appetite, causes bad breath, nausea, headaches, even dizziness in many people.

I find it incredible that Dr. Atkins proudly claims his plan causes ketosis. I've had many patients report these clinically concerning symptoms after trying his diet for even a short period.

On the other hand, a diet that is high in both complex carbohydrates and fiber will make you feel full. Unlike the consequences of low-carbohydrate diets and ketosis, you'll discover only health benefits when you reduce your appetite by eating high-fiber carbohydrates.

Health Concerns Associated with High-Protein and Low-Carb Diets

Are you beginning to get concerned about what these diets can do to your health? Good. You should be. My greatest concern is how many calories these diets would have you eat in the form of animal fat. Hundreds of dietary studies from around the world have shown a strong relationship between the amount of animal fat we consume and blood cholesterol levels. And study after study has demonstrated that high blood cholesterol levels are linked to heart attacks caused by coronary artery disease.

You don't have to be a dietician to know that high-protein/low-carbohydrate diet plans (such as Dr. Atkins') that encourage you to eat all the pork chops, bacon, steak and eggs you want are high in fat—particularly saturated fat, the type of fat that most significantly drives up your cholesterol.[6]

The following chart might help you better understand the physiological consequences of high-protein/low-carbohydrate diets. This health chart belongs to Steven, a forty-nine-year-old man who has come to the Meadow Brook Health Enhancement Institute since 1991 for comprehensive physical exams. For the past nine years, Steven's total cholesterol was no higher than 247mg%; in fact, it's been 237mg% or below since 1992.

But note the changes in his profile when he came to us in January 2000. Suddenly, his cholesterol had jumped to 290mg%! The difference? Steven had started Dr. Atkins' high-protein diet (against my recommendation) only three months earlier. His blood cholesterol level had jumped seventy points since his last evaluation.

Steven was shocked, thinking the diet would *lower* his cholesterol. He quit the Atkins program—particularly motivated by the fact that his father had died of a heart attack at the young age of fifty-five.

	9.3.91	10.6.92	10.31.94	4.9.96	4.3.98	6.26.98	1.11.00		
VITAL SIGNS									
Resting blood pressure	116/68	110/72	120/80	108/70	114/88 130/88	98/72 Post Ex	118/82 116/80		
Resting heart rate		53	51	58	72		60		
BODY COMPOSITION									
Weight (lbs.)	168	177	179	172	179	167	173.5		
Percent body fat M ≤ 15% F ≤ 25%					29.7		23.5		
Recommended Minimum					31.0		NC		
Weight Reduction					31.0 34.0		17.3 NC		
BLOOD ANALYSIS									
Glucose >70 ≤100	86	87	78	86	89	93	80		
Triglycerides ≤75		154	121	162	153	104	95		
Total Cholesterol <170	247	236	224	230	237	220	290		
LDL <100		165	166		159	158	225		
HDL >50	48	40	34	33	47	41	46		
Cholesterol/HDL ratio ≤3.4	5.1	5.9	6.6	7.0	5.0	5.4	6.3		

Steven's health profile chart, which identifies his cholesterol increase.

Had he lost weight? Yes, for a while. But was the weight reduction worth a 70-point jump in his cholesterol? Absolutely not. What good will it do for you to lose weight if (1) you haven't enhanced your health; and (2) you develop premature coronary artery disease from high blood cholesterol levels?

Would you be willing to make that trade?

So Why Do We Continue to Gain Weight?

It depends on whom you ask.

Have you ever heard supporters of high-protein/low-carbohydrate diets arguing that by trying to reduce fat consumption in this country, we've only created further problems with weight control.

How do they arrive at this conclusion? The fact is, some studies do suggest that Americans are consuming more calories in the last twenty years. But there's more to this story.

How We Substitute Foods

When we diet, we typically substitute one food for another. The choices we make, however, will often be our downfall.

In our attempts to reduce fat consumption, Americans frequently choose refined carbohydrates with reduced fiber content. These foods, often high in sugar, are absorbed rapidly in to your blood stream, which creates volatile blood sugars. And low blood sugar, created by refined carbohydrates, is a powerful appetite stimulant. That's right, it makes you *hungry*.

What's more, you can eat all the fat-free food you want, right? After all, we're told to watch our fat intake. Unfortunately, no. Many manufactured, fat-free foods also contain refined carbohydrates with reduced fiber content. Consequently, we feel hungry, ultimately resulting in a high total caloric intake.

At this point, it's important to point out that not all carbohydrates are equal. Many carbohydrates—vegetables, fruits and most grains—are high in fiber. Fiber reduces our desire to eat (this is called the satiety factor). This effect on our motivation to eat has been demonstrated both within and between meals.[7] These foods can help us prevent the major cause of death in the United States and should represent the foundation for any dietary plan intended to create long-term weight control.

Other high-carbohydrate foods, like many fat-free pastries and desserts, have predominantly *refined* carbohydrates. These foods contain carbohydrates that have been stripped of fiber. What's left are simple sugars (or carbohydrates) that are rapidly absorbed into your blood, resulting in an increased desire to eat. If you remove the fiber from carbohydrates, the health benefits associated with plant foods are substantially reduced.

We Forget the True Key to Long-Term Weight Loss

Whether or not you succeed in controlling your weight is strictly a function of calories. A diet low in fat and high in complex carbohydrates offers you the best prospect for controlling weight and preventing heart disease, strokes, cancer, hypertension and diabetes.

Another reason we've failed so miserably to control weight in this country is related to our sedentary lifestyle. Many Americans are reluctant to accept this well-established clinical observation—that the major cause of obesity in this country is lack of physical activity.

Without a commitment to a lifestyle that includes regular physical activity, it's unlikely that any dietary plan will be completely successful in solving your long-term weight-control problem. A physically active lifestyle is the true key to long-term weight loss.

3

A Basic Understanding of Carbohydrates, Fats, and Proteins

In This Chapter:
- ✔ Nutrition made simple
- ✔ The difference between carbohydrates, fats and proteins
- ✔ Blood insulin levels and obesity
- ✔ Causes of death linked to high fat consumption

This chapter probably isn't the most entertaining part of the book. But I'm going to ask you to bear with me, because you need a basic understanding of nutrition and physiology to be able to select the best nutritional plan. Once you understand these nutritional concepts, you'll be better prepared to scrutinize fad diets and recognize dietary nonsense.

Let's start with the basics.

Nutrients

Nutrition, in its simplest terms, refers to foods we supply to our body so it can maintain normal functions. Nutrients are specific food components such as carbohydrate, fat, water, protein, vitamins and minerals. Of these:

- You need protein, vitamins and minerals to build the body structures and chemical compounds necessary to sustain life.
- The only nutrients that supply calories are carbohydrate, fat and protein.
- Calories, in turn, provide energy to function.

Per given amount of these nutrients, fat contains more than twice as many calories as carbohydrate and protein:

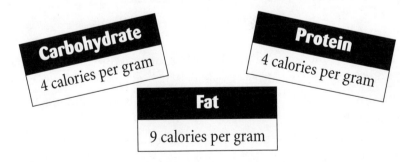

Carbohydrate
4 calories per gram

Protein
4 calories per gram

Fat
9 calories per gram

So, assuming the quantity of food you consume is the same, the meal containing the highest amount of fat will have the highest calorie content. Remember, it's important to understand the calorie content of these nutrients because your ability to change your body fat content is strictly a function of calories.

Let's look at the three nutrients supplying calories to the body—carbohydrate, fat and protein.

1. Carbohydrates

The primary purpose of carbohydrate is to provide energy for the body. The basic unit of a carbohydrate is called a *monosaccharide,* and the most common monosaccharide is glucose. When glucose molecules are combined, they create the most common carbohydrate in our diet—starch.

Glucose is stored in the body in the form of glycogen, and the glycogen supply in your body is stored with water. In fact, about three grams of water are stored with every gram of glycogen. That's why the significant weight loss you initially experience on a restricted carbohydrate diet is actually water.

For glucose to be used by your body, it must be transported through cells with the help of insulin, a hormone provided by your pancreas. After you eat a meal, your body's rise in blood glucose stimulates the pancreas to produce insulin. If your blood glucose level drops and your body becomes deprived of glucose, it will take fat and protein and turn them into glucose so the brain can continue to function. While most of the cells in your body can use both fats and carbohydrates for energy, the brain cannot; it's exclusively dependent on carbohydrates. When the supply of glucose to the brain is inadequate, the brain cells begin to die.

2. Fats

The building block of a fat is the fatty acid, and fats that are stored in your body are called triglycerides. Much of the fat in your body does not come directly from your diet but instead is manufactured in the body.

It's important to emphasize that fat, carbohydrate and protein are converted into body fat when your caloric intake exceeds your caloric expenditure (in other words, when you eat more calories than you burn). Here's the important link with glucose: When glucose is available, your body stops burning fat calories. As long as glucose is available, your body will prefer to use it for energy purposes rather than fat and protein.

High-protein/low-carbohydrate diet advocates have used this observation to suggest that by limiting your intake of carbohydrates, the body's fat stores would be depleted more rapidly and accelerate weight loss. While the concept may sound logical, there is insufficient research support to suggest that it will affect your ability to lose body fat. The amount of body fat metabolized is based on your calorie needs at the time. If you consume excess calories—be it in the form of carbohydrate, fat or protein—the extra calories will be stored as body fat.

3. Proteins

The third and last nutrient providing calories is protein, which makes up about 15 percent of your body weight. The basic building blocks of protein are called amino acids.

Your body uses protein to create cells and new tissues. Typically, you must get at least 30 grams each day to replenish the protein destroyed by the normal wear and tear your body experiences. When you eat more protein than your body needs, it's converted into carbohydrate and used for energy or stored as a body fat.

The pancreas and insulin

You should also understand the role of your pancreas and insulin as you formulate your dietary plan. The pancreas is a gland located just below your stomach that, as mentioned above, secretes insulin and controls your body's glucose use. Insulin released from the pancreas is also sensitive to protein levels in your blood.

Low-carbohydrate diet advocates have claimed that higher protein diets reduce blood insulin levels and, in so doing, increase weight loss. But research has clearly demonstrated that high complex-carbohydrate diets that create weight loss improve (lower) blood insulin levels. So it's actually weight loss that is most important in reducing blood insulin levels. It doesn't matter whether weight loss occurs due to restricting carbohydrate, fat or protein; blood insulin levels will improve if you reduce your body fat.

The High-Protein/Low-Carb Myth:
"Carbohydrates = High Insulin Levels = Obesity"

Academicians and clinicians sucked into the high-protein diet whirlwind have been most influenced by the claim that eating more carbohydrates leads to high blood insulin levels. I realize the next section of this chapter will be more technical, but it's brief—and necessary for you to understand the most important myth associated with diets like the *New Diet Revolution.*

Authors of these diet books claim that high blood insulin levels create obesity and prevent weight loss. What's more, they suggest that too many carbohydrates in your diet will accentuate blood insulin levels.

The truth is, many studies have shown that when you lose weight on a high-carbohydrate diet, you'll actually improve your blood insulin levels. A study by Piatti compared a high-protein diet—made up of 45 percent protein, 35 percent carbohydrate and 20 percent fat—to a high-carbohydrate diet—one that was 60 percent carbohydrate, 20 percent protein and 20 percent fat. The caloric content of both diets was the same at 800 calories per day.[1]

So what happened? Blood glucose levels remained unchanged and insulin levels decreased for individuals on both diets.

Other studies have also demonstrated that both high-protein and high-carbohydrate diets can improve insulin levels. So how can these authors claim that too many carbohydrates increase blood insulin levels when it's clear that too much protein has the same effect? This is a major physiological crack in the very foundation of these diets.

Remember, insulin is released from the pancreas in response to both carbohydrate and protein consumption. Recent research has demonstrated that consuming complex carbohydrates with high fiber content will improve insulin levels in people with an insulin problem. Obesity and lack of physical activity most frequently are the lifestyle causes of high insulin levels.

The suggestion that eating more carbohydrates causes blood insulin problems and ultimately obesity is not supported by research. Obesity causes insulin problems, regardless of whether your diet is high in carbohydrate, protein or fat. Therefore, balancing your caloric intake and expenditure on a daily basis is the key to preventing high insulin blood levels. Interestingly enough, foods with no carbohydrate at all cause fairly substantial insulin responses.

Where's the Beef?

Not necessarily in America. Despite the success of McDonald's and other burger joints in our country, beef consumption has actually declined in the United States over the last 20 years until 1999, when it increased by 3.5 percent. Over these two decades, we had the greatest drop in deaths from coronary artery disease *in the world.*

Wouldn't it be unfortunate to see death rates due to heart disease begin to rise in America because we're adopting these high-protein/low-carbohydrate dietary plans? Based on what we know about nutrition and heart disease, we can predict it will happen unless we expose the myths associated with these diets.

There's more bad news if you have adopted a high-protein/low-carbohydrate diet. In recent years, researchers have established a clear link between animal fat consumption and several serious chronic—and preventable—diseases.

Cancer

Research has documented a link between animal fat and the risk of several specific cancers including:

- Colon
- Kidney
- Ovarian
- Prostate
- Possibly breast

The American Cancer Society recognizes the connection, and now recommends that you limit animal products in your diet.

Osteoporosis

Animal protein has been linked to osteoporosis, a gradual weakening of the bones associated with a loss of calcium from your skeletal system. Recent research suggests that animal protein, such as meat, can cause calcium to be leached from bone. The building blocks of protein are amino acids, so in essence, protein metabolism (when your body breaks down the protein) is an acid-producing process.

The pH of your body (the measure of acidity and alkalinity) ranges from neutral to slightly alkaline (basic). Your body maintains an acid-base balance through a buffering system that involves the skeletal system (bones). Phosphorus in your bones combines with calcium to form alkaline phosphates, which helps your body neutralize the acid-producing protein (which would otherwise cause death). The calcium used in this complex biochemical process is taken from your bones and excreted by your kidneys.

The bottom line? The ultimate impact of a high-protein diet can be a loss of bone density and, ultimately, osteoporosis.

In fact, population studies have uncovered the strong link between bone fractures and protein:

- The African Bantu have a very low-protein diet and consume an average of 350 mg of calcium per day (Americans are asked to consume between 1,000 mg and 1,500 mg of calcium daily). Calcium deficiencies and bone fractures are rare with the Bantu.
- Eskimos consume a diet high in fat and protein and have the highest incidence of osteoporosis in the world, even though their diet is also very high in calcium.
- The Chinese have a diet much higher in carbohydrate and lower in protein and calcium, yet have one of the lowest rates of osteoporosis.[2]

In one study, young adults ate 48 grams of protein and 500 mg of calcium every day, yet researchers saw no net loss of calcium. On the other hand, subjects who ate 112 grams of protein and 1,400 mg of calcium per day lost substantial amounts of calcium in their urine.[3]

The *Nurse's Health Study* reported that women who consumed higher amounts of protein had a greater risk of forearm fractures.[4] The type of protein you eat appears to be an important factor in calcium excretion. For instance, research has demonstrated that soy protein does not stimulate calcium excretion, even when you eat high amounts.[5]

What's more, your body can better absorb calcium from plant sources than animal/dairy products. So vegetarians require less calcium in their diet than people who include animal products in their diet.

Kidney Concerns (Uric Acid, Gout, Kidney Stones and Kidney Function)

If you're thinking of trying a high-protein diet, you should also be concerned about elevated uric acid levels, which can lead to gout and kidney stones. Dr. John P. Foreyt, Director of the Nutrition Research Clinic at Baylor College of Medicine, is just one expert who has expressed concern about the effect of high-protein diets on long-term kidney function.

> *Too much protein can also tax the kidneys, which go into overdrive trying to process and excrete the nitrogen in protein.*[6]

Some reports suggest that residents of affluent nations lose kidney function as they get older, and link this concern to the amount of protein they consume.[7]

You should now have a good foundation for understanding the basic nutritional and physiological misconceptions associated with high-protein/low-carbohydrate diets. In the next chapter, we're going to address specific claims by the most popular high-protein/low-carbohydrate diet on the market—and we'll compare these claims to the body of research information.

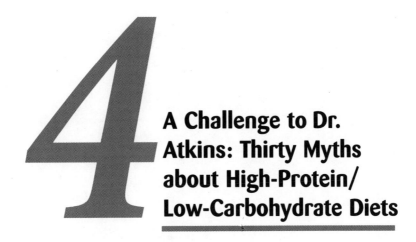

4 A Challenge to Dr. Atkins: Thirty Myths about High-Protein/Low-Carbohydrate Diets

In This Chapter:
- ✔ A summary of the Atkins plan
- ✔ Two reasons people turn to high-protein/low-carbohydrate diets

There's no question that high-protein/low-carbohydrate diets are currently the rage in American fad diets. And perhaps no author promoting these diets has sold more books than Dr. Robert C. Atkins. His dietary plan, *Dr. Atkins' New Diet Revolution*, is a runaway bestseller. He is clearly considered the guru and media darling of this type of diet.

A Review of the Atkins Plan

In his own words, Dr. Atkins' plan:

- Sets no limit on the amount of food you can eat

- Completely excludes hunger from the dieting experience

- Includes foods so rich that you've never seen them on any other diet

- Reduces your appetite by a perfectly natural function of the body (ketosis)

- Gives you a metabolic edge so significant that the whole concept of watching calories will become absurd to you

- Produces steady weight loss, even if you have experienced dramatic failures or weight regain on other diets

- Is so perfectly adapted to use as a lifetime diet that, unlike most diets, the lost weight won't come back

- Consistently produces improvements in most of the health problems that accompany overweight.[1]

Some interesting claims by Dr. Atkins.

Now consider the food selections for breakfast, lunch and dinner that Dr. Atkins includes in his "Typical Induction Menu" (shown on the following page, using Dr. Atkins' own words).

Breakfast
Eggs, scrambled or fried
Bacon, ham, sugarless sausage or Canadian bacon
Decaffeinated coffee or tea

Lunch
Bacon cheeseburger, no bun
Small tossed salad
Seltzer water

Dinner
Shrimp cocktail with mustard and mayo
Clear consommé
Steak, roast, chops, fish or fowl
Tossed salad (choice of dressings)
Diet Jell-O with a spoonful of whipped, artificially sweetened heavy cream[2]

Fad Diets: What's New and What's True?

I'm particularly concerned with the number of physicians who have either tried the diet themselves or advocated it for their patients. Physicians tend to make medical decisions based on clinical trials, yet the fact that Dr. Atkins has failed to report research to support his claims seems to be of little concern and is ignored. I'm even more concerned about the number of cardiac and diabetic patients who are considering or have already started a high-protein/low-carbohydrate diet.

Through my work at Oakland University's Meadow Brook Health Enhancement Institute and during speaking engagements across the country, I've received hundreds of requests to provide my perspective on *Dr. Atkins' New Diet Revolution*. Even within the university at which I work, people seem to be talking about a family member, friend or colleague who is on the diet. Many I've spoken with are concerned about a spouse, child or friend who is on the diet. Intuitively, they seem to know they should be concerned about any dietary plan that encourages unlimited amounts of meat and other animal products.

While Dr. Atkins is not the sole proponent of such plans, he is one of the most visible, so we will expose his dietary theories by addressing specific claims he has made in interviews, on my radio show and in his book. I hope this information will also help the many physicians and other health care providers who need to be able to explain why Dr. Atkins' diet is based on a series of fallacies.

Remember, there are two important reasons why we fall prey to fad diets:

- Often, we've failed many times to lose and maintain weight loss on other dietary programs. This makes us more vulnerable to the latest fad diet.

- Dr. Atkins has created a weight loss theory that sounds so logical it becomes seductive to the chronic dieter.

Let's scrutinize thirty of Dr. Atkins' positions or statements, and analyze them based on current research.

Fallacy #1: *"A person who has trouble gaining weight requires fat."*[3]

Reality Check: You can gain weight by increasing your lean body weight or adding to your body's store of fat (adipose tissue). But you can only gain weight by eating more calories than you burn off. Whether the extra calories come in the form of fat, protein or carbohydrate is irrelevant.

Dr. Atkins is a cardiologist, so the recommendation that anyone should eat more fat is quite surprising, as it contradicts the dietary guidelines developed by the American Heart Association and the American Medical Association and can lead to degenerative diseases.

Fallacy #2: *"A person with an unstable blood glucose will learn that the only one of the three major food groups that stabilizes blood sugar is fat."*[4]

Reality Check: The fundamental cause of Type II diabetes, seen so frequently in the United States, is physical inactivity and too much body fat.[5] The insulin resistance that develops in this form of diabetes has been linked nutritionally to a high-fat diet.[6] As long you remain overweight and inactive, you simply can't stabilize your blood glucose by eating more fat.[7]

Based on well-supported research, diabetics who add more fat to their diet most likely will increase their blood cholesterol level and further accelerate atherosclerosis. In fact, diabetics frequently die prematurely of plaque-narrowed arteries.[8] The average diabetic will develop atherosclerosis 8.3 years earlier than non-diabetics. How can eating more fat possibly be helpful?

Interestingly enough, eating more fiber (carbohydrate) is a nutritional element that can *lower* insulin levels. Recently, in one of the world's most respected medical journals, researchers concluded that "high-fiber diets may protect against obesity and cardiovascular disease by lowering insulin levels."[9]

Fallacy #3: *"The whole idea that egg yolks and meat are dangerous is totally without evidence. Let's just go back to the 1920s. Dr. Paul Dudley White ... reported that he had not seen a single heart attack—even though he had an EKG machine—between 1921 and 1928. Back then people ate plenty of egg yolks and plenty of meat. The fat that they used was mainly lard. They used butter, they used tallow, and they didn't use polyunsaturated fats. And they had no heart disease. Therefore, the burden of proof would be on the person who says that foods that were consumed in the 19th century cause heart disease."[10]*

Reality Check: Hundreds of respected scientific studies have linked meat and animal products to coronary artery disease.

Atkins' claim also makes the erroneous assumption that all things are equal between the early twentieth century and the present, even causes of death and life expectancy.

You see, in the early 1900s, the major causes of death were infectious. Americans died more frequently from influenza, pneumonia and tuberculosis than heart disease. Also, coronary artery disease most often manifests itself after the age of 50, but life expectancy in 1900 was only forty-seven years. So at the turn of the century, the average American died before reaching the age when heart attacks are most likely to occur. Perhaps Dr. White didn't see heart attacks because his patients were not living long enough to develop coronary artery disease!

Today, life expectancy is approximately seventy-six years. As we live longer, heart disease has become a more common cause of death. (It's now number one in our nation.)

In the late 1960s, the United States, along with several other nations, led the world in deaths due to coronary artery disease. At the same time, more than 40 percent of the calories in the American diet came from fat. Research observation suggests that these two statistics are directly linked.

Since then, we have led the world in decline in deaths due to coronary artery disease. Over the same three decades:

- The percentage of calories we consume in the form of fat has decreased from 40 percent to approximately 33 percent.

- Death rates due to heart attacks have plummeted by more than 60 percent.

- Strokes caused by narrowed arteries in the brain have also dropped more than 60 percent.

- Average cholesterol levels have decreased from about 235mg% to the current 205mg%. Studies have demonstrated that for every percent blood cholesterol decreases within a population, deaths due to coronary artery disease drop by two percent.

Many studies have concluded that the drop in blood cholesterol levels we've seen in the United States has been due to reduced fat consumption.

Fallacy #4: *"In our center, when people are put on the low-carbohydrate diet, they are able to go off the cholesterol-lowering medications they come to us with. We allow them to eat bacon and eggs and butter and cheese and meat. And we end up with a better lipid profile without the medication than they had when they were taking it and trying to follow a low-fat diet, albeit one as foolish as the American Heart Association version."*[11]

Reality Check: The truth is, studies around the world have demonstrated an unequivocal relationship between blood cholesterol levels and the percentage of calories you eat in the form of fat.[12]

This claim by Dr. Atkins is one of many he bases on *observations* of his patients. Yet he has never presented data collected in an acceptable scientific method, nor has he provided such data to any scientific group.

If you're trying to lower your cholesterol level and avoid coronary artery disease, both research and common sense suggest the stakes are too high to accept such a radical position and to begin eating more animal fat. Animal studies, population studies and clinical trials all have demonstrated that your cholesterol level will rise as you eat more fat calories. (Remember Steven, my patient from chapter two?)

Lastly, new medications that lower blood cholesterol levels have also dramatically reduced death rates due to coronary artery disease. They are quite literally saving lives. It is irresponsible to suggest that people who adopt the *Dr. Atkins' New Diet Revolution* can eliminate the need for cholesterol-reducing medication by eating more animal fat.

Fallacy #5: *"Word of mouth has gotten my book up to five million readers ... Is the observation of 60,000 patients with before and after results unscientific?"* [13]

Reality Check: Yes, it is absolutely unscientific.

How does Dr. Atkins know that 60,000 patients have benefited from his diet? There is simply *no way* to make such a claim without analyzing data. And if he has truly determined that 60,000 patients have benefited from his diet, why doesn't he present the information like most responsible clinicians do? This point is extremely important because of the long-term health implications high-protein/low-carbohydrate diets could have on the health status of the American population.

Many people I have talked to indicate that they believe Dr. Atkins, as a cardiologist, couldn't possibly recommend a dietary plan that was not in their best interest. They've been strongly influenced by the fact that he is a physician. And clearly, any physician who chooses to tell people they can reduce their risk of heart disease while eating unlimited amounts of bacon, cheese, hamburgers and eggs is likely to sell a lot of books.

Fallacy #6: *"There are only two kinds of medicine—proven and unproven. I'm happy to say that the unproven medicine could easily be the one that works better."* [14]

Reality Check: Are you ready to ignore research and medical fact? Are you willing to be the one who will try this "unproven medicine" without knowing the true long-term impact on your health?

When you consider Dr. Atkins' slam on traditional medicine, you should also remember that the United States is *the envy of the world* with respect to medical advances.

As I mentioned earlier, life expectancy over the last century has increased from forty-seven years to seventy-six years. Our advances in medicine have generally resulted from clinical trials and research. To demean this system that has increased our life expectancy and vastly improved our quality of life appears to be an attempt to appeal to vulnerable people who have not achieved health benefits from traditional medicine.

Fallacy #7: *"Obesity is not an accidental accumulation of extra ounces, it is a basic metabolic disorder intimately related to ill health."* [15]

Reality Check: How does this explain the epidemic of obesity across our country? The United States is made up of people from all over the world, so is Dr. Atkins suggesting that all of the obesity genes and metabolic problems have migrated to the United States?

As you saw in the last chapter, Dr. Atkins' claim that carbohydrates in the American diet have created metabolic abnormalities leading to obesity is not supported by research, especially when you consider the populations around the world that consume even more carbohydrate and less protein than we do and yet are much leaner. No, the major reason we struggle with our weight in this country is much simpler and less controversial—inactivity. Again, any weight loss plan that fails to include an exercise component is unlikely to be effective.

In advanced nations, people don't have to be as active physically to earn a living. The Pima Indians, described in chapter two, offer us one of the best examples of how advancing technology and less physical activity lead to obesity.

Fallacy #8: *"When I wrote my original bestseller, Diet Revolution, twenty years ago, I was chiefly concerned about showing people how to lose weight quickly, easily, and without much pain or bother."* [16]

Reality Check: Fad diet authors frequently use phrases such as "lose weight quickly, easily, and without pain or bother." But people who lose weight rapidly tend to have a higher failure rate in the long run.

Given our technologically advanced society, controlling weight through physical activity will continue to require more determination and effort. Past generations were forced to be more physically active because they didn't have the time-savers and effort-savers we enjoy today—luxuries like cars, power tools and vacuum cleaners. Nowadays, people have to schedule time for regular exercise to make up for our occupational and social inactivity. Those who don't will suffer health problems linked to inactivity.

Fallacy #9: *"[The Atkins Diet] sets no limit on the amount of food you can eat."* [17]

Reality Check: Suggesting that we can eat unlimited amounts of food simply fails to take into consideration why Americans too often choose to eat.

Unfortunately, we don't always eat just when we're hungry. We eat because of environmental factors, physiological circumstances or external cues. For example, many of us eat when we're stressed or depressed. Others eat from boredom or link food with TV or sports watching. In modern America, eating is interwoven with our social activities and cultural priorities. There are ways to modify our eating behaviors, and we'll discuss them in a later chapter.

The American Medical Association has expressed concern about any diet that advocates an unlimited intake of saturated fats and cholesterol-rich foods, because of the long-term concerns for increasing death rates due to stroke and heart attacks.[18]

Limits are a healthy and vital part of our lives. Be wary of anyone who tells you to ignore the limits you know are right within your life.

Fallacy #10: *"[The Atkins Diet] reduces your appetite by a perfectly natural function of the body."*[19]

Reality Check: The high-protein/low-carbohydrate diet advocated by Dr. Atkins actually creates an UNNATURAL physiological state called ketosis in which the body actually thinks it is starving to death. Ketosis can cause bad breath, lightheadedness, dizziness, fatigue and fainting. Starvation is not natural. It's so unnatural, in fact, that many physicians who understand the health consequences of being in ketosis will actually recommend that you be under medical supervision if you implement this type of diet.

Fallacy #11: *"A carbohydrate-restricted diet is so effective at dissolving adipose tissue that it can create fat loss greater than occurs in fasting."*[20]

Reality Check: Studies have consistently demonstrated that populations consuming the highest amount of complex carbohydrates tend to be the leanest people in the world. They also tend to have the highest caloric expenditures. We know that all weight control is a function of calories, so to imply that restricting carbohydrate will mysteriously promote the loss of body fat is not supported by research.

In one study, for example, women were placed on three different 1,200-calorie diets and followed for ten weeks. The diets consisted of 25 percent, 45 percent or 75 percent carbohydrate, with variations in fat and protein. While weight loss occurred on all three diets, no significant difference was noted on any of the diets.[21]

Fasting, while not recommended as a weight control approach, is the most restrictive way to reduce calorie intake and decrease adipose (fat) tissue. I know of no research that supports the claim that a carbohydrate-restricted diet will produce greater fat loss than fasting. Body fat loss occurs in a predictable manner based on caloric intake, regardless of the composition of nutrients.[22]

Fallacy #12: *"It's not that calories don't count, it's just that you can, in fact, sneak them out of your body, unused or dissipated as heat."*[23]

Reality Check: Dr. Atkins suggests that his dietary plan defies the physical law of thermogenesis. If you could figure out how to sneak calories out of your body, that secret alone would make you a very rich person indeed!

Fallacy #13: *"People with a less than average degree of metabolic resistance will lose anywhere from 8 to 15 pounds in two weeks on the diet; people with an average level, somewhat less."*[24]

Reality Check: Suppose you were able to go a week without consuming even one calorie. How much *body fat* would you lose? Surprisingly, only about four pounds for the entire week. So an 8- to 15-pound weight loss in two weeks, promised by Dr. Atkins, would be predominantly water loss, if it occurred at all. As mentioned in chapter two, your body stores carbohydrate as glycogen. For every gram of glycogen you deplete by restricting carbohydrates, you lose three grams of water.

Fallacy #14: *"When your body is releasing ketones—which it will do in your breath and your urine—that is chemical proof that you're consuming your own stored fat."*[25]

Reality Check: You don't have to be in ketosis to burn body fat. Any time you experience a caloric deficit, your body will take energy from stored body fat.

Fallacy #15: *"I've treated people who, on 700 or 800 balanced calories a day, couldn't lose weight.... And yet they lost weight when they were placed on ketogenic diets of even more calories."*[26]

Reality Check: Of course they lost weight initially—because of water loss. When we start talking about losing body fat, studies clearly demonstrate that it's directly proportional to caloric intake, regardless of the nutrients you're eating (note the study referenced in Fallacy #11).[27]

Fallacy #16: *"In other words, this diet will give you an edge, what in scientific lingo would be called a metabolic advantage. That's what will enable you to lose weight on the Atkins diet eating the same number of calories you used to gain on."*[28]

Reality Check: Weight loss on his diet occurs because of water loss and burning more calories than you consume.

It would be easy for Dr. Atkins to demonstrate the credibility of this claim by simply presenting data collected from his clinic in a scientifically accepted method. He is either unwilling or unable to do so.

It's important to remember that you can lose weight with any dietary plan that restricts caloric intake. Ultimately, however, you have to consider the health consequences and benefits of that plan.

Unfortunately, Americans have demonstrated, time after time, that they are willing to sacrifice their health to achieve weight loss goals. This is best demonstrated by the popularity of medications people take to lose weight, even though they ultimately result in adverse health consequences. Too many people say, "Give me a pill or a no-effort way to lose weight and I'll be ready to start my weight loss program."

Fallacy #17: *"I hate to be so cynical as to suggest that proper diet might adversely affect the thoroughly profitable administration of insulin and oral diabetic drugs, but I will certainly say that if sugar and high-carbohydrate diets were denounced from the scientific pulpits as if they were sin, it would seriously compromise a mutually supportive food and pharmaceutical industrial cartel."* [29]

Reality Check: To suggest such a conspiracy in the face of scientific evidence is outrageous. But speaking of profits, read on.

Fallacy #18: *"I have made a delicious, very low-carbohydrate, high-protein energy bar available to my patients and the public. Called The Atkins Diet Advantage Bar™, it contains a small amount of glycerine, which makes it ideal for getting people 'over the hump' when the blood sugar needs to be stabilized."* [30]

Reality Check: Dr. Atkins is able to get away with this claim because his Advantage Bar is considered a "food supplement." If the FDA regulated the product, he would be required to demonstrate that the suggested benefits could be measured.

Fallacy #19: *"I wish I could invite you all to study the case records of the Atkins Center."* [31]

Reality Check: The implication here is that the patient files within the Atkins Center contain proof of all the claims of health benefits associated with the Atkins diet. The Atkins Center has never presented data to trained researchers who could validate the benefits in a scientifically acceptable method.

Fallacy #20: *"I actually treat cardiac patients with probably more success on this diet as Dr. Dean Ornish claims (I'm sure truthfully) for the patients whom he treats on a wildly different diet, an extreme low-fat, vegetarian diet."* [32]

Reality Check: Dr. Dean Ornish, to his great credit, has published his results in professional journals. If anyone was forced to overcome great odds in challenging traditional medicine, it was Dr. Ornish. He undertook the proper research necessary to support his dietary plan. Dr. Atkins, on the other hand, asserts that working with patients is equivalent to conducting research.

How is it that a vegetarian diet—the opposite of the Dr. Atkins diet—has demonstrated such remarkable cardiovascular benefits? Dr. Atkins, with a diet that's unsubstantiated scientifically, is actually claiming many of the benefits that Dr. Ornish *confirmed* with his research. The vast majority of research conducted worldwide supports the observation that Dr. Ornish has made—deaths from heart attacks and its complications will decrease as we eat less animal fat.

Fallacy #21: *"The nutritional pharmacology is part of the reason behind our patients' success, as is chelation therapy."*[33]

Reality Check: The American Heart Association has reviewed the available literature on the use of chelation (EDTA, or ethylenediamine tetra-acetic acid) in treating atherosclerotic heart disease. They found no scientific evidence to demonstrate any benefit from this form of therapy.[34]

Stephen Barrett, M.D., a national expert on medical quackery, has warned about the dangers of treating atherosclerosis with chelation therapy.[35]

Fallacy #22: *"Insulin—the hormone that makes you fat."*[36]

Reality Check: Several theories have been used to promote high-protein/low-carbohydrate diets. One such theory suggests that consuming carbohydrate will increase your blood insulin levels, causing insulin resistance and preventing glucose from being converted into energy. This process would ultimately transfer the glucose (carbohydrate) into stored fat and lead to obesity. At this point, according to Dr. Atkins, your body would like to slim down but has become a fat-producing machine.

To support their positions, high-protein/low-carbohydrate diet advocates, including Dr. Atkins, have cited research conducted by Dr. Gerald Reaven, Professor of Medicine at Stanford University.

Interestingly enough, when Dr. Reaven was asked if insulin resistance causes obesity, he replied, "Absolutely not. Years ago, we put people with different degrees of insulin resistance on dramatically different diets—in one study, carbohydrates were either 85 percent or 17 percent of calories. The only thing that affected their weight was how many calories they ate. More recently, we've published long-term studies showing that weight gain is unrelated to how insulin-resistant people were when the studies began. And weight loss with low calorie diets is also unrelated to the degree of insulin resistance. So there's not one shred of evidence that insulin resistance causes obesity." [37]

Fallacy #23: *"Add to that [antioxidants] the vita-nutrients known to be useful for each of the myriad medical problems my patients face, and you'll see why many of them take over 30 vitamin pills each day."*[38]

Reality Check: Can you imagine taking thirty pills a day? Just think of the potential negative interaction among supplements. It is far better to consume the fruits, vegetables and grains in their natural form rather than supplements, which contain extracted nutrients.

In their own wonderful way, plants offer great health benefits because they have the ability to biochemically integrate nutrients, something science has never been able to replicate in supplements. Maybe that's why one respected nutritional scientist once said to me, "If you want to consume one of the best supplements for health benefits, eat a strawberry."

Fallacy #24: *Referring to the Atkins Diet: "As a rule, people eat considerably less fat on a ketogenic/lipolytic diet than they do on their usual diet."*[39]

Reality Check: Dr. Atkins does not provide an analysis of his diet based on nutritional content. However, *The Nutrition Action Health Letter* used the recommended menu plans in his book and calculated that a whopping 55 percent of the calories in Atkins' diet are from fat—25 percent of those saturated. According to that report, you would also consume 880 milligrams of cholesterol each day using his menu plans.[40]

Fallacy #25: *"Satiety, after all, is not a matter of fooling your stomach, it is a matter of humoral (blood constituent) factors. You eat less on a low-carbohydrate diet than you do on a low-fat diet."*[41]

Reality Check: Actually, it's been shown that you will eat less on a high-carbohydrate (or high-fiber) diet because fiber suppresses appetite. Dr. Atkins diet reduces hunger as well, but with the potential for health consequences.

We can create the same result but without the negative effects on your health. The American Journal of Clinical Nutrition reports:

> *"Evidence suggests that when given in equal volumes, carbohydrate and fat have similar effects on hunger, satiety and subsequent food intake. "...the best dietary advice for weight maintenance and for controlling hunger is to consume a low-fat, high-carbohydrate diet with a high fiber content."*[42]

Fallacy #26: *"The same flawed epidemiology we saw with heart disease applies to cancer. No one really knows what it is in our highly complex environment—including our nutritional environment— that is most directly contributing to our explosive cancer rates. But there is good evidence that it may not be fat."*[43]

Reality Check: The evidence linking diet to cancer has, in fact, been based on population studies. For example, up to 80 percent of breast, bowel and prostate cancers have been attributed to dietary factors with a strong positive association with meat consumption.[44]

Lack of fruits and vegetables has been linked repeatedly to cancers of the mouth, larynx, esophagus, cervix and bladder. A similar association has been demonstrated between cancers of the breast, ovary, prostate and possibly colon.[45]

The American Institute for Cancer Research has published its dietary recommendations, based on current research that has linked specific dietary factors to cancer. According to the AICR, a healthy diet should:

- be based on plant products

- emphasize vegetables and fruits; you should eat 400 grams each day to provide at least half of your energy needs

- minimize sugars; they should comprise less than 10 percent of your calorie intake

- minimize meat; eat no more than 80 grams each day, preferably fish or poultry.[46]

The most respected institutions creating guidelines for cancer prevention have established nutritional guidelines that consistently recommend a diet low in animal fats (meat and whole dairy products) and high in fruits, grains and vegetables.

Fallacy #27: *"Sugar is the Western world's most frequently consumed carcinogen."*[47]

Reality Check: Sugar causing cancer? Dr. Atkins provides no data or references to support this claim. While you should limit your sugar consumption for other health reasons, there is inadequate evidence that sugar is linked to cancer.

Fallacy #28: *"Certainly a significant percentage of the metabolically resistant have underactive thyroid function."*[48]

Reality Check: Research has failed to provide support for this claim. Thyroid function can influence metabolic function, but it only applies to a small percentage of Americans.

Fallacy #29: *"The essential fact you must know for this chapter is that the best doctors I know actually treat their patients with vita-nutrients.... Let me simply list what I prescribe. I make no claims that the nutrients below have a direct therapeutic effect on the conditions for which they are used. The effects they have are accomplished through nutritional pathways. Since I have been prescribing in this manner, my patients show clinical improvements four or five times more frequently than they did when I practiced a very competent brand of orthodox internal medicine."*[49]

Reality Check: No direct therapeutic effect from taking nutritional supplements? The effects they have are accomplished through "nutritional pathways"? Dr. Atkins does not explain the difference (if indeed there is one) between direct therapeutic effect and nutritional pathways.

The 1994 Dietary Supplement Health and Education Act (DSHEA) established specific guidelines for FDA regulation of dietary supplements. These include vitamins, minerals, herbs, botanical and other plant-derived substances, as well as amino acids and concentrates, metabolites, constituents and extracts of the substances. However the FDA's requirement for pre-market review of dietary supplements is less than that of other products it regulates, such as drugs and many additives that are used in conventional food.

Because dietary supplements are not considered drugs, supplement producers cannot claim to cure, treat or prevent disease. A dietary supplement whose label claims a new treatment or cure for specific diseases or condition is considered unauthorized and thus illegal. Moreover, FDA review or approval of supplement ingredients and products is not required before marketing.

Dr. Atkins says he makes no claims about his recommended nutrients. But consider these recommendations he has made:

- For hypoglycemics, he recommends Atkins Formula HF-12

- For diabetes, he recommends Atkins Formula DM-17

- For lowering cholesterol, he recommends Vita-Nutrient

- For hypertension, he recommends Atkins Essential Oils Formula

- For coronary artery disease, he recommends Atkins Formula AA-5.

Fallacy #30: *"There is neither clinical nor epidemiological evidence that people who consume a high-protein diet develop more osteoporosis; so we should place this complaint into the 'Needs More Evidence' category."*[50]

Reality Check: No evidence? Clinical research has clearly demonstrated that the high intake of animal protein increases calcium excretion in the urine, which in turn can lead to osteoporosis.[51] In fact, epidemiological studies have demonstrated a strong link between protein intake and bone fractures.[52]

II

A BETTER WAY—*THE GOOD NEWS* DIET PLAN

5

Now, the Good News: Nutrition Can Prevent—Even Reverse—Disease

In This Chapter:
- ✔ What can we learn from the Chinese?
- ✔ Four major causes of death—and how your dietary habits can reduce your risk
- ✔ How your lifestyle can induce hypoglycemia
- ✔ Plant-based foods that make a difference in your health

Get ready for some good news. Now that you understand that losing body fat is strictly a matter of creating a "caloric deficit"— taking in fewer calories than you burn off—it's easy to see how you can lose weight on any dietary plan, as long as it restricts your caloric intake.

The next step, then, is to start a nutritional program that not only will decrease your caloric intake but also provide long-term health benefits. Why not adopt a weight-control dietary plan that can actually help to prevent the major causes of death and disability in the United States—and could actually *reverse* the disease process.

Well, it's nutritionally possible. There are foods that act as the proverbial garlic clove, keeping chronic degenerative diseases at bay. In fact, four of the seven leading causes of death in the United States (heart disease, cancer, stroke and diabetes) are linked to what you eat. So, let's develop a nutritional plan that, based on extensive research, can significantly increase your life expectancy, energy levels and and general feeling of well-being.

Diet and Chronic Degenerative Diseases in China

We're so used to our fast-food chains and meat-and-potato traditions that we don't recognize the health benefits of a different approach to eating. Actually, we can learn a lot by examining the lifestyle and dietary habits of other cultures. Observations regarding the Pima Indians were insightful; the same can be said of the Chinese.

A comprehensive survey of the diet, lifestyle and death rates of 65 counties in rural China showed that eating *any* amount of beef, chicken or other animal-based food products can significantly increase their risk of cancer and cardiovascular disease.[1]

The China Project, which began in 1983, is a collaborative effort among nutritional researchers in America and China. Together, they surveyed 10,200 people who were genetically similar and tended to eat the same diet for their entire lives. This ongoing research project provides a compelling link between nutrition and the major causes of death in the United States.

The Chinese average 15 percent of their calories in the form of fat; Americans average 33 percent (and as we said earlier, that figure was over 40 percent at the height of the epidemic of heart disease in America). The Chinese eat far less protein; most of what they do consume comes from plant sources rather than animals. Also, their diet is rich in vegetables and grains (high-starch foods like rice, wheat, corn and sweet potatoes). In fact, the diet of the study's Chinese subjects was about 70 percent to 80 percent carbohydrate.

Researchers observed that within the group being studied, cancer death rates (leukemia, liver, colon, rectum, lung and brain) increased as their cholesterol levels increased. So did heart disease and diabetes.

More impressively, the researchers recorded less disease when the subjects ate more plant-based foods—no matter how small the amount—or when they decreased their fat intake even a small amount. The conclusion? Even minor amounts of animal food products are linked to significant increases in blood cholesterol levels which, in turn, can cause a higher risk of heart disease, cancer and other chronic degenerative diseases.

The implications? Reducing your consumption of animal products, even moderately, can reduce your risk of dying from one of the major causes of death in America. Even if you're not ready to become a vegetarian, adding plant-based foods to your diet can provide additional disease prevention benefits.

More findings from the study:

- People living in more affluent areas of China ate more animal products—and died more often from chronic degenerative diseases.

- The Chinese people in the study had a lower rate of osteoporosis compared to Western nations. Surprisingly, they consumed almost no dairy products and very low amounts of calcium.

- The higher the fiber content of the Chinese diet, the lower the rate of colon cancer. It's been estimated that the Chinese eat three to four times more fiber than Americans.

- The Chinese men in the study had very low advanced prostate cancer rates (one in every 100,000 men) while Chinese Americans living in San Francisco have a rate that is nineteen times higher.

Overwhelming research evidence from around the world suggests that as fat consumption increases, particularly animal fat, blood cholesterol levels go up—and so does the risk of developing a chronic degenerative disease. So let's examine the research evidence linking specific nutritional factors to the major causes of death in the United States: coronary artery disease, cancer, stroke and diabetes.

Eat to Live: Preventing Four Killer Diseases

1. Coronary Artery Disease (Heart Attacks)

The year was 1945. The world was deep into the second global war; meat and other animal products were scarce—and Europe experienced a drop in deaths due to heart attacks.

Animal fat and protein

Years later, researchers would study this phenomenon and hypothesize a relationship between animal products and heart attacks.[2] Since then, metabolic ward studies have demonstrated "unequivocally" that diets high in saturated fats increase your blood cholesterol level.[3] In turn high blood cholesterol levels increase your risk of coronary artery disease.

That's not all. Eating less fat improves your blood cholesterol levels. Numerous studies have clearly established that reducing blood cholesterol levels *reduces* your chance of dying from coronary artery disease.[4]

Yes, we now have overwhelming evidence that indicates the high-fat diets of affluent nations, such as America, cause coronary artery disease; and reducing dietary fat, especially saturated and hydrogenated fats, lowers your risk.[5]

You might be surprised how much of a difference your diet can make. Some studies suggest the United States could lower its heart attack death rate by up to 20 percent if all Americans would decrease their fat intake to less than 30 percent of their total calories.[6]

That's especially encouraging when you realize that coronary artery disease is the number-one cause of death in America.

You have the option of selecting a dietary plan—like the one I will present to you in the next chapter—that has only 10 percent fat. If we would adopt this dietary approach as a nation, the average blood cholesterol level would likely drop to 150mg% and we would see an even more dramatic drop in deaths due to coronary artery disease—perhaps to the point where the number-one cause of death in the United States could be eliminated as a public health issue.

Fruits, vegetables and grains

Although there is general agreement on the benefit of reducing fat consumption, particularly saturated and hydrogenated fats, researchers still disagree on which nutrient should replace those fats. Some studies support reducing total fat intake to 10 percent of your total caloric intake.[7] Those plans replace fat with complex carbohydrates such as fruits, grains and vegetables. Other research supports a Mediterranean-style diet, which substitutes vegetable fats.[8]

Clearly, a vegetarian diet provides advantages in your attempts to prevent coronary artery disease. People who eat higher amounts of animal products are more likely to die from coronary artery disease than vegetarians.[9]

Those who have developed coronary artery disease should be encouraged by research that suggests that a low-fat vegetarian diet as part of a comprehensive healthy lifestyle has the potential to reverse even severe atherosclerosis.[10]

Fiber

Fiber can also be a powerful health enhancer. Foods rich in soluble fiber have been shown to lower blood cholesterol levels, especially when you also reduce saturated fat and cholesterol.[11]

Population studies suggest that eating complex carbohydrates and dietary fiber is associated with an inverse risk of heart attack. In other words, eat more and lower your risk; eat less and increase your risk. What's more, long-term clinical trials have demonstrated that by eating more fiber, as part of a low-fat diet, you can drop your blood cholesterol level 3 percent to 5 percent below that of a low-fat, low-cholesterol diet.[12]

So, based on global research, we can best prevent coronary artery disease by maintaining a diet that is:

- Low in animal fat and protein

- Rich in fruits, vegetables and grains

- High in fiber content.

Common Plant-Based Foods

It's not hard to include plant-based foods in your diet. Just pick your favorites, or to add variety, try something new. They fall in basically three categories:

GRAINS
(AND THEIR DERIVATIVES):
amaranth
barley
buckwheat
millet
oat
quinoa
rice
rye
soy/tempeh
spelt
wheat

MORE COMMON GRAIN
SOURCES:
bagels
bread
crackers
pasta
rice
rolls/biscuits
tortillas

VEGETABLES:
broccoli
cabbage
carrots
cauliflower
corn
green pepper
lettuce
mushrooms
onions
parsnips
peas
potatoes
radishes
sweet potatoes
turnips

FRUITS:
apples
apricots
bananas
blackberries

blueberries
cantaloupes
cherries
clementines
cranberries
grapes
guavas
kiwifruit
mangoes
nectarines
oranges
papayas
peaches
pears
persimmons
pineapples
plums
prunes
strawberries
tomato (yep, it's a fruit)
watermelon

Can You Really Prevent a Heart Attack?

In twenty-five years, we have tested thousands of patients at Oakland University. And over this quarter-century, we've yet to record even *one* heart attack due to coronary artery disease in the people who have maintained the following health and lifestyle profile:

- A cholesterol/HDL ratio of 3.4 or less or total blood cholesterol of 150mg% or less (this refers to the amount of fat in your blood and how it is transported)

Food, Nutrition and the Prevention of Cancer

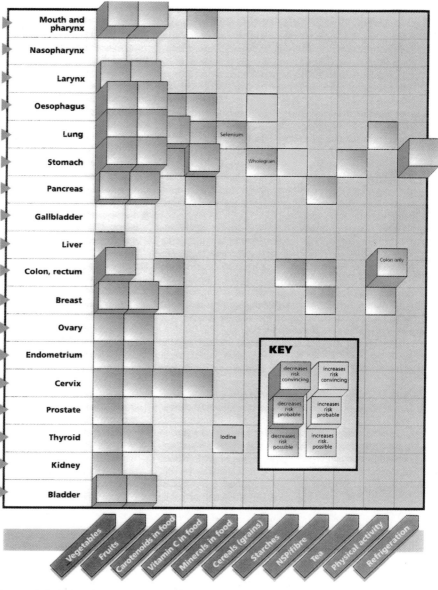

The matrix is designed as a convenient reference. The rows specify the individual cancers. The columns on the left-hand page show aspects of diet that decrease the risk of cancer and those on the right-hand page indicate aspects that increase the risk of cancer.

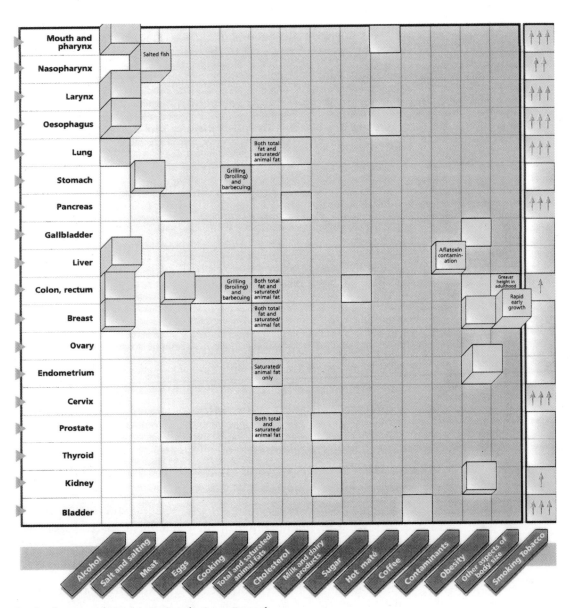

Reprinted courtesy of American Institute for Cancer Research

- A blood pressure of 120/80mm/Hg or less (the pressure in your blood vessels and arteries)

- No tobacco products

- A normal fasting blood glucose (the sugar level in your blood)

- A regular aerobic exercise program.

The number-one cause of death in the United States is virtually *unseen* in our patients with this profile. Shouldn't you compare your current health and lifestyle profile to one this successful in preventing coronary artery disease?

The Institute's nutritional program, which stresses high fiber consumption and the avoidance of animal fat, has helped hundreds of individuals achieve this profile. It's our belief that nearly every American is capable of achieving this health profile through appropriate lifestyle changes and, when necessary for genetic reasons, pharmacological intervention.

2. Cancer

The relationship between diet and cancer is undeniable. One of the most comprehensive worldwide reviews of diet and cancer has concluded that diet and other lifestyle changes could prevent up to *four million* cases of cancer every year.[13]

This report was the result of three years of work by a panel of more than 150 scientists who reviewed and evaluated 4,500 research studies. The report concludes that nutrition plays an important role in preventing cancer.

Perhaps most important, the report recommends that you choose a diet that is predominantly plant-based with a variety of vegetables, fruits and grains. This recommendation is consistent with that of the National Cancer Institute, the National Academy of Sciences, the American Cancer Society and the Surgeon General of United States, all of whom have recommended that Americans eat fewer meats, dairy products and fats and more fruits, vegetables and grains.

The dietary recommendations made by these professional groups are a serious indictment of the high-protein/low-carbohydrate diets on the market today. Can you really afford to adopt a high-protein/high-fat/low-carbohydrate program that is not consistent with cancer prevention?

Let's examine how certain foods influence your risk for particular cancers, according to the American Institute for Cancer Research. Why was your mother right when she told you to eat your vegetables? They can help prevent more than a dozen cancers, especially of the colon, stomach, lung, esophagus, even mouth and pharynx.

Fruits? They're associated with a reduced risk of at least twelve cancers, especially stomach, lung, esophagus, mouth and pharynx.

Grains and starches are associated with a reduced risk of stomach, colon and rectal cancers.

Foods high in vitamin C reduce your risk of six cancers, stomach in particular.

Review the previous table, developed by the American Institute for Cancer Research, which shows how diet is linked to particular cancers. You might also consider making a copy and posting it on your refrigerator as a reminder.

In summary, based on current research, you can reduce your risk for developing cancer if you:

- Eat less animal fat and protein

- Avoid alcohol

- Eat more plant-based foods. Plant foods contain fiber plus hundreds of vitamins, minerals and other substances that research suggests can help prevent cancer

- Eat five or more servings of fruits and vegetables each day, as well as other plant-based foods such as breads, cereals, grain products, rice, pasta or beans several times each day, as recommended by the American Cancer Society.

3. Strokes

Stroke deaths in America have dropped almost 60 percent in the last three to four decades. And the most important explanation for this decline is the treatment of high blood pressure (hypertension).[14]

Your lifestyle can profoundly influence your blood pressure. And yes, nutrition can play a role in determining your susceptibility to hypertension. A diet rich in fruits and vegetables, coupled with reduced saturated and total fats, can substantially lower your blood pressure.[15] Studies have demonstrated that fruits and vegetables actually help *prevent* stroke through antioxidant mechanisms.[16]

Hydrogenated and saturated fats increase blood cholesterol levels. In turn, decreasing animal fat and hydrogenated fat can reduce the risk that you'll develop atherosclerosis leading to plaque-forming strokes. (Four out of five strokes are caused by plaque formations in the arteries of the brain; these are called ischemic strokes.)[17]

The dietary factors that will most likely reduce your risk of hypertension or strokes include:

- Eat fruits and vegetables daily

- Eat less animal fat

- Minimize hydrogenated fats (margarine, shortening, etc. Also sometimes included in baked products; typically, you'll find them listed on a product's ingredient panel)

- Consume less than 2,000 mg of sodium per day

- Minimize alcohol.

4. Diabetes

Diabetes is a clinical condition in which your blood glucose, or blood sugar, level is elevated. Your body regulates glucose through a hormone called insulin, which transports glucose into your body's cells. Diabetes develops if you don't produce enough insulin or if the insulin is ineffective in transferring glucose from the blood to your body's cells.

There are two types of diabetes. Type I, also called insulin-dependent diabetes mellitus, affects about 5 percent of diabetics, mostly children and young adults. With Type I, the pancreas is unable to provide enough insulin to remove the glucose from your blood. Type II diabetes, striking more than 90 percent of diabetics, is often referred to as non-insulin dependent diabetes mellitus. The major causes are excessive body fat, physical inactivity and poor dietary habits.

Nations that enjoy greater affluence typically begin to experience more Type II diabetes. With affluence comes technology and an ever-increasing sedentary lifestyle. The Westernization of nations also brings about dietary changes such as higher animal fat and less fiber consumption. Many of the commercially created food products found in emerging societies have a reduced fiber content because of processing. It's been our clinical experience that the majority of Type II diabetics would achieve normal blood sugar (fasting blood glucose) levels if they would simply modify their diet, achieve their recommended body fat content and maintain an active lifestyle.

Because carbohydrate increases blood sugar levels, it was assumed for many years that we should avoid carbohydrates. Research now suggests that a high-fiber diet, especially of the soluble variety, helps to improve carbohydrate metabolism and reduce blood glucose levels.[18]

In addition, diabetics are more likely to suffer atherosclerosis. Thus, diabetics who hope to avoid premature heart attacks and strokes must minimize animal fat in their diet.

Based on current research, Type II diabetes is best prevented by following these dietary guidelines:

- A high-fiber diet, especially soluble fiber (typically found in oat bran, rice bran, fruits, vegetables and legumes such as beans, lentils and peas)

- A diet with low-glycemic index foods (carbohydrates that don't significantly increase blood glucose levels). Many dietetic associations around the world recommend this dietary approach for diabetics. However, diabetics should never alter their diet without consulting their physician

- Fewer animal, hydrogenated and saturated fats. This dietary emphasis will help lower your caloric intake and control your blood lipid values, essential steps in preventing heart disease and strokes. In addition, you are likely to consume fewer calories, thereby helping to control body fat content.

The glycemic index of foods is a method used to quantify how rapidly carbohydrates enter the bloodstream. The lower the index value, the slower the rate of absorption.

While so many popular diets today encourage you to eat more protein and fat, studies from around the world continue to link protein and fat to higher cancer, heart disease, diabetes and stroke rates. Those same studies demonstrate that vegetables, fruits, grains and other plant-based foods help prevent the same diseases.

What should concern you the most about the proponents of these diets—from Atkins to Sears—is their lack of research support.

Functional Hypoglycemia

There's yet another health concern and quality of life that has been linked to diet: hypoglycemia, or low blood sugar. In the United States, hypoglycemia often is caused by personal lifestyle choices, leading to a physiologically reduced quality of life.

Symptoms of hypoglycemia include fatigue, lack of concentration, headaches, anxiety, depression, changes in heart rhythm, trembling, sweating and hunger. People with these symptoms often report they constantly feel sick and have for years.

Many of our patients at Oakland University's Meadow Brook Health Enhancement Institute say they had forgotten what it was like to feel good—until they started our dietary and lifestyle plan. Over and over, patients who stick with the program tell us they finally feel healthy and energized.

Most people with hypoglycemia induce these symptoms by the lifestyle they've chosen. Obesity and lack of physical activity contribute to this condition, while reducing or eliminating caffeine, nicotine and alcohol can dramatically improve this condition.

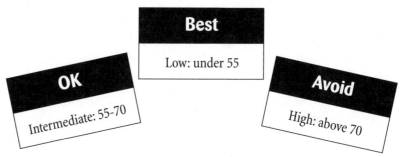

These glycemic index guidelines are from The Glucose Revolution, *Miller et al., Marlow and Company, 1999*

Equally important in your attempts to reduce your blood sugar volatility is maintaining a diet that's high in both complex carbohydrates and fiber, and low in refined carbohydrates. If you make these nutritional objectives the basis of your diet, you'll enhance your feeling of well-being. And believe me, you *will* notice a difference!

Glycemic Index of Selected Foods

FOOD	GLYCEMIC INDEX
Kidney beans	27
Peach	30
Fettuccine	32
Apple	38
Spaghetti	41
Snickers™ candy bar	41
Oatmeal (old fashioned)	49
Carrots	49
Brown rice	55
Sweet corn	55
Popcorn	55
Whole wheat bread	69
Short grain white rice	72
Bagel	72
Corn chips	72
Vanilla wafers	77
Wafer cracker	78
Jelly beans	80
Kellogg's Corn Flakes™	84
Baked potato	93

If you're one of the millions of Americans who have a reduced quality of life because of hypoglycemia, adopting these nine lifestyle changes can send you on the road to recovery:

- Eat at least 25 grams of fiber each day
- Follow a high-complex carbohydrate diet
- Avoid refined carbohydrates (sugars)
- When eating foods individually (a snack for example), choose low-glycemic index foods

- Spread your calories over the course of the entire day; eat at least every two hours

- Eat less fat to control your calorie intake

- Eliminate caffeine, nicotine and alcohol

- Achieve your recommended weight based on body composition studies (see chapter 8)

- Maintain a regular program of cardiorespiratory exercise (see chapter 9).

If you have lifestyle-induced hypoglycemia and adopt these nutritional recommendations, you won't believe how much better you'll feel and function in just *two weeks*. I cannot emphasize enough the number of people who have personally told me how their quality of life improved within a few weeks of implementing these steps.

And that *is* good news.

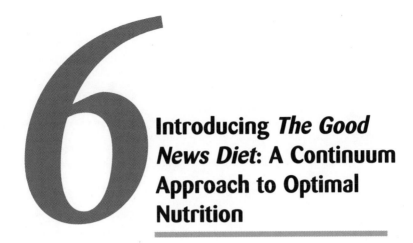

Introducing *The Good News Diet*: A Continuum Approach to Optimal Nutrition

Are you tired of weight control failure? Tired of experts who suggest that one specific approach to weight loss will be effective for everyone?

Let's face it: We're not all the same. We're different in age, body type, size, height—you name it. We come from different cultures and have different physiological and psychological makeups. Some of us are better able to withstand food temptation than others. You might eat only when you're hungry; others eat when they feel stressed. For those simple reasons, dietary plans have to be adaptable.

Wouldn't you like to adopt a dietary plan you are responsible for creating? Maybe you're committed to achieving the best possible health profile and want to begin with a nutritional program that gives you the best chance of achieving this goal—becoming a vegetarian. Or perhaps you want to hang on to your favorite chicken or beef dishes two to three times a week, but you're willing to consider other dietary options to achieve an enhanced health status.

By placing nutrition on a continuum, from a plan that is most likely to increase your risk of a health problem to one that is most likely to be preventive, you can decide on a dietary plan that fits the priority you place on health.

You're ready for *The Good News* Diet.

In the past few chapters, I've demonstrated that a high-protein/low-carbohydrate diet is not consistent with achieving optimal health. (Is the call of those Sirens fading in the distance?) We've also analyzed worldwide research on the relationship between disease prevention and what you eat. Now, let's engineer a nutritional plan that's customized for you—one that helps you achieve and maintain your recommended weight and is also likely to increase your life expectancy.

Sound good so far?

Be assured that if you make the right nutritional decisions along with other lifestyle changes I'm going to recommend, you have the potential to *feel better than you've ever felt before.* I don't care if you're age twenty, fifty or eighty; you can enjoy a better quality of life than you could imagine.

Have you established specific health goals for yourself? Maybe you want to lose weight. Or maybe you'd like to really feel good for the first time in years. Perhaps your goal is to stay healthy enough to play with your children or grandchildren later in life, or to maintain a high level of well-being that allows you to enjoy retirement. Is your priority to look as good as a friend or neighbor? Or is it to avoid the heart attack, cancer or stroke that has taken others in your family?

Whatever your specific health goals may be, you should feel motivated by knowing you are more likely to achieve all of your other priorities in life by reaching the enhanced state of health and well-being this lifestyle plan can offer.

Intrigued?

Then let's get started!

Is Your Diet Plan Like Conquering Mt. Everest?

Sir Edmund Hillary is known for becoming, in 1953, the first person to reach the summit of Mount Everest. In the sport of climbing, that's unquestionably a "10." But do you know how many smaller mountains he scaled first?

He actually started mountain climbing in his native New Zealand, then went on to the Alps and finally the Himalayas, where he climbed eleven different peaks above 20,000 feet.

By this time, Hillary was ready to confront the world's highest mountain. Lying between Tibet and Nepal, Mt. Everest certainly was no piece of cake, though (pardon the nutritional pun). Seven major expeditions had failed to reach the peak in the 32 years prior to Hillary's conquest.

In 1951, barely thirty-one years old, he joined a New Zealand party to survey a route up the southern flank of Mount Everest. After his success in 1953, he admitted, "We didn't know if it was humanly possible to reach the top of Mt. Everest. And even using oxygen as we were, if we did get to the top, we weren't at all sure whether we wouldn't drop dead or something of that nature."

Do you see any similarities between Sir Edmund Hillary and your dietary history? He began by studying the intricacies of mountain climbing, much as you probably have researched diet and nutrition in your quest to enhance your health.

Hillary then climbed progressively more difficult peaks before finally tackling the greatest of all, Mt. Everest. He didn't know if was humanly possible—but he did it anyway.

Every time Hillary topped one of the smaller peaks, did he feel like a failure for not having conquered Everest? Or did he savor those smaller victories and gradually learn from those experiences to make sure his next challenge was a success?

I'm sure that at times your goal of weight control and good health seems as impossible as reaching the summit of Mt. Everest. Many of you may want to consider an incremental approach to health enhancement—a series of progressive lifestyle changes.

(By the way, Sir Edmund remained fit and continued to take on new challenges in New Zealand at the young age of eighty-one.)

This approach means you simply cannot fail because *you're* choosing the health goals. And you'll discover how to successfully reach peak after peak, progressively improving, on your way to optimal health (a "10").

I'm going to demonstrate how you can create a dietary plan designed to enhance your health that you alone are responsible for and comfortable with. You'll have the basic knowledge necessary to make informed nutritional decisions. And you'll be prepared to make choices based on a continuum of nutritional options that range from least desirable to most optimal.

The Good News Diet—A Summary

The Good News Diet represents a continuum of nutritional options that, if progressively followed, has the potential to increase your life expectancy and feeling of well-being. This nutritional program allows you to choose how close to an optimal diet you would like to get. I won't tell you what to eat; instead you'll have the responsibility of selecting your own diet based on a continuum, from the least desirable to optimal.

It's been my experience that most people simply haven't been given the opportunity to gain the health benefits of an optimal diet because their physician assumed they wouldn't make the necessary dietary changes. What a terrible mistake. Your doctor's responsibility is to define what represents the best dietary plan for you to achieve your personal health goals—and then to let *you* decide what changes you're willing to make.

As you make your nutritional decisions in implementing *The Good News* Diet, you should be guided by these health goals:

- Achieving and maintaining your recommended weight
- Increasing your life expectancy through food selections associated with disease prevention
- Improving your feeling of well-being and experiencing less fatigue, more energy, higher productivity, less anxiety, better concentration and fewer mood swings

You can apply the continuum concept to these three health goals as well. You can choose to: (1) make nutritional and lifestyle decisions that have the potential to radically enhance your health status but require a significant commitment to change, or (2) take smaller steps in achieving long-term health enhancement.

The choice is yours.

The Good News Health Enhancement Continuum

POOR QUALITY OF LIFE;	MODERATE QUALITY OF LIFE;	OPTIMAL
HIGH RISK FOR POOR HEALTH	AVERAGE AMERICAN	QUALITY OF LIFE

1 —————————————→ 5 —————————————→ 10

Consider this health continuum:

Where would you like to be on the continuum? Probably not a "1" and probably not a "5". But a "10" may seem too daunting. Maybe you're not ready for that kind of lifestyle commitment. Perhaps a "7" or "8" seems a little more reachable for now.

It's your decision, and it's important that you take responsibility for establishing your health goals. Don't assume your physician will keep you healthy. Our health care system is so focused on the curative aspects of medicine that we often forget to emphasize the potential for preventing disease or enhancing our well-being if we're not "sick."

Ultimately, your life expectancy and quality of life will be driven, most importantly, by the lifestyle you choose. And of all the lifestyle changes you can make, nutrition is one of the most important in your quest to achieve the health goals you establish.

The Good News Diet is *not* one of deprivation. Eating for weight control and optimal health can be an extremely enjoyable experience, even though you'll have to make choices along the nutritional continuum that may require change. In addition, most people gain an enhanced feeling of well-being while on this plan, and this will motivate you to experiment with foods. You'll find yourself wanting to move along the health continuum by continually making better nutritional and lifestyle choices.

Finally, recognize that many of your eating preferences are conditioned responses. As you make better nutritional choices, you'll be surprised to find that many of the foods you once enjoyed or craved will no longer be as desirable. Later, I'll help you identify ways to manage your environment and behavior so that you can achieve better eating patterns and food preferences.

Now, get your gear. We're ready to begin our ascent.

7

The Six Nutritional Principles of *The Good News* Diet

In This Chapter:

✔ *The Good News* Diet
✔ *The Good News* Food Pyramid
✔ Getting all your vitamins
✔ Socially accepted drugs

*T*he *Good News* Diet that I have presented in this book is based on six basic nutritional principles:

1. Limit fat consumption to no more than 25 grams per day

2. Eat at least 25 grams of fiber per day

3. Follow the food groups and recommended servings from *The Good News* Food Pyramid

4. Limit animal products (meats and dairy selections)

5. Avoid refined carbohydrates. When consuming foods individually, choose foods with a low glycemic index

6. Minimize alcohol and caffeine intake.

Understanding these principles is a little like the essential preparation Sir Edmund Hillary undertook before climbing a mountain: You need to map out the face of the mountain. By understanding the trails you must follow, and the deceptive crevices to avoid, you're more likely to successfully reach the summit.

Let's address these principles one by one. (This would be a good time to get out a highlighter, so you can emphasize specific points.)

PRINCIPLE #1
Limit Fat Consumption to No More Than 25 Grams of Fat Per Day

"Twenty-five grams of fat per day? Are you crazy?"

Now, don't overreact. Take a deep breath. You're going to be surprised to discover just how easy it can be.

For almost thirty years, I've asked patients at Oakland University's Meadow Brook Health Enhancement Institute to restrict fat consumption to no more than 25 grams per day. Of the 25 grams they consume, I ask them to minimize saturated and hydrogenated fats.

Of all the dietary changes I've asked people to make, limiting fat consumption has had the most dramatic impact on weight loss and reducing their risk for a chronic degenerative disease.

Here's a simple illustration of a continuum of choices you can make to restrict fat consumption:

There's a lot of confusion and misinformation about the degree to which fat consumption should be restricted. Unfortunately, it can come from some very credible sources. Dr. C. Everett Koop, former Surgeon General of the United States, has done a commendable job of raising our awareness of and support for national health issues. His current website offers a tremendous scope of health information, but it also encourages far more fat consumption than can be supported by research.

A colleague recently visited the site, which provides a fat intake calculator. Dr. Koop's calculator recommended that this man—at thirty-seven years old, 5'6", with a medium build and moderately active lifestyle—consume 82 grams of fat per day! If this same person had an active lifestyle, he was allowed 88 grams. For a sedentary lifestyle the recommendation dropped—to 70 grams per day.

As I pointed out earlier, the United States has led the world in reducing deaths due to heart attacks over the last forty years. Lower blood cholesterol levels have contributed substantially to this decline. In turn, the single most important factor in improving blood cholesterol levels has been the reduction of fat consumption by almost 25 percent, as a nation. Despite this improvement, the average American still consumes a whopping 73 grams of fat per day (assuming an average intake of 2,000 calories per day). That's actually down from several decades ago, when the United States led the world in deaths due to coronary artery disease; at that time, Americans consumed more than *100 grams of fat* per day.

The American Heart Association (AHA) recommends a further reduction in the amount of fat Americans eat, to 67 grams per day. Unfortunately, the AHA hasn't recognized that decreasing fat consumption from 73 to 67 grams per day isn't enough to cause a further

Daily Fat Consumption for a Person Consuming 2,000 Calories Per Day

HIGH RISK FOR DISEASE		AVERAGE AMERICAN	AHA		OPTIMAL
1 ——————————→		5 ——————→	6 ——————————→		10
100+ grams/day		73 grams/day	67 grams/day		25 grams/day

dramatic reduction in death rates due to coronary heart disease and other chronic degenerative diseases.

AHA representatives have often acknowledged the benefits of restricting fat consumption much more dramatically, but they say the average American simply would not comply. If Americans are unaware of the health benefits of further reducing fat, it is unlikely that blood-cholesterol levels will continue to improve.

On the other hand, many people will seek an optimal diet—and reap the benefits—if they're presented with the nutritional research facts. Many patients at our Institute who have adopted my dietary plan, for example, *no longer need medication to treat their high blood cholesterol or hypertension.* I can't tell you how often people have told me they were never given the opportunity to go on a dietary plan that restricts fat to 25 grams per day. Too often, they were simply placed on the AHA dietary plan, which in most cases reduced their fat intake only minimally.

They assumed that a plan recommended by the AHA would give them the *best* chance for avoiding medication and preventing coronary heart disease. Unfortunately, despite the positive impact the AHA has had on preventing heart disease, the association hasn't been aggressive enough in providing low-fat nutritional guidelines.

Differences in Fats

A rose may be a rose, but fats in your diet simply are not the same. I'd like to present the differences, and suggest which ones you should include in your dietary plan.

All fats are made up of a specific percentage of saturated, monounsaturated and polyunsaturated elements (fatty acids). Researchers generally agree that fats with a higher percentage of saturation are least helpful in preventing chronic degenerative diseases. Where they disagree is whether to emphasize monounsaturated or polyunsaturated fats. The Mediterranean diet contains fats such as olive oil (which are higher in monounsaturated fats), and has been advocated for the prevention of coronary heart disease.

Some researchers have noted that a low-fat diet, while decreasing total blood cholesterol levels, will also reduce HDLs—the transporters of cholesterol which ultimately help the body rid itself of cholesterol (sometimes erroneously referred to as the "good cholesterol"). These researchers argue that the benefits of a low-fat diet are offset by this *decrease* in beneficial HDLs. There is, in fact, research that suggests monounsaturated fats, rather than polyunsaturated fats, can help prevent HDLs from dropping when you adopt a low-fat diet.

I should point out that the Mediterranean-type diet is higher in total fat content than *The Good News* Diet (or others, like the Ornish plan). In populations where fat consumption is low and heart disease rare, total blood cholesterol levels are low, but so are HDLs. It may simply be that HDLs play a more important role in preventing coronary artery disease prevention within populations that eat high-fat diets and have high blood cholesterol levels.

Don't assume that lowering your total blood cholesterol level is as easy as adding monounsaturated fats to your diet. Adding olive oil to your salad, for example, will likely have the opposite effect.

Hydrogenation is the chemical process of making fat more saturated. Watch for partially hydrogenated fats when selecting your 25 grams of fat each day. Unfortunately, current labels do not identify the amount of hydrogenated fat in food products. Fats that have been hydrogenated will be identified under ingredients but are not quantified.

Don't assume "low cholesterol" products are preferable. Some patients come to our institute on a low-cholesterol diet, yet have a difficult time understanding why their blood cholesterol levels don't improve. The fact is, you'll see many products advertised as "low in cholesterol" or "cholesterol-free" that also contain a significant amount of fat, much of it saturated.

One of my favorite stories involves a cardiac patient who baked chocolate chip cookies for me one day. He was eager for me to try them because he had discovered a way to make them with little cholesterol in the recipe. The product that allowed him to make the cookies was Crisco. This product is advertised as having no cholesterol. When I asked the patient to read the nutritional information on the label, he was shocked to find it was 100 percent fat, much of which had been hydrogenated and, therefore, saturated.

The most important fats influencing your blood cholesterol level are saturated. While dietary cholesterol can increase your cholesterol level, saturated fats are significantly more concerning.

Fatty Acid Composition of Selected Oils and Fats

Saturated	Monounsaturated	Polyunsaturated

Canola Oil (Puritan Oil)

| 6 | 62 | 32 |

Safflower Oil

| 9 | 13 | 78 |

Sunflower Oil

| 11 | 20 | 69 |

Corn Oil

| 13 | 25 | 62 |

Olive Oil

| 14 | 77 | 9 |

Soybean Oil

| 15 | 24 | 61 |

Peanut Oil

| 18 | 48 | 34 |

Sockeye Salmon Oil

| 20 | 55 | 25 |

Cottonseed Oil

| 27 | 19 | 54 |

Lard

| 41 | 47 | 12 |

Palm Oil

| 51 | 39 | 10 |

Beef Tallow

| 52 | 44 | 4 |

Butterfat

| 66 | 30 | 4 |

Palm Kernel Oil

| 86 | 12 | 2 |

Coconut

| 92 | 6 | 2 |

Proportions (%) of saturated, monounsaturated and polyunsaturated fats in selected dietary fats.

So, of the 25 grams of fat recommended each day on *The Good News* Diet, select the most *unsaturated* choices. The table on the previous page identifies the percentage of saturated fats (those of greatest concern), as well as monounsaturated and polyunsaturated that contribute to the dietary source of fat.

In the next chapter, I will present a weight-loss plan that has helped thousands of people decrease their body fat content and enhance their overall health status. Nutritionally, you'll limit fat, the most concentrated source of calories in your diet (there are nine calories per fat gram compared to four calories per gram in carbohydrate and protein).

You'll want to obtain your 25 grams of daily fat from whole foods rather than oils. By consuming the fat as it exists in the plant, you'll also gain beneficial vitamins, minerals and fiber. Oils are 100 percent fat without the associated nutrients that promote good health. If you eat a sufficient variety of whole foods, you won't have to worry about eating too little fat or, for that matter, protein.

The following table will help you compare *The Good News* Diet to the average American diet, the AHA diet and Dr. Atkins' diet.

Percent of Calories and Grams of Protein, Fat and Carbohydrate in Selected Dietary Plans*

	PROTEIN % OF CALORIES/GRAMS	FAT % OF CALORIES/GRAMS	CARBOHYDRATE % OF CALORIES/GRAMS
The Good News Diet	10–15/50–75	10/22	75-80/375-400
American Heart Association	15/75	≥30/≥67	55-60/275-300
Average American	17/85	33/73	50/250
Atkins Diet†	22/110	60/122	18/190

Percent of calories and grams of protein, fat and carbohydrate on The Good News *Diet, the average American diet, AHA diet and Atkins Diet (assuming an average caloric intake of 2,000 calories/day).*

* Based on an average American's caloric intake of 2,000 calories per day.
†Estimates based on analysis from "Nutrition Action Health Letter," March 2000, Vol. 27, No. 2, Pg 6.

PRINCIPLE #2
Consume at Least 25 Grams of Fiber Per Day

Earlier, I indicated that dietary fiber has important health benefits for disease prevention and weight control. Dietary fiber is a non-digestible form of complex carbohydrate that comes from plant cell walls. For generations, our parents and grandparents referred to this as roughage.

Fiber is made up of diverse components including cellulose, hemicellulose, lignin, gum and pectin. It's found in whole grains, vegetables, fruits, nuts and seeds. Meat, dairy products, eggs and fish contain no fiber. Therefore, high-protein/low-carbohydrate diets are inevitably deficient in fiber.

The typical American diet has a low fiber content because so many of our carbohydrate sources have been refined.

Low-Fat Shouldn't Mean Low-Fiber

Over the last forty years, much of the fiber found in grains has been reduced as a result of the refinement process.

Much of the bran found in the wheat kernels in whole wheat was removed and made into white flour. The same process is used to convert brown rice into white rice.

Because of the recent interest Americans have had in low-fat foods, a glut of products have been produced that have no fat but also have been stripped of their fiber content. In many cases, fat-free products have actually become less beneficial in preventing health problems because they create a new problem—fiber deficiencies in the American diet.

Low-Fat Foods that are Deficient in Fiber		
FOOD	QUANTITY	GRAMS OF FIBER
Cookies	20	0.7
Graham Crackers	4	0.8
Rice Cakes	5 mini	0.3

Fiber Intake Continuum for a Person Consuming a Diet of 2,000 Calories Per Day		
HIGH PROTEIN/LOW-CARB DIET	AVERAGE AMERICAN	OPTIMAL
1 ⟶ 5 ⟶ 10		
Less than 5 grams/day	10-15 grams/day	At least 25 grams/day

Fiber Content of Complex Carbohydrates vs. Refined Carbohydrates

COMPLEX CARBOHYDRATES		REFINED CARBOHYDRATES	
FOOD	GRAMS OF FIBER	FOOD	GRAMS OF FIBER
Apple, Medium	3.7 gm	Apple Juice, 6 oz	0.2 gm
Whole Grain Bread, 1 oz	2.0 gm	Bread, 1 oz	0.7 gm
Whole Wheat Pasta, 1 cup	6.3 gm	Pasta, 1 cup	2.2 gm
Brown Rice, 1 cup	3.5 gm	Rice, 1 cup	0.6 gm
Whole Grain Flakes – Cereals, 1 cup	5.2 gm	Wheat Flake Cereal, 1 cup	3.0 gm

Examples of high-fiber foods and refined products in which much of the fiber content has been removed. Note the dramatic nutritional difference between complex and refined carbohydrate choices.

Reducing fat consumption is clearly a high nutritional priority, but it's a mistake to assume that artificially created low-fat food products can substitute for the naturally low-fat advantages of eating fruits, vegetables and whole grains.

PRINCIPLE #3
Select the Food Groups and Recommended Servings from *The Good News* Food Pyramid

If you grew up with the USDA's Basic Four food groups as your model for optimal nutrition, the health benefits of lower meat and dairy consumption may surprise you. Likewise, the dairy industry convinced an entire nation that nutritionally, its products were nearly optimal. Once research began to offer evidence that dairy products and other animal foods were associated with many major health problems, the USDA revised its dietary recommendations and created the Food Guide Pyramid.

The newer guideline reduced the serving suggestions for animal products. While this is a substantial improvement over the Basic Four plan, eating these foods regularly is not optimal and is associated with an increased health risk.

If you eat fewer animal products and fat than the USDA Food Guide Pyramid recommends, you can expect further health benefits. The American Dietetic Association has concluded that scientific data demonstrates a positive relationship between a vegetarian diet and lower risk for obesity, coronary artery disease, hypertension, diabetes and certain cancers. Given the research support for a vegetarian diet, isn't it interesting that national diet gurus so infrequently recommend it? Instead, they turn to one of the main culprits for poor health and death in the United States—fat.

I've trained physicians in preventive medicine for the last twenty years and, sadly, less than one in a hundred has been exposed to the benefits of a vegetarian diet. It's simply not part of their repertoire of treatment plans. It's not surprising that the incredible potential vegetarianism offers in the prevention and treatment of common health problems is not appreciated because we've embraced a curative model of medicine in the United States.

So, you have to assume this responsibility. Make no mistake,

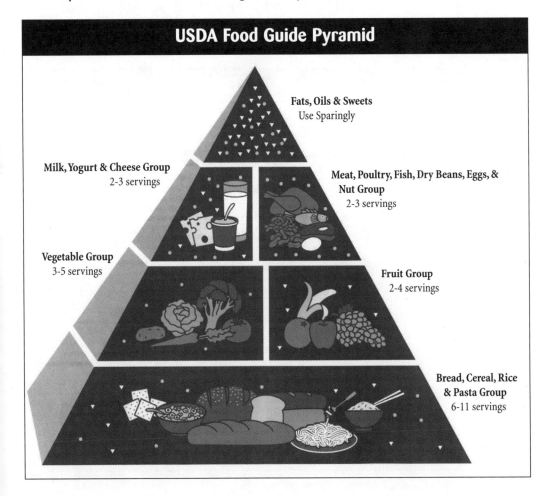

when all other lifestyle factors influencing health status are equal, the healthiest people in the world are vegetarian.

A New Look for an Old Pyramid

Given current research on the relationship between nutrition and disease prevention, I have modified the USDA Food Guide Pyramid. Selecting food groups and recommended servings from *The Good News* Food Pyramid will give you the best opportunity to achieve optimal health.

Nutritional points of emphasis for this revised food pyramid include the following:

- At the foundation of the pyramid, whole grains are emphasized. I recommend six or more servings a day of bread, rice, pasta, hot or cold cereal, corn, millet, barley, bulgur or tortillas. Most of your servings and calories should come from these selections. Whole grains

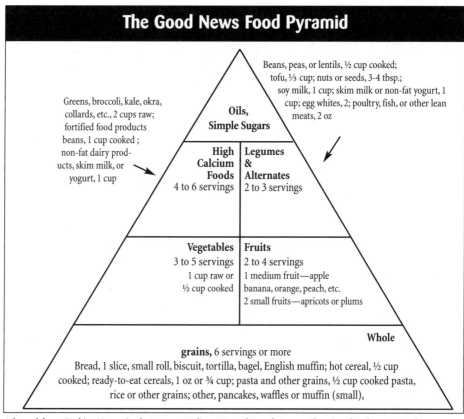

Adapted from *Cooking Vegetarian* by Vesanto Melina, RD, and Joseph Forest, Chronimed/Wiley 1998 and *Becoming Vegetarian* by dieticians Vesanto Melina, Brenda Davis, and Victoria Harrison, Book Publishing Co., 1995.

are rich in fiber and other complex carbohydrates. A serving size would represent a half-cup of hot cereal, one ounce of dry cereal or one slice of bread.

- Three to five servings of vegetables are recommended each day. Vegetables are loaded with vitamins, minerals and fiber. A serving size would be equal to one cup of raw vegetables or a half-cup of cooked vegetables.

- Consume two to four servings of fruit daily. Fruits are high in fiber, with nutrients like vitamin C and beta-carotene. At least one of your servings should be citrus fruit, melon or strawberries. It's better to select whole fruit than fruit juices to ensure you're getting a higher quantity of fiber.

- Eat two to three servings of legumes or other protein sources every day. Options include lentils, black-eyed peas, soybeans, chickpeas, kidney beans, pinto beans or black beans. Nuts, seeds and peanuts also can provide one or more servings; however, they're also high in fat. If you adopt *The Good News* Diet, you can choose fish and skinless poultry, selected wild game, egg whites or no-fat dairy products as less than optimal options. Serving size examples include a half-cup of cooked beans, a half-cup of tofu, eight ounces of soy milk, one cup of yogurt or skim milk, two egg whites or two ounces of poultry, fish or other lean meat.

- Consume four to six servings of foods high in calcium. Plants are preferred calcium sources and include greens such as broccoli, collards, kale and okra (one cup cooked); fortified food products such as soy milk, rice milk and orange juice; tofu; beans and figs. If you decide to implement *The Good News* Diet, a less optimal serving choice would be non-fat dairy products.

If you avoid all animal products, make sure you get vitamin B-12 daily from fortified food products or a multipurpose nutritional supplement. Also, on a vegan (one who eats no animal products, including dairy) dietary plan, you'll need vitamin D each day; you can obtain this vitamin from sun exposure, fortified food products or a multipurpose nutritional supplement.

Oils and simple sugars, at the top of this food pyramid, receive the least emphasis.

PRINCIPLE #4
Limit Animal Products (Meats and Dairy Selections)

In previous chapters, I discussed the benefits of avoiding animal products. The benefits of a low-fat vegetarian diet cannot be denied when you study populations from around the world. People in less-affluent societies tend to be vegetarian and heart disease, cancer, diabetes and other chronic degenerative diseases are much less common.

So we can create a continuum of health benefits when comparing animal to plant-based diets:

Two Common Misconceptions About Reducing Animal Fat

A number of reasons have been given for the importance of including meats and dairy products in the American diet. Based on my clinical experience two misconceptions are most commonly associated with minimizing animal products in your diet.

MISCONCEPTION #1: You need the protein.

The American Dietetic Association, in a position paper on vegetarian diets, stated that plant sources of protein are adequate if your diet is sufficiently varied and meets your energy needs.[1]

Animal- vs. Plant-Based Dietary Continuum				
ANIMAL PRODUCTS INCLUDING MOST MEATS	AVERAGE AMERICAN	AHA DIET	FISH, POULTRY & NON-FAT DAIRY	LOW FAT AND VEGETARIAN
1 ⟶	5 ⟶	6.5 ⟶	8 ⟶	10
Increased risk of a chronic degenerative disease				Optimal; low risk of a chronic degenerative disease

In previous chapters, I made a strong argument that animal protein contributes to many of our chronic degenerative diseases. Most meat-eaters consume too much protein, increasing their risk of cancer, a heart attack or one of the other major causes of poor health in the United States.

Many people who exercise regularly, who participate in athletics or who are trying to increase muscle mass assume they need higher amounts of protein. By consuming more calories to offset the higher caloric expenditure, however, your body's protein needs are being adequately met. When you eat additional calories in the form of protein, they're stored as fat if your caloric intake is greater than your caloric expenditure.

MISCONCEPTION #2: Vegetarians don't get enough vitamins and minerals.

The only type of vegetarian who would have difficulty consuming all the recommended vitamins and minerals would be a vegan. If you've chosen to eliminate all animal products, then consider this nutritional information:

Iron

Plant foods contain only nonheme iron, which theoretically can limit your body's iron absorption. While the vegetarian diet has a typically higher iron content than the nonvegetarian, iron stores

Iron Content of Selected Plant Sources

FOOD	SERVING SIZE	IRON CONTENT
Tofu	½ cup	6-13 mg
Lentils	½ cup	3.3 mg
Kidney, garbanzo & pinto beans	½ cup	2.2-2.6 mg
Soy milk	1 cup	1.4 mg
Cream of Wheat	¾ cup	9-11 mg
Bran flakes with raisins	¾ cup	4.5 mg
Whole wheat bread	1 slice	0.9 mg
Baked potato	1	2.8 mg
Peas	½ cup	1.2 mg
Broccoli	½ cup	0.9 mg
Tomato	1 medium size	0.6 mg
Dried apricots	10	1.5 mg

appear to be lower in vegetarians. However, the clinical significance of this observation is questionable because vegetarians and nonvegetarians have very similar rates of iron deficiency anemia.

Recommendation: 10 to 12 mg daily for men; 10 to 15 mg for women; and 6 to 15 mg for infants and children.

Vitamin B-12

Vegans do not have a reliable source of this vitamin. Fortified foods or a multipurpose nutritional supplement is recommended if you plan to eliminate all animal products from your diet.

Calcium

Calcium requirements haven't yet been established for people who eat less animal protein. It is my position that vegetarians need less calcium because they maintain a more alkaline diet, which has been shown to create a calcium-sparing effect (less calcium is leached from your bones, reducing the need for calcium in the diet).[2] Calcium is well-absorbed from many plant sources and even the vegan option can provide adequate calcium.[3]

If you adopt *The Good News* Diet and consume 25 grams of fiber with 25 fat grams or less each day, coupled with a variety of foods,

Plant Sources of Calcium

FOOD	SERVING SIZE	CALCIUM CONTENT
Tofu (made with calcium)	¼ cup	430 mg
Navy beans	½ cup	64 mg
Pinto beans	½ cup	41 mg
Almonds, dry roasted	1/3 cup	120–170 mg
Broccoli, cooked	1 cup	178 mg
Okra	1 cup	176 mg
Kale	1 cup	94 mg
Rutabaga	1 cup	72 mg
Orange	1, medium size	54 mg
Strawberries	½ cup	16 mg
Apple	1, medium size	10 mg
Collards	½ cup	144 mg
Spinach	½ cup	84 mg
Pancake	1 (4" diameter)	116 mg
Tortilla, corn	1 (6" diameter)	60 mg
Bran muffin	1	57 mg

it's unlikely you'll be nutritionally deficient (unless you choose a vegan option from *The Good News* Diet, where fortification or supplementation is recommended). Compare your current diet for the food pyramid above to fine-tune it into an optimal plan.

Recommendation: National recommendations for calcium intake for people on a plant-based diet have not been determined.

Vitamin D

Most diets have the potential to be deficient in this vitamin. You need vitamin D in your diet only when sun exposure is limited. The sun's exposure to your hands, arms and face for as brief as five to fifteen minutes each day appears to adequately provide for your vitamin D needs. If your exposure to the sun is inadequate, you may need a nutritional supplement or fortified foods.

Zinc

The bioavailability of zinc may be lower when it's obtained from plants. Some studies suggest that most vegetarians have zinc intake similar to nonvegetarians. Also, zinc levels in various body tissues of vegetarians is similar to nonvegetarians.

Recommendation: 12 to 15 mg daily for adults; 5 to 15 mg for infants and children.

Selected Plant Sources of Zinc

FOOD	SERVING SIZE	ZINC CONTENT
Adzuki beans	½ cup	2.0 mg
Tofu	½ cup	1.0 mg
Garbanzo beans	½ cup	1.3 mg
Lentils	½ cup	1.2 mg
Legumes (average)	½ cup	1.0mg
Pumpkin or flax seeds	¼ cup	2.6 mg
Pecans	¼ cup	1.5 mg
Walnuts	¼ cup	0.8 mg
Brown rice, cooked	½ cup	0.6 mg
Oatmeal, cooked	½ cup	0.6 mg
Whole wheat bread	1 slice	0.4-0.6 mg
Peas	½ cup	1.0 mg
Baked potato	1	0.6 mg
Avocado	1	0.7 mg

Comparing plans

So we've now established a nutritional foundation that will help you reach and maintain your recommended weight, increase your life expectancy and improve your feeling of well-being. If you choose the most optimal position on *The Good News* Diet (a "10"), the percentage of calories you eat in the form of carbohydrate, fat and protein will be approximately 75 to 80 percent carbohydrate, 10 percent fat, and 10 to 15 percent protein.

Here is a quick comparative summary of the differences in foodstuffs between *The Good News* Diet and the Dr. Atkins Diet.

	Protein	Saturated Fat	Mono and Poly Unsaturated Fat	Total Fat	Carbs
Dr. Atkins' Diet vs. The Good News Diet					
Dr. Atkins*	22%*	25%*	35%*	55%*	18%*
Good News	10-15%	0-2%	8-10%	10%	75-85%

Based on analysis from the Nutrition Action Health Letter.[3]

PRINCIPLE #5
Avoid Refined Carbohydrates; Choose Foods with a Low Glycemic Index

A high-fiber diet helps to prevent the rapid absorption of simple carbohydrates. Carbohydrates are made up of sugar molecules that are connected together in varying lengths and numbers. The glucose in your blood is a single sugar, while table sugar (sucrose) has two sugars attached to each other. Foods that are high in starch have literally thousands of sugars connected to each other.

The greater the number of sugar molecules attached to one another, the more difficult they are to break down in your digestive system and ultimately get absorbed into your bloodstream. If the chain of sugars is long enough, little (if any) absorption takes place, as is the case with fiber.

Simple carbohydrates (sugars), then, are quickly absorbed into your blood. The rapid absorption of glucose (sugar) is followed by a rapid reduction in blood sugar.

This physiological response is the body's overreaction to the rapidly absorbed sugar. The result is an over-secretion of insulin, which frequently culminates in low blood sugar (functional hypoglycemia). In turn, low blood sugar can create unpleasant side effects including lack of concentration, fatigue, sleepiness, shakiness, nausea and lightheadedness. Caffeine and alcohol accentuate this hypoglycemic response.

The rapid absorption of simple carbohydrates can also influence your ability to control your weight. Low blood sugar is one of the most powerful appetite stimulants. The absorption of complex carbohydrates (many sugars connected together) is a much slower process and less likely to stimulate your appetite.

One of the reasons I've asked you to eat 25 grams of fiber every day is that fiber slows sugar absorption, which helps keep your blood sugar more stable. Also, your appetite is more likely to be suppressed and during the day, physiological ups and downs in your energy level (due to fluctuations in blood sugar levels) will be less common.

Fruit sugars vs. table sugar

Q: Are fruit sugars any better for you than table sugar?

A: If you extract the fruit sugar from apples, grapes or berries, the answer is no. By extracting the sugar from a sugar beet, you eliminate the fiber and other important nutrients such as vitamins.

Don't be fooled into believing that a food product sweetened with a fruit sugar provides any health benefit; it's no different than being sweetened by table sugar.

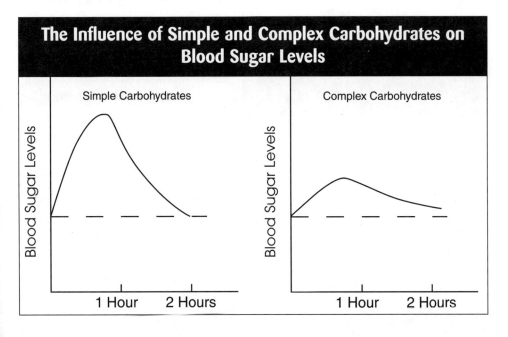

The Influence of Simple and Complex Carbohydrates on Blood Sugar Levels

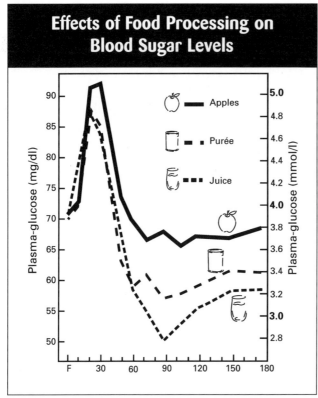

Effects of Food Processing on Blood Sugar Levels

Adapted from *The Lancet,* Oct 1, 1977, p. 680

Sugar Found in Plant Sources

When sugar is found naturally in fruits, grains and vegetables, it's usually associated with fiber, which significantly blunts the possibility that the sugar will be absorbed rapidly. It's only when you extract the sugar from the plant and discard the fiber, vitamins and minerals that nutritional dilemmas develop.

Types of Fiber

Dietary fiber is frequently classified as either soluble or insoluble; both provide distinctive health benefits.

Insoluble fiber, which does not dissolve in water, is found in wheat bran, whole grains and vegetables. Insoluble fiber absorbs water, increasing the fecal bulk. That's one reason constipation, diverticular disease and hemorrhoids are less likely in people who consume adequate amounts of insoluble fiber. Also, colon cancer is less of a risk, perhaps because foods pass more rapidly through the digestive system when you eat higher amounts of insoluble fiber.

Soluble fiber dissolves in water and is found in beans, oats, barley and some fruits and vegetables. Evidence suggests this type of fiber helps prevent the absorption of cholesterol and reduces the rate of sugar absorption into the bloodstream.

Sources of Soluble and Insoluble Fiber

SOLUBLE	INSOLUBLE
Oat bran	Wheat bran
Rice bran	Vegetables
Beans	Fruits
Lentils	Corn
Peas	Rye
Fruits	Barley
Vegetables	Brown rice

What About Fiber Supplements?

While fiber supplements can provide some health benefits, they are no substitutes for the fiber found naturally in fruits, grains and vegetables.

PRINCIPLE #6
Minimize Alcohol and Caffeine Intake

Before you begin *The Good News* Diet, there are several other nutritional concerns to consider.

Caffeine

Americans consume more caffeine than any other population in the world. The use of this socially accepted stimulant (drug) is a reflection of American priorities. Because, as a people, we're motivated by jobs and money, we frequently use stimulants in an attempt to become more productive.

Caffeine is a form of "artificial energy," which in the short term can stimulate mental function, relieve fatigue and drowsiness, and elevate mood in general. My clinical experience has taught me, however, that most people who borrow energy from a drug typically have to make some form of unwelcome payback.

Do you have any of the symptoms in the list (right)? Is it possible caffeine is the source?

Your body has remarkable internal mechanisms that prevent you from becoming overly stressed and ultimately anxious. Too often, unfortunately, we seem willing to disregard body signals (like fatigue, irritability, lack of concentration and anger) that if properly interpreted would result in disengagement from the stressful situation.

Without the use of stimulants, we might not be able to complete a project or meet a specific deadline. But we would also be much less susceptible to stress-induced symptoms and health problems.

Symptoms Associated with the Use of Caffeine

1. Nervousness
2. Irritability
3. Headaches
4. Tachypnea (rapid breathing)
5. Tremulousness
6. Insomnia
7. Restlessness
8. Tachycardia (rapid heart rate)
9. Dysrhythmia (irregular heart beat)
10. Nausea
11. Diarrhea
12. Heartburn
13. Irritable Bowel

The single most important factor influencing your feeling of well-being is your ability to manage stress effectively. If you don't manage it well, your quality of life goes south. Haven't you noticed a relationship between stress and your feeling of well-being in your own life? When your anxiety levels are well-controlled, you probably feel great.

It's been my clinical experience that much of the depression and many of the anxiety disorders that we see in the community surrounding our Institute is affected, if not induced, by socially accepted drugs like caffeine, nicotine and alcohol.

When you optimize your diet and make other lifestyle changes that enhance your quality of life, you won't need to use stimulants.

Caffeine Content in Selected Beverages, Foods and Medications

SOURCE	CAFFEINE CONTENT
Coffee (5-oz cup)	
Drip method	110-150 mg
Percolated	64-124 mg
Instant	40-108 mg
Tea (5-oz cup)	
1-minute brewed	9-33 mg
3-minute brewed	20-46 mg
Instant	12-28 mg
Chocolate	
6-oz cup of hot cocoa	2-8 mg
1-oz milk chocolate	1-15 mg
Soft Drinks (12-oz can)	
Mountain Dew	54 mg
Coca-Cola/Diet Coke	46 mg
Dr. Pepper	40 mg
Pepsi Cola	38 mg
Diet Pepsi	36 mg
Stimulants and Pain Relievers	
No-Doz Tablets	100 mg
Vivarin	200 mg
Anacin	32 mg
Excedrin	65 mg

Alcohol

Traditional medicine today defines "alcohol moderation" as one or two drinks per day. That's unfortunate. This definition suggests to people that having fourteen scotch and waters each week is moderate consumption.

While alcohol appears to provide some cardio-protective benefits, it's unconscionable to encourage people to reduce their risk of heart disease by drinking alcohol, especially when the potential for other health problems increases. If everyone began to drink wine to prevent heart attacks, we would experience significant increases in alcoholism, social drinking problems, cancer death rates, gastro-intestinal complaints, hypertension, obesity and other related health problems.

It's best to abstain from alcohol if your goal is to reduce your overall health risks and maintain a high quality of life. If you choose to drink alcohol, maintain at least five days of abstinence each week, while limiting your quantity to no more than three ounces of pure alcohol per week (28 to 30 ounces of wine, three to four mixed drinks or six 12-ounce beers).

Sodium

Many authors overstate their concern that virtually all people should limit their salt consumption. Too many of our patients have emphasized restricting sodium intake over achieving other nutritional goals.

For the most part, patients with hypertension (high blood pressure) need to be most concerned with restricting sodium. But not all patients with hypertension are sensitive to sodium, so limiting their intake has little impact on their clinical status.

Sodium Content of Selected Foods

FOOD	SERVING SIZE	SODIUM CONTENT
Bacon	1 strip	71 mg
Frankfurter	1 frank	627 mg
Sausage	3½ oz	740 mg
Cheddar cheese	½ cup	350 mg
Peanut butter	3 tbsp	291 mg
Macaroni and cheese prepared from package	1 cup	574 mg
Frozen turkey pie	8 oz	1020 mg
Whole wheat bread	1 slice	121 mg
Corn flakes	1 cup	251 mg
Shredded Wheat	1 cup	2 mg
Noodles, spaghetti	1 cup	2–3 mg
Milk	1 cup	122 mg
Orange juice	6 oz	Trace
Catsup	1 tbsp	156 mg
Pickle, dill, 3" long	1	928 mg
Salt	1 tsp	2132 mg
Soy sauce	1 tsp	440 mg

Larry's pseudo-heart attack

Larry, 29, woke up one morning sweating and with his heart racing. He was convinced he was having a heart attack.

He ended up seeing several physicians and undergoing many cardiac tests. The results were all normal and each of the physicians concluded his heart was fine. Every time a physician would tell Larry his heart was healthy, his anxiety level would decrease for about 12 hours. Then he would start to worry all over again that the physician had missed something. How else could he explain his recurring chest pain?

Finally, Larry came to see me at Oakland University's Meadow Brook Health Enhancement Institute, unable to go to work because of extreme fatigue and lack of concentration. After he finished providing me with his health history, I asked what he was doing on the day and evening before he woke up thinking he was having a heart attack. He said he had planted trees that day and was chewing tobacco the entire time. That night he was extremely tired and while he did paperwork, he began drinking diet soft

Here's what you need to know about restricting sodium from your diet: If you have high blood pressure, limit your sodium intake to 2,000 mg per day. (The average American consumes between 4,000 and 6,000 mg per day.) That's it. If you are among the one-in-five individuals who has high blood pressure and is sensitive to sodium intake, this level of restriction is usually necessary to reduce your blood pressure.

Decide on Your Plan of Action

Are you ready to determine your specific nutritional goals for reducing body fat, preventing disease and enhancing your feeling of well-being?

Good. Here again is a quick summary of the six principles that serve as the foundation for *The Good News* Diet:

- Limit fat consumption to no more than 25 grams of fat per day

- Consume at least 25 grams of fiber per day

- Select food groups and recommended servings from *The Good News* Food Pyramid

- Limit animal products (meats and dairy selections)

- Avoid refined carbohydrates. When consuming foods individually, choose foods with a low glycemic index

drinks with caffeine and eating chocolate. As his fatigue levels increased week after week, he found himself requiring more stimulants (caffeine) to overcome his fatigue.

That night, when Larry thought he was having a heart attack, he was really experiencing what Dr. Claire Weeks calls a fatigue or collapse of his nervous system. When Larry and I reviewed the weeks and months preceding the event, he realized it wasn't something that "happened out of the blue." It had been building for many months, but he didn't recognize the signals his body was sending him.

Chewing tobacco results in a rapid absorption of nicotine. Combined with the caffeine in his soft drinks and chocolate, his nervous system simply couldn't take anymore.

This story has a happy ending. I gave Dr. Weeks' book, *Hope and Help For Your Nerves* to Larry. He quit using all stimulants and gradually regained his good health. Once he understood how devastating the fatigue of his nervous system could be and made healthy lifestyle changes, he was on his way to recovery.

• Minimize alcohol and caffeine intake.

And remember that *The Good News* Diet is based on a continuum of nutritional options. You now have the responsibility for determining the specifics of your diet, based on the priority you have placed on health enhancement.

Be assured that if you follow *The Good News* Diet, you will significantly improve your chances of achieving your recommended body fat percent and reducing your risk of a chronic degenerative disease.

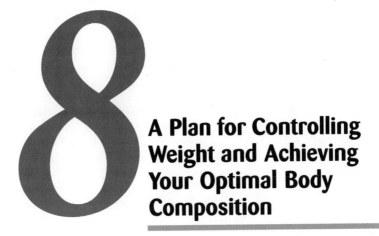

A Plan for Controlling Weight and Achieving Your Optimal Body Composition

In This Chapter:

✔ Body type, optimal weight and genetic limitations

✔ Measuring your body fat content

✔ Three approaches to lowering your body fat content

If I asked what you thought you should weigh, based on the goal of achieving your optimal health, what would you say? Maybe you think you need to lose 20 pounds; maybe 40 or even 80. What would you base your decision on?

Now, draw a picture in your mind of the body contour (figure) you would like to have. What would it look like?

Many times, the body shape and appearance you desire may not be consistent with your genetic limitations. Also, achieving a body composition (or a weight) that is associated with optimal health may not match with the body contour you'd like to have. In other words, your optimal weight for health enhancement purposes may not result in the body shape you want. Remember, while everyone is capable of achieving a low percentage of body fat, not everyone can have the body appearance they would like.

Unfortunately, too many people decide what they should weigh based on height and weight charts or body mass index tables. Although these references correlate with your ability to prevent heart disease, cancer, strokes and diabetes, it's not a *strong* correlation.

Also, height and weight tables don't provide information about the *type* of body you have, making it impossible to determine the genetic limitations you'll face in trying to create your ideal body contour. Too often, the body contour we strive for is based on a "model" used in an advertisement, rather than genetic reality.

For these reasons, you should have your body composition assessed when beginning a weight loss program. Every year, I see many people who have misconceptions about the body type they have, what they should weigh and the genetic potential they have to create a specific body shape and weight.

Completing body composition studies can clear up the confusion. Without it, you're vulnerable to outrageous advertisements claiming you can create any type of body you want. Remember the Sirens we talked about? You'll find them in these ads, too. Their attractive models will seduce you into believing you can have the perfect body by buying their product.

Sorry, it doesn't happen that way. Instead of wishing for a body type you can't achieve, stay focused on what you should weigh for optimal health.

Measuring Fat Through Body Composition Studies

Body composition studies help differentiate between the types of body tissues you have. Two people of the same sex, height and weight can vary substantially in the amount of body fat they have.

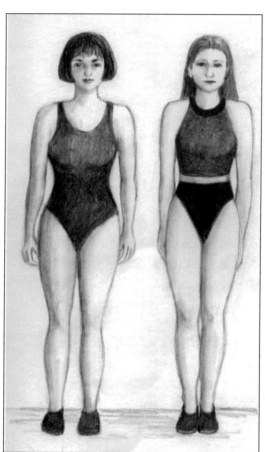

Height and weight charts tell you how *big* you are compared to people of a similar height, not how *fat* you are. It's not necessarily un-healthy to weigh more than other people of the same height. You should be more concerned with your percentage of body fat. Carrying extra amounts of body fat, no matter how tall or heavy you are, increases your risk of developing a major health problem.

Clinically, body composition measurements are more meaningful than height and weight charts. The reason is, your weight is made up of a combination of both lean tissue (muscle and

	SUBJECT A	SUBJECT B
Weight	150 lbs	150 lbs
Height	5 feet, 7 inches	5 feet, 7 inches
Body Fat	32%	25%
Body Fat	48 lbs	37.5 lbs
Lean Body Weight	102 lbs	112.5 lbs
Recommended Max. Weight	136 lbs	150 lbs

bone) and fat tissue. So you need to determine your optimal weight based on the amount of body fat you have.

At Oakland University's Meadow Brook Health Enhancement Institute, we recommend the following body fat percent ranges:

Men		Women
9% to 15%		19% to 25 %

We've seen many patients achieve these body-fat percent values and none of them—not one—has experienced a health problem that was linked to his weight. And while you can reach a lower body fat percentage than what I recommend, we have not been able to demonstrate further health benefits of doing that. Any decision to further reduce your body fat content would have to be based on how you want to look or feel.

Assume you're a male weighing 160 pounds and your body composition study indicates you have 25 percent body fat. Let's figure the maximum weight we would recommend for you.

According to the above standard, your maximum body fat as a male should be 15 percent; your lean body weight, of course, should remain the same (I don't want you to lose any muscle or bone weight). So, you should reduce your body fat from 25 percent to 15 percent, while maintaining lean body weight.

Your body composition results would be:
Weight = 160 pounds
Fat percent = 25
Fat content = 40 pounds (25% of 160 pounds)
Lean body weight = 120 pounds
Recommended maximum weight = 141 pounds
Recommended minimum reduction = 19 pounds
   (160 pounds - 141 pounds)
In this example, you would have to lose 19 pounds of body fat.

Hydrostatic (water) weighing is the most accurate way to determine your body composition and recommended weight. Best of all, it's painless. We ask you to change into a swimsuit and then immerse your body in a water tank.

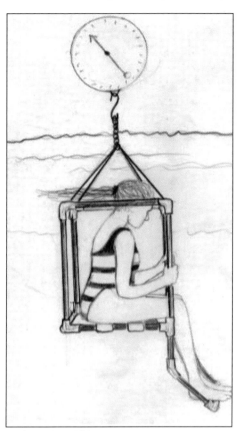

Hydrostatic weighing

The principle is simple: muscle sinks in water but fat will float. The heavier you are underwater, the leaner you are. That's because as body fat decreases or lean body mass increases, your underwater weight increases.

Skinfold analysis is a simplistic way to measure body fat, but it provides a good body composition estimate when administered by a technician with experience. This technique uses a hand-held, tong-like instrument that painlessly "pinches" fat at selected sites on your body, allowing the technician to measure fat content at each spot.

The technician can develop a good estimate of your body composition through skinfold analysis because most of your body fat is directly under the skin. Equations have been developed, based on underwater weight observations, that estimate the percentage of your total body fat.

Lower Your Body Fat Content and Reach Your Recommended Weight

You should lose weight only by losing body fat. However, it's possible to lose lean mass and body fluids through a variety of weight loss procedures—all of them undesirable. The program I've outlined below will help you lose weight safely and effectively.

Body Fat and Energy Balance

As indicated in previous chapters, body fat changes are a function of the energy balance equation. Your body fat content won't change if you take in and burn off the same amount of calories.

IF your caloric intake = caloric expenditure,
THEN body fat content is unchanged

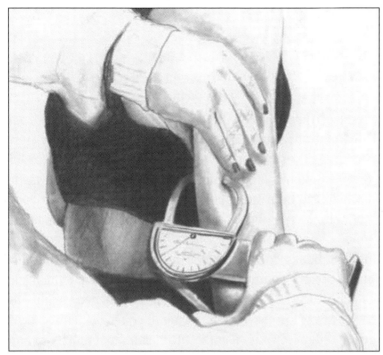

Skinfold analysis is a simple way to measure body fat.

Your body fat content will change any time there's an imbalance in this simple formula. Eat 2,000 calories and burn off 1,800? You'll end up with more body fat. Take in 1,500 and expend 2,000? Now you're losing body fat. Either way, you're changing the fat content of your body.

You can take three approaches to lower your body fat content:

- Diet: Take in fewer calories than your daily energy requirements

- Exercise: Burn more calories than your daily energy requirements

- Develop a program that combines exercise *and* diet.

Even small changes in this daily energy balance equation can dramatically influence your weight over time. You could gain an extra ten pounds of body fat over the course of a year, for example, just by consuming a hundred calories a day above your caloric expenditures. That amounts to one extra light beer or a medium-sized apple per day.

Example

An additional apple or light beer per day = 100 calories

100 calories x 365 days = 36,500 calories

One pound of body fat contains about 3,500 calories

36,500 calories / 3,500 = 10.4 pounds

At the end of the year, you would wonder where that extra ten pounds came from and what you did differently. Without a good understanding of just how many calories you take in and burn off every day, it would be hard to point to that daily beer or apple as the culprit. Obviously, even small changes in your diet or activity patterns can dramatically affect your body fat content over a long period of time.

Most diet books don't recognize the importance of a complete program of weight control. We have failed miserably to halt our nation's epidemic of obesity because we've approached weight loss almost exclusively through dietary means. If you hope to lose weight and then maintain it, your weight control plan *should* include more than just the most recent fad diet.

Despite the difficulty you may have in losing body fat or keeping it off, be encouraged by the fact that *everyone* is capable of achieving one's recommended weight. It may mean you'll have to work harder than others—or maybe you won't.

It all depends on your personal commitment to the three weight control steps I'm going to outline for you in the next chapter—your three keys to finally getting rid of unwanted body fat.

Phil discovers the benefit of body composition studies

Recently Phil, a diabetic patient, came to our institute for a body composition study. His physician had recommended he reach a certain weight based on height and weight charts. By using hydrostatic (water weighing) measurements, we determined that he should lose an additional 30 pounds of body fat beyond his doctor's target weight.

Based on this recommendation, he lost the additional weight—and no longer takes medication for his diabetes.

Body fat content is a powerful risk factor for adult onset diabetes. If you have diabetes or a family history of it, body composition analysis becomes even more important.

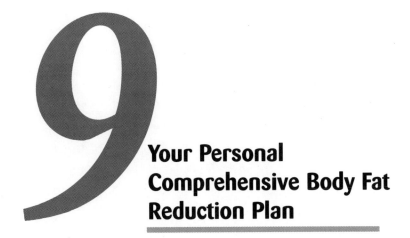

9
Your Personal Comprehensive Body Fat Reduction Plan

In This Chapter:
- ✔ The top ten benefits of exercise
- ✔ An exercise prescription for reducing body fat
- ✔ Seven tips for exercise success
- ✔ The importance of reading food labels
- ✔ Keeping your food diary

The body contour you would like to have may not be realistic given your genetic limitations. However, the most important goal when reducing body fat content is to achieve optimal health— the highest level of good health and quality of life that you can personally reach.

This goal is well within your reach, assuming you make weight loss a priority and follow your own personal comprehensive body fat reduction plan.

In chapter seven, I presented to you the six principles that form the foundation for *The Good News* Diet. This dietary plan will be part of a comprehensive program for reducing body fat content that includes the following components:

- Exercise that burns at least 2,000 calories each week above the energy needs of your normal recreational and occupational activity

- The 25/25 nutritional plan that limits fat to 25 grams per day and includes at least 25 grams of fiber a day

- A strategy for behavior modification.

Your Exercise Plan for Reducing Body Fat

The major cause of latent weight gain in the United States is lack of physical activity.[1] Over the last century in America, we've actually *decreased* the amount of calories we take in. In fact, some estimates suggest we now eat up to 10 percent *fewer* calories than a few years ago.[2] So why are we more obese? Quite simply, we live more sedentary lifestyles.

Many studies suggest exercise is more effective than dieting if your goal is long-term control of body fat content.[3] Our nation's technological explosion has made us the economic power of the world, but it's also been a health curse.

Think of all your daily tasks that are less demanding physically thanks to our technological boom. Instead of shoveling snow, you use a snowblower. You ride a lawnmower rather than push it (and if you still walk behind one, it's probably self-propelled). Electric washing machines, clothes dryers and dishwashers are as common as televisions. There are thousands of additional examples of how Americans today actually program physical activity *out* of their lives. Is it any wonder we face an epidemic of obesity as a nation?

Take a minute to count how many ways you've become less active over your lifetime. Maybe it's time to build an exercise program back into your life before you face the inevitable result: a protruding abdomen and weight gain.

Given this trend toward less daily activity, it's unrealistic to expect to lose body fat—and keep it off—without making a commitment to regular exercise. Already, I can hear the collective groan out there, along with common excuses and complaints:

> *"But I don't like to exercise."*

> *"Who has time? Between work and kids, I barely have time to sleep."*

> *"I just don't have the energy anymore."*

> *"Can't you give me an easier way?"*

While you may see exercise as an unpleasant requirement right now, it can actually become the highlight of your day once you get going. The hard part is taking that first step. Regular exercise pays great dividends in your quest to achieve optimal health. Motivate yourself by thinking about these health benefits that are associated with regular exercise.

As you develop a plan for optimal health, one of your priorities should be to improve your ability to function. Many people can actu-

---

The Top 10 Benefits of Regular Exercise

1) Lower risk of death from heart attacks

2) Lower risk of death from strokes

3) Lower risk of death from cancer

4) Lower risk of diabetes

5) Lower risk of osteoporosis

6) Lower risk of hypertension

7) Lower risk of obesity

8) Lower risk of depression

9) Lower anxiety levels

10) Better overall functionality: strength, flexibility, muscular endurance, cardiorespiratory endurance

ally reach age 100 if they live an optimum lifestyle. But it won't mean much if you increase your life expectancy yet lose your ability to function physically and experience a lower quality of life.

Personally, I've set as goals to achieve a longer life expectancy and a high quality of life, and that's why I've made exercise my most important lifestyle priority.

How Activity Affects Your Appetite

Exercise can influence your appetite, but it depends on the type and duration of the activity.

If your job requires you to burn a lot of calories, your appetite will probably be stimulated. Construction workers and lumberjacks can burn so many calories that they require a higher calorie intake to maintain their weight. Under these situations of extreme caloric expenditures, the body seems to compensate with a stimulated appetite. But these are extreme physical examples. When you exercise regularly and burn the equivalent of 2,000 calories each week, most people will experience a reduced appetite.

Keep in mind that exercise affects each person's appetite differently. However, most patients I've worked with have less of an appetite after beginning a regular exercise program.

Here's another great tip: Use physical activity as a substitute behavior when you find yourself in an environment that typically stimulates appetite. For example, watching television is frequently associated with eating. Going for a short walk before watching your favorite TV show, though, can reduce your motivation to eat.

Love to snack while watching a ball game? Take a bike ride just beforehand or lift weights during the first inning. You'll be surprised how your appetite decreases.

Find yourself eating more on lazy Saturday afternoons? Start every Saturday with a family walk, a bike ride through the neighborhood or yard work. You'll tend to want to eat less during the day.

How Much Body Fat Will You Lose from Exercise?

Most people have no idea what to expect from their exercise program.

I've trained more than five hundred physicians in preventive medicine, and I continue to be amazed at how reluctant they are to make exercise recommendations that their patients might perceive as overly demanding. I'm also surprised at their misconceptions about exercise and weight control, such as the amount of body fat patients can expect to lose from prescribed exercise programs.

One of our physicians, currently in training, prescribed for Susan, a 150-pound female, a one-mile walk to be completed in 20 minutes, four times each week. Susan was asked to return three months later to evaluate her progress.

Before leaving, Susan asked how much body fat she could expect lose in three months from this exercise prescription. The question took our physician-in-training by surprise. His answer was that if she would keep her caloric intake constant, she should lose about 15 pounds by her three-month appointment.

After hearing this, I asked him to actually calculate the amount of body fat she would lose. Using a standard energy expenditure table, you can see that a 150-pound woman burns 5.4 calories per minute while walking. Susan was asked to walk one mile in 20 minutes; this creates a caloric expenditure of 108 calories.

Susan's prescription was to walk three times a week for three months. So each week, she would burn 324 calories (108 calories times three) and in twelve weeks, or three months, she would burn 3,888 calories (324 times 12). One pound of body fat equals 3,500 calories, so if she keeps her calorie intake the same, Susan can expect to lose about 1.1 pounds of body fat in three months.

When your top health priority is to lose weight, there's a world of difference between 15 pounds and 1 pound. Obviously, Susan would have become very discouraged if the discrepancy between her actual weight loss and the physician's expectation was so substantial.

I need to make several important points regarding the above example:

- It's unrealistic to expect significant reductions in body fat content in a short period of time. Even in running a marathon, most people will only lose one pound of body fat (even though they many lose many pounds of weight due to fluid loss).

- Don't confuse this slow process of losing body fat with the long-term answer to weight control: regular exercise. You can lose 10 pounds of weight in a year by walking just one extra mile every day. (That's more than Susan; remember, she was only asked to walk three times a week for three months.) Make exercise a way of life rather than an activity that you skip when other priorities come up.

- Energy expenditure table references are available that can allow you to create your own exercise prescription for reducing body fat content. You'll know exactly how much weight you can lose, based on the duration and frequency of the activity you select.

Don't Break Your Stride

It's important that you follow a reasonable progression of physical activity as you begin your program. This is particularly true if you're carrying too much body fat and have been inactive for a long time. While it's important to talk with your physician before implementing an exercise program, it has been my clinical experience that most people can tolerate an exercise program that burns 900 calories per week.

The key in starting is to make sure the intensity of your effort is appropriate in the early stages of your exercise program. Start with a program that burns 900 calories per week, and be consistent by exercising on most days during the week. Three months into your program, most people can begin to add 100 calories of activity every week until reaching the goal of burning (expending) 2,000 calories per week.

Your Exercise Prescription to Reduce Body Fat

Ideally, assessing your work capacity by completing a stress test can create the most appropriate exercise prescription. This objective assessment of your ability to work allows you to individualize your program.

Consider these five prescription components when you create your exercise program designed to reduce body fat content:

A. Type of exercise

B. Duration

C. Intensity

D. Frequency

E. Caloric expenditure.

A. Type of exercise

The activity you select should involve large muscle groups and be an activity that is continuous and rhythmic. Try walking, using a treadmill, jogging, dancing, cycling, rowing and other forms of continuous exercise that can be tolerated orthopedically and controlled cardiovascularly. The physiological intensity of these activities should be fairly consistent as you perform the exercise.

Racquetball, basketball and other court sports can be intense cardiovascular activities; I don't recommend them if you're just starting your conditioning program. While these sports burn plenty of calories and can be great activities in your future plans for exercise, make sure you're well-conditioned first to avoid injuries.

The exercise I most frequently recommend is walking. In most cases, you don't need a facility to walk and the only investment you have to make is in a good pair of shoes. Injury rates are low and it has great social benefits. You can walk with a neighbor, relative, pet or friend—or take the opportunity to make a new friend.

Ultimately, the form of exercise you choose for body fat reduction should be a personal preference. Just decide on an activity you enjoy. Choosing an activity you dislike or find boring makes it unlikely you'll continue a lifetime program of physical activity.

Get involved in several different activities; maybe walking one day and cycling the next. You'll enjoy the variety and gain additional benefits by exercising multiple muscle groups.

B. Duration of exercise

So how long should you exercise? Ten minutes? An hour? It depends on the type of exercise you choose as well as the health and performance goals you establish.

If your primary goal is to lose weight, then you'll want an activity you can do for longer periods (and one you'll be able to tolerate orthopedically and control cardiovascularly). The duration of your exercise is the single most important variable that determines caloric expenditure for an individual workout session and, thus, how much body fat you lose. It's very simple: The longer you can exercise, the more calories you'll burn.

Exercises such as walking, using the treadmill, swimming, cycling and rowing generally allow you to exercise for longer periods with a lower risk for an overuse injury.

I encourage you to begin your exercise program, with some form of continuous activity, for at least thirty minutes per session. At Oakland University's Meadow Brook Health Enhancement Institute, even our sixty- and seventy-year-old participants are able to continuously exercise for at least thirty minutes, with the appropriate exercise intensity.

Two months after you begin your conditioning program, add one minute per exercise session per week until you reach one hour of continuous exercise per session.

If you decide you can't or don't want to exercise continuously for at least one hour per day, you can do thirty minutes in the morning and thirty in the evening. You'll burn essentially the same number of calories, whether you exercise all at once or in multiple sessions.

Here's a sample schedule:

	MONDAY	WEDNESDAY	FRIDAY	SUNDAY
Weeks 1–8:	30 min.	30 min.	30 min.	30 min.
Week 9:	31 min.	31 min.	31 min.	31 min.
Week 10:	32 min.	32 min.	32 min.	32 min.
Week 11:	33 min.	33 min.	33 min.	33 min.

… and so on, until you reach sixty minutes per session. Also, make it your goal to exercise on most days of the week, but three at a minimum.

C. Intensity of exercise

Now you need to determine the intensity of your exercise. And the best way is to use your body's built-in exercise monitor—the heart.

Your heart rate (number of heartbeats per minute) provides an excellent indication of how hard your body is working. For example, you'll have a higher heart rate for a specific level of activity on a hot and humid day, when exercise is more challenging. In other words, this built-in monitor signals through your heart rate that the work has become more difficult physiologically.

To enjoy a safe and effective exercise program, then, you need to learn to record your pulse rate.

If you are a healthy person, you should be able to tolerate exer-

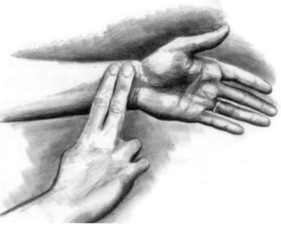

(Right) Pulse-counting from the radial artery.
(Below) Pulse-counting from the carotid artery.

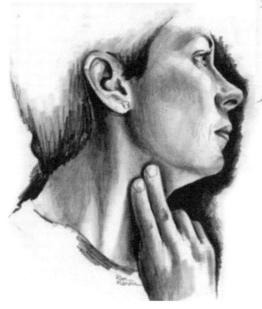

cising at 70 percent to 85 percent of your maximum heart rate, recorded immediately after exercise. This level of exercise intensity will enhance your cardiorespiratory fitness and produce a caloric expenditure that you should be able to sustain. If you've completed a stress test, your maximum heart rate should have been recorded at the peak of the stress test, when you were unable to keep up with the treadmill. Find out what that maximal rate was by requesting the information from your physician.

As an example, if your maximum heart rate is 180 beats per minute, then most people would be encouraged to achieve an exercise heart rate of at least 126 beats per minute.

As you begin to exercise, stop and check your pulse. Take it for six seconds and add a zero to the rate you obtained to determine beats per minute. If your heart beats 12 times in six seconds, add a zero to the 12 to get your heart rate: 120.

Counting your pulse for longer than six seconds may not provide as good an indication of the heart rate you achieved during exercise.

In this example, if your heart rate was less than 126 beats per minute, you may want to increase your exercise intensity.

It's not necessary to exercise above 85 percent of your maximal heart rate to achieve significant health benefits and a significant caloric expenditure.

You can estimate your maximum heart rate, even if you have not completed a stress test or fitness evaluation. Just subtract your age from 220. For instance, if you are fifty years old, we can estimate your maximum heart rate to be 170 (220 - 50 = 170). The recommended range while exercising would still be 70 percent to 85 percent of this number.

Age: 50
Estimated maximal heart rate: 220–50 = 170
170 x 70 percent = 119 beats per minute
170 x 85 percent = 145 beats per minute
Recommended range for exercise: 119 to 145 beats per minute

Remember that when using the equation (220 minus your age) to estimate your maximum heart rate, it is just that—an estimate. Your maximum heart rate can be different from that of someone else your age. Also, certain medications and health problems can affect your heart rate during exercise.

You can also use the following Borg Scale to determine an appropriate exercise intensity. This scale quantifies your perception of exercise intensity.

The Borg scale of perceived exertion

You don't need to exceed a 12 or 13 on the Borg Scale to lose weight, or to gain most other health benefits, for that matter. Forget what the TV infomercials say; exercise doesn't have to be hard to create a significant caloric expenditure. Here's a simple test for whether your activity is too intense: You should be able to carry on a conversation while you exercise. If you can't, the intensity is greater than it needs to be.

You can estimate which types of exercise will burn the most calories based on your heart rate response. Generally, the higher your heart rate, the more calories expended. Remember, though, that early in your exercise program, you should emphasize long-duration, low-intensity activities.

In other words LSD—Long, Slow, Duration.

The Borg Scale of Perceived Exertion

6
7 very, very light
8
9 very light
10
11 fairly light
12
13 somewhat hard
14
15 hard
16
17 very hard
18
19 extremely hard
20

D. Frequency of exercise

So, how serious are you about achieving optimal health? Do you *really* want the best opportunity to lose body fat?

If so, exercise on most days. This is the best approach to losing body fat and to achieve the greatest overall health benefit.

At a minimum, consider committing to exercising at least every other day. Any exercise will burn calories, but if you exercise fewer than three times a week, you're not likely to lose a significant amount of body fat or to reach an enhanced cardiorespiratory fitness level.

The longer you are into your exercise program, the easier it will get. By committing to a more frequent exercise program, the more health benefits you will likely experience—and the easier it will be to make it a priority in your life.

E. Caloric expenditure

Initially, expend nine hundred calories per week. After three months of conditioning, burn an additional one hundred calories per exercise session per week—an extra mile of walking for example—until you're expending two thousand calories.

5-Step Exercise Prescription for Reducing Body Fat

A. Type of exercise: Continuous exercise that can be tolerated orthopedically and controlled cardiovascularly (walking, treadmill exercise, cycling, stair climbing, swimming, jogging, etc.)

B. Duration: Initially, 30 minutes; eventually 60 minutes or more per exercise session (remember to follow the progression described above)

C. Intensity: 70 percent to 85 percent of your maximum heart rate (recorded immediately following exercise)

D. Frequency: Preferably, cardiorespiratory exercise most days; minimally, every other day

E. Caloric expenditure: At first, burn 900 calories per week. After three months of conditioning, burn an additional 100 calories per exercise session until you are using 2,000 calories per session.

Seven Tips for Exercise Success

Now that you have a prescription for exercise, I have a few final suggestions for getting started—and for maintaining your program.

1. Find the Right Time

Take the first week or two to determine your most desirable time to exercise. Maybe you need to get up an hour early, before work and before getting the kids up. I meet at 7 a.m. to jog with a dozen or so people every weekday morning. It's built right into our workdays.

Maybe your lunch hour works. I know a hospital CEO who jogs for 30 minutes at lunchtime and then has a quick healthy lunch. He invites employees and colleagues to join him; it ends up being a great time to discuss business and to become more social. If a busy hospital executive can commit to exercising every day at lunch, maybe you can too.

My wife is a night person. She prefers to exercise in the evening. The idea of getting up early to exercise doesn't motivate her.

2. Make It a Family Affair

Who says you have to go it alone? Get your family to go with you. Start healthy habits in your children, or rebuild your romance over racquetball. Exercise can be built into many family activities. Make it fun by including the whole family.

Make it simple, too. Take the family for a 30-minute walk every day after dinner. Take a scenic bike ride every evening. Go for a hike by a nearby lake. Include other activities, from in-line-skating to ice skating together. Come on, use your imagination!

3. Find a Buddy

Sometimes it's tough to stick with it when you exercise alone. So try the buddy system. Get someone to join you. It could be your spouse, neighbor, father, daughter, friend, co-worker, boss, pastor—anyone you think is as committed to exercise and health enhancement as you are.

A colleague of mine has told me that he finds it hard to stay with a regimen of working out. So he and his wife joined a gym together. On days he doesn't want to go, his wife motivates him. On other days when she's feeling lazy, he motivates her. Together, they're able to stay with a consistent exercise program.

4. Get the Right Equipment

You'll stay more committed and avoid injury if you invest in the right equipment. If you're planning to walk or jog, invest in a good pair of shoes. Find a store that specializes in footwear for walkers and joggers. This experience in helping you make your selection can be the difference between maintaining your program or developing an injury.

Whether it's racquetball, soccer, cycling or rowing, you need to make sure you have high-quality equipment. If you do, you're more likely to enjoy exercise and less likely to develop an injury.

5. It's OK to Switch

Just because you start on a cycle and end up bored doesn't mean you have to quit exercising altogether. If you don't like cycling, try walking. If you don't like in-line skating, get a bike. If racquetball isn't your game, maybe basketball is.

If your initial type of exercise doesn't grab your interest, find something that does. Also, this is another good reason to include multiple types of exercise into your weekly plan.

Just remember you can't fail unless you quit.

6. S-T-R-E-T-C-H

Start each session with moderate stretching and warming-up exercises. Stretch the muscles you'll be working that day, and warm up by jogging in place or walking at a slow to moderate pace for a few minutes.

7. Give It Time

Don't expect miracles right away. It takes time to lose body fat, and it takes time to get into the exercise groove. If you've been exercising regularly for a month and it still doesn't feel like a habit, don't worry. You need to give it more time.

How long does it take to break a habit? How long would it take to stop smoking or quit using caffeine? Some people can go cold turkey, but most of us take a few weeks, even months to put it behind us. Likewise, for exercise to become a way of life, give it a little more time.

Stick with it. The health payoff can be incredible.

25/25: Your Dietary Plan To Reduce Body Fat

The nutritional foundation for your dietary plan to reduce body fat was presented in chapter seven.

You may recall that there are two practical approaches to implementing this plan. The first requires you to count the number of fat and fiber grams you consume each day. The second option involves following a specific menu plan that has been prepared for you, that provides less than 25 grams of fat and at least 25 grams of fiber every day. To make it easier to remember, we'll call it the 25/25 approach.

Counting Fat and Fiber Grams

What could be more practical than a diet that lets you choose the foods you like to eat?

That's the major advantage with *The Good News* Diet. You have the flexibility to select foods that are consistent with your eating preferences. That means you can develop a plan—*your* plan—that is practical and more likely to be maintained.

If you're willing to follow the 25/25 recommendation and keep track of how much fat and fiber you consume, the chances are *excellent* that your diet will help reduce your body fat content.

Even though all weight loss is directly related to calorie intake, I won't ask you initially to count calories. (I hear a sigh of gratitude out there.) For most people, just quantifying fat and fiber (25/25) grams will result in a caloric deficit without the need to count calories. Remember, to achieve your recommended weight, you need to combine this dietary plan with other elements of your comprehensive body fat-reducing program—exercise and behavioral modification.

The nutritional tables found later in this book provide fat and fiber content for numerous foods. They'll be an excellent reference as you keep track of your grams of fiber and fat each day.

The Importance of Reading Food Labels

Your ability to read a food label will be essential to your success in quantifying fat and fiber intake. Here are the keys to label-reading:

Serving size

An often-overlooked label item is the serving size. In the example (on page 130), the serving size of this cereal product is a half-cup. My canary eats more than a half-cup of almost anything.

Food producers are notorious for low-balling serving size. Don't be deceived by this technique. Take the time to learn how much of a

Nutrition Facts

Serving Size ½ cup (114g)
Servings Per Container 4

Amount Per Serving

Calories 90   Calories from Fat 30

	% Daily Value*
Total Fat 3g	**5%**
Saturated Fat 0g	**0%**
Cholesterol 0mg	**0%**
Sodium 300mg	**13%**
Total Carbohydrate 13g	**4%**
Dietary Fiber 3g	**12%**
Sugars 3g	
Protein 3g	

Vitamin A	80%	•	Vitamin C	60%
Calcium	4%	•	Iron	4%

* Percent Daily Values are based on a 2,000 calorie diet. Your daily values may be higher or lower depending on your calorie needs:

		Calories	2,000	2,500
Total Fat	Less than		65g	80g
Sat Fat	Less than		20g	25g
Cholesterol	Less than		300mg	300mg
Sodium	Less than		2,400mg	2,400mg
Total Carbohydrate			300g	375g
Fiber			25g	30g

Calories per gram:
Fat 9 • Carbohydrate 4 • Protein 4

More nutrients may be listed on some labels.

A food label.

food product is in a cup, tablespoon or ounce. Initially, you'll have to measure containers and quantities, but soon you'll be able to judge by sight and experience.

For instance, my cereal bowl contains a cup-and-a-half of the cereal, so I would be consuming three servings of the cereal described on the label. As for fat and fiber content in this example, multiply the amount on the label on the left (grams of each) by three to determine the total amount you have eaten. If you've done the math correctly, you would have determined that there would be 9 grams of fat and 9 grams of fiber in my bowl of this cereal. (This example doesn't include the fat content of any milk that you add to the cereal.)

Calories

Most people will end up eating fewer calories by restricting fat consumption to 25 grams a day while eating 25 grams of fiber. That's good news, considering that your ability to decrease body fat content depends on calorie consumption.

How does the 25/25 program lower your calorie intake? Well, remember that eating more fiber will suppress your appetite. Also, you'll reduce the highest calorie nutrient in your diet—fat.

If you reach a body fat reduction plateau—you stop losing body fat before reaching your ideal weight target—counting calories at that point may be required.

Total carbohydrate

When you examine food labels for carbohydrates, be sure to emphasize fiber content since you're trying to consume 25 grams a day.

Also, try to reduce your consumption of simple carbohydrates (sugars). Remember, you want your carbohydrate sources to be primarily unrefined, with as little simple sugar added as possible.

Dietary fiber

One basic question: Does the food product you're considering contribute to your fiber goal of 25 grams per day? If not, can you find a better substitute?

Protein

Most Americans eat too much protein, particularly animal protein (meat and dairy). Yet we're constantly told to make sure we get plenty of protein in our diet.

Don't worry about getting enough protein; just make sure you get it from the right sources and that you're using *The Good News* Food Pyramid in making food selections. Preferably, your protein sources would be beans, grains and cereals.

Vitamins and minerals

Keeping track of all the vitamins and minerals you need on a daily basis is almost impossible. You don't need the legion of supplements and vitamin combinations that clog pharmacy shelves. Vitamins and minerals will take care of themselves, if you are guided by *The Good News* Diet Food Pyramid and eat the recommended servings for each food group.

Total fat

Check the labels on your food choices. How much fat do they contribute toward your goal of eating no more than 25 grams per day?

Saturated fat

Saturated fat is the major nutritional culprit that elevates your blood cholesterol levels and increases your risk of coronary artery disease. Of the 25 grams of fat or less in your daily diet, ideally no more than five grams would be saturated.

Cholesterol

Most people, including physicians, place too much emphasis on reducing dietary cholesterol. The most important nutritional factor related to your blood cholesterol level is your saturated fat and hydrogenated fat intake.

If you have chosen to reduce your fat intake to no more than 25 grams a day and your food selections are guided by *The Good News* Diet Food Pyramid, your cholesterol intake will take care of itself.

Sodium

As discussed in chapter seven, restricting sodium intake is primarily a concern for people with high blood pressure. Most people should focus on eating less fat and more fiber, rather than restricting sodium.

If you are salt-sensitive or have high blood pressure, restrict your intake to no more than 2,000 milligrams per day. There are few other clinical reasons your physician may ask you to limit your salt intake. Remember, most of the sodium in your diet doesn't come from the saltshaker; it's hidden in the foods you choose.

Daily value

The percent of daily value on your food labels is based on the USDA food pyramid. If you adopt *The Good News* Diet, these daily values will not be meaningful.

Behavioral Modification Considerations in Reducing Body Fat

Can you think of a reason you eat when you're not hungry?

Almost everyone finds themselves eating for reasons other than hunger. For me, watching a football game on TV stimulates my desire to eat. Surprisingly, this urge to eat can come right after finishing a very large meal.

Much like Pavlov's dog, which was trained to salivate whenever a bell would ring (even in the absence of food), there are many behavioral reasons why we choose to eat. Make no mistake, it will take time and effort for you to understand and ultimately change the behavioral factors that prevent you from sticking with healthy dietary guidelines. It can be difficult to change the role of food in your life, but it can be done—if you have a plan.

At the Institute, we've developed a weight management program that emphasizes behavioral modification. Participants are asked to keep diaries of their eating habits, similar to the one on the next page.

You'll find sample pages of the *The Good News* Food Diary in the back of this book. Use it if you're finding it difficult to comply with the dietary recommendations for your body fat reduction plan.

Record what you eat and how much. You'll be surprised how this information alone will influence your eating behavior. So many times people in our weight management class have told us they were

Food Diary

TIME	MINUTES SPENT EATING	DEGREE OF HUNGER - SCALE FROM 1-5 (1-not hungry) (5-very hungry)	ACTIVITY WHILE EATING	LOCATION WHILE EATING	DESCRIBE FOOD, TYPE & QUANTITY (BRAND NAMES WHERE POSSIBLE) PLEASE BE SPECIFIC (one per line)	AMOUNT	FAT GRAMS / FIBER GRAMS
7:00	10	2	driving	car	blueberry muffin	1 med	
					vanilla cappucino	1 large	
12:15	25	5	talking	cafeteria	turkey sandwich on	4 slices	
					white bread &	2 slices	
					provolone, lettuce	1 piece ea.	
					tomato	1 slice	
					mayo, honey mustard	2 tbl ea.	
					potato chips	sm. bag	
					Coke	16 oz	
4:00	10	3	working	office	M&M's	sm. bag	
6:00	30	4	t.v.	family rm	spaghetti &	2 cups	
					tomato sauce &	1 cup	

TIME	MINUTES SPENT EATING	DEGREE OF HUNGER - SCALE FROM 1-5 (1-not hungry) (5-very hungry)	ACTIVITY WHILE EATING	LOCATION WHILE EATING	DESCRIBE FOOD, TYPE & QUANTITY (BRAND NAMES WHERE POSSIBLE) PLEASE BE SPECIFIC (one per line)	AMOUNT	FAT GRAMS / FIBER GRAMS
					meatballs	3 large	
					garlic bread	2 slices	
					water	12 oz	
10:30	10	2	t.v.	family rm.	mixed nuts	2 handfuls	

totally unaware of the amount, and in some cases the specific foods, that they were eating. Do you sometimes find it hard to recall specific foods you've eaten during the day?

There's an added benefit to the diary. The simple fact that you have to write down every food you eat will reduce your interest in the snack you were thinking about.

You'll also want to keep track of the conditions that may be affecting your eating habits:

- the time of day
- where you were eating

- with whom you're eating

- your emotional state at the time

- your degree of hunger

Start by deciding to complete your *Good News* Food Diary for two weeks (make copies of the diary if needed). Remember, keeping this eating behavior diary will require diligence and commitment.

Your motivation: The potential to gain lifelong skills that will help you control your eating behavior and ultimately your body fat content.

Your "Top 10 List" for Analyzing Your Diary

If you choose to keep *The Good News* Food Diary, here are 10 suggestions for analyzing the results:

- People eat in the most unusual places. Designate the kitchen (or dining room) as the only place in your home where you'll eat.

- Avoid putting food items in clear containers or in places where you constantly see them. And avoid bringing foods in the house if they aren't in your dietary plan. You can't eat what you don't have. Why tempt yourself? It's amazing how often healthy foods get eaten when they fill your cupboards and kitchen. This is particularly relevant to children. One of the greatest gifts you can give your kids is exposure to a healthy lifestyle. Condition them to practice dietary habits that will give them the best chance to become healthy adults. Kids eat what they find in the home. If the likes and dislikes of your children are determining your family's eating habits, take back control. Someday, they'll give you a healthy thank you.

- Always have a time delay between servings. If you're still hungry after your first serving, wait at least 15 minutes before asking for seconds. In most cases, I'll bet you won't ask for the other serving. Of all the behavioral changes people have reported to me, this one has had the greatest impact on reducing the amount of food they ate.

- Create substitute behavior for the cues that stimulate you to eat. One of the best substitutes is exercise. When I find myself wanting to eat while watching a football game, I do a quick set of push-ups or sit-ups to reduce my interest in food. (Yes, it works!) As you review your diary, identify the circumstances you tend to associate with eating. Your favorite hobby can be a substitute activity.

- Identify the times when you're most likely to eat. If you tend to eat again after dinner, instead get into the routine of going for a walk, even a short one. This also gives you a chance to talk with your spouse or friend, or to enjoy a pet. Whatever you plan as a substitute behavior, make sure it helps break the cycle of conditioned eating that is influenced by time.

  Recently, a relative was visiting us in our home. We asked if he was hungry, and he replied by asking the time. When my wife indicated it was noon, he said, "Yes, I think I'm hungry." The implication, of course, is that his eating decisions are based on the time of day rather than hunger. Reliance on these types of external cues can keep you from gaining control of your weight.

- Don't go grocery shopping when you're hungry. You're more likely to make poor food choices.

- Your desire to eat should be driven by hunger. Don't be misled into believing you need a certain number of meals at specific times every day for proper nutrition (unless you have a specific medical condition that requires a specific eating pattern). Eating more rather than less causes most of our nutritional health problems.

- Many of us had parents who told us to clean our plates. It's time to break that habit. Fight the guilt you feel from leaving food on your plate. We live in era where our health is being threatened by an epidemic of obesity. Take smaller portions if you have a choice; otherwise, leaving food on your plate suggests you are eating for the right reasons.

- We often eat for self-gratification, stress management or other emotional reasons. If you find a relationship between eating and your mood, develop a strategy of lifestyle change that will improve your feeling of well-being. Avoid caffeine, alcohol, nicotine and sugar-binges; they influence how you mentally and physiologically deal with food. Relaxation techniques and exercise are great ways to alter your mood without seeking solace in food.

- Slow down the overall eating process. Just like our patient Ted, put your utensils down between mouthfuls. Some people even count bites between each mouthful, a sure-fire way to make sure you're not eating too fast. If you're successful, you'll be less likely to overeat.

Ted discovers his appetite cues

Ted is a medical student who found himself quickly gaining weight as he continued his education. Recogniz-ing his inability to control his eating, he came to the Meadow Brook Health Enhancement Institute to begin a body fat-reducing program that included modifying his behavior. We made several important observations when we analyzed his eating behavior diary:

Ted ate dinner every day at 6 p.m., typically in a recliner while watching the evening news. He always ate the same amount of food, even when he felt less hungry. It became clear that the TV, evening news and recliner were the cues stimulating him to eat, so we asked him not to eat while watching TV and to eat only in the kitchen. While it was tough for him to change his evening dinner ritual, his calorie intake dropped dramatically once he did.

Ted always ate in less than ten minutes. He scooped up another mouthful of food before he finished chewing the previous one. We asked Ted to put down his spoon or fork after every bite. That made Ted spend more time with each meal, so eating became less of a compulsion. He actually began to enjoying eating more, even though he ate less.

These types of behavioral changes, along with exercise and better nutrition, helped Ted regain control of his body fat content. Do any of his behaviors resemble your eating habits?

Be motivated by your goal of finally achieving your recommended weight. You *can* lose body fat if you follow this plan. Most importantly, you're likely to maintain your weight reduction. You *will* look and feel better about yourself. You *will* enjoy a greater feeling of well-being.

Remember your other important objective. As mentioned in chapter seven, you'll be following a nutritional plan that can increase your life expectancy.

Remind yourself that we, as a nation, are in the middle of an epidemic of obesity—but that you can set yourself apart. We have failed to stem our country's ever-increasing obesity problem through the proliferation of diet books. If weight loss and weight control were simple, we wouldn't have to fight this battle of the bulge. This comprehensive approach to body fat reduction is the solution that will finally help us gain control of the American waistline—not to mention *yours*.

Summary of Your Dietary Plan to Reduce Body Fat

1. Limit fat consumption to 25 grams per day
2. Eat 25 grams of fiber per day
3. Select foods based on *The Good News* Diet Pyramid

III

STARTING YOUR PHYSICAL CONDITIONING

10

Ten Myths About Losing and Gaining Body Fat

In This Chapter:
- ✔ Ten myths about altering body fat content
- ✔ Can you spot-reduce body fat?
- ✔ How to lose cellulite
- ✔ Does sweating help you lose body fat?
- ✔ How much body fat can you expect to lose in a week?
- ✔ Are starchy foods more fattening?

O ver the course of my professional career, I've spent a significant amount of time debunking misconceptions about weight loss and reducing body fat content.

This was the focus of *Fitness and Fallacies*, a book I co-authored in 1990 with Rich Delorme, M.A., M.S. In it, we discussed popular myths used to promote useless exercise equipment, products and methods.

Weight loss is a multibillion-dollar industry in the United States, so there's fierce competition for your dollars. The Food and Drug Administration (FDA) has been unable to regulate the barrage of weight-loss products and claims that lack scientific scrutiny, partly because of lack of legislative authority and partly because of insufficient resources. This means charlatans often feel safe in targeting the public's naivete.

Laypeople aren't the only ones who accept these weight-loss misconceptions. I've mentored hundreds of physicians as they completed rotations in preventive medicine, and it's clear they've perpetuated many of these myths by passing them on to their patients.

My hope is that after you read this chapter, you'll be able to identify false product claims and weight-loss scams that can waste your money and potentially cause health problems.

As you read these myths, keep track of how many you were aware of and we will grade you at the end of the chapter.

Myth #1
You can reduce fat from a specific area of the body.

This may well be one of the most common misconceptions associated with weight loss. So many times we hear that you can spot-reduce a specific area of the body. Don't like your belly? You should focus on exercises that trim your midsection, right? Many products and methods are sold on the premise that they can somehow remove the fat from the body protrusion you'd like to reduce.

The truth is, many studies have shown that you lose body fat from the last place it was deposited when your weight gain was occurring. In other words, if you last gained weight by adding fat under your chin, that's where you'll lose fat first when your caloric expenditure is greater than your intake.

People have the misconception that regional deposits of fat can somehow be **spot reduced** by exercising, massaging or applying a reducing agent—such as creams of various chemical content—to the body protrusion. There is no known product or method that will allow you to spot-reduce fat other than surgery (liposuction).

For instance, many women would like to reduce the size of their thighs. Through an examination, we can determine whether the excess size is from fat or muscle. If it's from fat that's directly under the skin (subcutaneous), then you have the potential to reduce your thighs through weight loss. However, you're not guaranteed to lose weight from the area you want to reduce. You just have to hope the reduction occurs from the body area you want to change.

If I asked you where your most recent fat gain was deposited, you probably could tell me. That spot will be the first area reduced when you take in fewer calories than you burn. So while it may seem logical to attack a specific area with exercises targeted at that spot, it really doesn't work that way.

Don't confuse spot reduction attempts with muscle-building techniques that target a specific muscle group. You can strengthen particular body regions through exercise, but you can't spot-reduce body fat.

I should point out that in the example above, a thigh examination occasionally reveals a protrusion that's essentially muscle. Some women have what is called "pear" shapes: big legs and small upper bodies. Unfortunately, women with this body contour have limited ability to reduce their larger thighs. So regardless of the advertising claims that guarantee any body shape you want just by using their products, the fact is that genetics play an important role in determining body shape—shapes that many times can't be altered.

Some people assume that a body protrusion or an area of their body that lacks a desirable shape is due to poor muscle tone. Rarely—if ever—is this true. Don't misunderstand, many people lack muscle tone and can benefit from regular, targeted exercise.

However, the benefit associated with regional exercise is unlikely to alter in any significant way the shape of the body area you're trying to change.

Remember, exercise is critical to achieving your overall body fat-reducing goals. You simply can't attack a region of your body and hope to reduce that spot.

Another associated misconception is that you can convert fat into muscle and muscle into fat. Biologically, fat and muscle are two different types of tissue. It is not possible to convert one into another. It would be like trying to change an apple into an orange. You can't do it.

As you review various weight-loss and exercise claims made in advertisements, see how often spot reduction is promised. Hopefully, you'll no longer be susceptible to these scams.

If I'm Exercising, I Must Be Losing Weight or Improving My Body Contour—Right?

I have conducted research evaluating two pieces of equipment, both promising to reduce abdominal fat. One was a weighted belt worn around the abdomen all day. The manufacturer recommended that you perform sit-ups while wearing the belt, implying that the compression would create a spot-reducing effect. The other piece of equipment was an exercise table with hinges in the middle, which supposedly would help you complete sit-ups. My study evaluated changes in waist measurements that included fat content and circumference in inches.

The results? The study failed to demonstrate any change in the measurements of the abdomen. Interestingly, many study participants were shocked to discover we were unable to measure changes. They were absolutely convinced they had lost inches. You can see how the power of the placebo effect can sell a lot of worthless products.

Are You Losing Weight or Getting Leaner? Or Neither?

Many people in weight-loss programs believe they are losing waist-line inches, despite the fact their overall weight hasn't changed. This claim is rarely valid. In most cases, the person is experiencing a placebo effect from their program or they are trying to rationalize their lack of success in losing weight.

Another excuse for not losing weight on an exercise program? "I'm increasing my lean body weight."

You may think your muscle mass is significantly increasing, but you have limited potential to increase your lean body weight through a cardiorespiratory exercise program, even if you were previously inactive. The average person may gain a pound or two of lean tissue, but not much more.

Exercise physiologists and dieticians are some of the most common perpetuators of this misconception. Either they are misinformed, feel sorry for their clients' lack of success or are rationalizing their failure to deliver the weight loss that was promised or expected.

Winning the Battle of the Bulge:
Lose Those Love Handles

Men tend to disproportionately accumulate abdominal fat, and will go to almost any extreme to reduce these unsightly bulges. How many devices have you seen that promise to reduce your waistline through spot reduction?

You can do spot exercises like sit-ups until your belly turns blue, but your waistline is unlikely to change. Sit-ups improve abdominal muscle tone, strength and endurance but have little effect on the real reason your abdomen protrudes. The fat lying directly beneath the skin simply wiggles while you complete the sit-ups. Likewise, products that imply you can spot-reduce your bulging abdomen (creams, belts, vibrators, stimulators, etc.) are rip-offs.

Go Ahead, Jiggle a Little

Don't laugh, it's true. One of the best ways to determine the nature of your protruding abdomen is to take off all your clothes, stand in front of a full-length mirror and jump up and down.

If your abdomen wiggles like Jell-O gelatin, your problem is not a weak muscle; it's a major fat deposit. Unfortunately, you can't tone fat. You've got to get rid of the fat by producing an overall weight loss and hope that some of the reduction comes from your waist.

Remember, if your most recent weight gain increased your waistline, then you should lose fat from this same area when your caloric expenditure exceeds your caloric intake.

Myth #2
It's impossible for some people to achieve their recommended weight.

It is impossible for some people to achieve their *ideal body shape*, but everyone is capable of getting to their recommended weight.

Your body shape is influenced genetically by the amount of muscle tissue you have, as well as how you distribute both your muscle and fat tissues. Your recommended weight, on the other hand, is determined by your relative amount of body fat (a lower percentage of body fat is associated with a reduced risk for numerous health problems).

Your susceptibility to accumulating body fat and your ability to lose it is influenced by genetics. However, this doesn't mean you can't achieve your recommended percentage of body fat. Some people simply have to work harder than others to reduce body fat. It may not seem fair that some people struggle with weight control while others seem to eat anything they want without gaining weight, but we can all achieve a healthy body fat content if we are sufficiently motivated.

Walk Your Way to Good Health

Some years ago, I worked with a woman who found it almost impossible to reach her recommended weight, despite a low-calorie diet and daily exercise. Jan had lost more than forty pounds on our 25/25 fat and fiber dietary plan, and walked an hour every morning. But she had reached a fat-loss plateau; her weight wouldn't budge.

Jan's difficulty was caused by a low basal metabolic rate (the rate at which you burn calories while at rest). As you lose weight, the decrease in body mass can lower your metabolism, making further fat loss more difficult.

For Jan, eating fewer calories wasn't an option because she wouldn't get enough vitamins and minerals. So, despite reservations on the part of my staff, I told her the only option was to burn more calories. Jan agreed to walk an hour in the evening, in addition to the hour she already walked every morning.

Guess what? At the time of her next physical exam, she had achieved her recommended weight. She reached a weight consistent with 25 percent body fat (the percentage recommended for females to best prevent a chronic degenerative disease).

Jan has one of the most depressed metabolic rates I've ever seen, yet she was able to reach her recommended weight. Obviously, she had to be motivated to reach her goal. By the way, Jan says that once she started her twice-daily exercise program, she looked forward to each walking session and never felt better.

While the fat reduction plan we created for Jan may seem extreme, her health was greatly enhanced in the end. Most importantly, increasing Jan's walking program was the only viable option to further reduce her body fat content. Unfortunately, many Americans who are susceptible to weight gain or who have difficulty losing weight choose unhealthy options—surgery, severely restricted calorie diets or supplements. Each of these has poor long-term success and can jeopardize your health.

Few people will have the extreme metabolic problem Jan has. The lifestyle changes I recommend are practical and can only improve your feeling of well-being. And once you adopt this lifestyle, you'll never want to go back to your previous eating habits or sedentary existence.

Myth #3
Cellulite is a special kind of body fat, requiring a unique approach to eliminate it.

The term "cellulite" originated in Europe and describes the fat deposits that appear as dimples in certain areas of the body, especially women's thighs. Some people have claimed this dimpled appearance is a different type of fat that requires special techniques to eliminate it. It has even been suggested that cellulite is an accumulation of toxic wastes in the body!

Because this dimpled fat tends to be unattractive, people will do almost anything to get rid of it. Enter the charlatans with their ineffective products and ridiculous cellulite-removing methods—sponges, cellulite-removing washcloths, creams, vitamins, minerals, herbs, rollers, enzyme and hormone injections, massage devices, vibration devices and so on.

So, what is cellulite? It's the same fat you'll find in other parts of your body. The dimpled appearance comes from the fibrous tissue that envelopes, or covers, the fat in certain body regions, such as women's thighs. As you gain weight, these pockets of fat create a dimpled appearance.

The way to eliminate this dimpled fat is the same as reducing your body's overall fat content. Getting rid of fat deposits can only occur as a result of an overall weight-reducing plan. The unique way your body deposits fat is controlled by your genetics. This doesn't mean you can't significantly alter the shape of your body; it simply means that your chances of achieving what you think of as the most desirable body shape are, unfortunately, limited.

Myth #4
Sweat-producing products help you lose body fat.

Plastic suits and rubber garments have been used for years to induce weight loss through sweating. Unfortunately, sweat-producing methods and products can be both dangerous and useless in your attempts to reduce body fat. Several people have actually died from dehydration and excessive body temperatures while using these products.

Weight reduced by sweating is simply water loss. Within 24 hours, you'll regain any weight lost from dehydration.

Myth #5
Losing weight is harder as you get older, because aging lowers your metabolism.

You're more likely to gain weight as you age because your metabolism can change. But what causes the decrease in your metabolism?

Aging isn't the key culprit; loss of lean body tissue is. As you get older, inactivity results in a loss of muscle tissue. Lean tissue is more metabolically active than fat tissue, so losing it causes a lower resting metabolism and a greater susceptibility to weight gain.

Is this primarily an aging effect? No, it's more related to your decision to be less active as you get older, resulting in muscle atrophy and a loss of lean tissue. A lower metabolism then becomes inevitable.

With a consistent exercise program, most seniors can minimize lean body tissue loss. Therefore, your susceptibility to weight gain as you get older can also be minimized.

Should You Actually Weigh Less As You Age?

Many physicians have decided it's inevitable and acceptable for you to gain weight as you get older. This mind-set is driven by the misconception that metabolism decreases simply because you get older.

Also, since so many senior patients gain weight with age in America, it has become a typical expectation. Instead of defining what *should* happen relative to weight gain and aging, we base standards on the average American. How unfortunate!

Your lean body weight typically decreases as you age, so you're likely to be getting fatter—if your weight stays constant. As you get older, then, your weight should actually *decrease* if your goal is to maintain good health. While some loss of lean body tissue is inevitable, you can minimize muscle atrophy through an appropriately designed exercise program (see chapter eleven).

Myth #6

The calories you eat just before going to bed are more likely to be converted into body fat.

It doesn't matter when you consume your calories. Changes in your body fat content are strictly related to your total caloric intake for the entire day, regardless of the time you eat them. So the related theory that exercising after a large meal prevents calories from becoming body fat is also a misconception. Those calories will turn into body fat only if they exceed your caloric expenditure for the day.

Myth #7

You won't lose weight with exercise because it makes you hungry.

As mentioned in the last chapter, most exercise programs suppress your appetite. While there are some exceptions to this rule, most people I've worked with report a diminished appetite when they include exercise in their weight-control program.

It's only when caloric expenditure becomes very high, as with a job that requires significant physical labor, that your appetite may be stimulated. Exercise can also be an excellent behavioral substitute for activities you might link to eating, such as watching television.

Myth #8
You can lose five pounds of body fat in a week.

You may lose five pounds, but it probably won't all be body fat.

Remember, weight change can be due to water as well as fat loss. To lose one pound of body fat, you have to burn 3,500 calories more than you eat. That means over the course of a week, you would have to create a caloric deficit of 17,500 calories to lose five pounds of body fat!

Just consider the numbers. The average American consumes about 2,000 calories a day, so even if you fasted for the entire week, you would only eliminate 14,000 calories (2,000 calories a day times seven days). Assuming you also burn an average of 2,000 calories a day, you would expend 14,000 calories during that week. You would still be 3,500 calories short of achieving a 5-pound fat reduction, and that's without eating the entire week! How many weeks can you do that?

That said, it *is* possible to lose five pounds in a week. Part of that, however, must be due to water loss. You can apply these same calculations to weight gain. It would be almost impossible to gain five pounds of *body fat* in a week.

The reason weight fluctuates significantly over a short period of time is usually related to sodium intake. If you weigh yourself on a regular basis, for example, which day of the week are you likely to weigh the most? For most people, it would be Monday because we tend to eat more on weekends. Inevitably, when we increase our food intake, we also consume more sodium. Water is retained in the process, creating a weight gain and a feeling of being swollen or bloated.

How Much Body Fat Can You Really Lose in a Week?

I have evaluated the body composition of patients immediately after a holiday like Thanksgiving. They're surprised to see significant increases in *body weight* without measurable changes in *body fat content*. The reason? Water retention. Typically, within two or three days of taking the measurements, much of the water gain they experienced is lost. Has this happened to you?

Most responsible clinicians will recommend a one- to two-pound weight loss per week. Losing body fat at this rate is a reasonable expectation. The calculations above don't lie or defy the laws of thermodynamics.

So, don't be duped into believing you can lose seven to fourteen pounds of body fat in a week or two. You'll be more likely to maintain your lifestyle changes if you experience a consistent one- or two-pound body fat loss each week.

Myth #9

To lose body fat through exercise, you have to work at a high intensity.

The difference in caloric expenditure between walking and jogging a mile is very small. It takes you longer to walk a mile than to jog, but it doesn't necessarily burn significantly more calories.

Working harder does burn more calories, but I encourage you to emphasize lower intensity exercise if your goal is to reduce body fat. Injuries are less likely and exercise is often more enjoyable when you're not experiencing a PTA session (pain, torture and agony).

So ex-athletes, or anyone else, don't have to run through a wall or feel pain to benefit from exercise. While high-intensity exercise is necessary to achieve the highest level of human performance, you can reduce your body fat content by participating in physical activities that are enjoyable.

Myth #10

Starchy foods like potatoes and pasta are fattening.

Which has more calories, a medium-size potato or a cup of cooked pasta?

Surprisingly, they both contain about 150 calories. Assuming you consume 2,000 calories per day to maintain your weight and you eat only potatoes or pasta, you would have to eat 13 potatoes or 13 cups of pasta to maintain your weight.

Do you think that's possible? Eating more than a bag of potatoes per day? Of course not. It would be almost impossible for you to maintain your weight on a diet so high in starch, because changes in your body fat content are strictly a function of calories—how many you eat and how many you burn.

Now, if you open up the potato and spoon on the sour cream or butter, the added fat doubles or even triples the calorie content. Fatty creams and sauces on pasta also create the caloric problem. But it's not the starch content of the pasta or potato itself, it's the added fat.

Time to score yourself

All right, how did you do? How many of the ten myths did you know were truly myths? Score yourself on this scale:

0 to 3: Watch your wallet! You're a good target for a health-related scam artist.
4 to 6: Not bad, but you might get fooled by a good salesman.
7 to 9: Now, that's a reasonable score. Nice job on a tough quiz.
10: You're a star! Congratulations for being so well-informed.

11

Developing Muscle Strength, Endurance and Flexibility

In This Chapter:
- ✔ Developing a comprehensive program of physical conditioning
- ✔ Being physically fit is more than walking, jogging or swimming
- ✔ How to start your comprehensive conditioning program
- ✔ Ten common exercise myths

Good ideas often come right out of left field. This one came from a flat tire.

It happened many years ago when John, a 63-year-old patient at Oakland University's Meadow Brook Health Enhancement Institute, heard his tire blow in a snowstorm. John pulled over to the side of the road and tried to change it himself. He ended up physically exhausted and actually hurt himself in the process.

What I haven't told you is that John was a cardiac patient.

Not long ago in Michigan, and throughout much of America, cardiac patients were typically discouraged from engaging in physical activity that might "stress" their hearts. So, along with several colleagues, I established one of the first cardiac rehabilitation programs in Michigan. We hoped to improve the risk profile and quality of life for cardiac patients.

We discovered that with an appropriate exercise prescription, many of these patients were able to do more cardiovascular work after rehabilitation than before their heart attack. Some of these patients actually went on to run marathons after recovering from a heart attack.

John was a participant in our cardiac rehabilitation program, so his inability to change a flat tire helped us recognize that our program simply wasn't comprehensive enough. Our cardiac rehabilitation program, at that time, primarily emphasized cardiorespiratory fitness— strengthening the heart muscle through endurance exercise.

Thanks to John, we realized that endurance exercise was important, but not sufficient. Even though some of our cardiac patients were ultimately able to run a marathon, we hadn't conditioned them to perform many daily tasks. And that's why John couldn't change that tire.

Based on the need to condition people for most daily and recreational activities, we incorporated other forms of conditioning into the program, including resistance training and flexibility exercises. Our cardiac program became a total fitness package.

...But Dr. Stransky, I Don't Have Heart Problems.

Maybe so, but what we learned from these cardiac patients can change your physical life, too. That's because living a long life isn't as meaningful if you can't function at a level that makes life exciting and worthwhile.

And what's the single most important lifestyle factor related to increasing your life expectancy and improving your quality of life? Regular exercise. That's what current research tells me. Moreover, researchers have estimated that only a third of your physical and half of your mental fitness later in life is genetically controlled. What you do now will make the difference.

Whether you have a healthy heart or a recovering heart, the commitment you make to regular exercise may determine how well you function in your senior years. In addition, if you are a twenty-, thirty- or forty-year-old, your quality of life will skyrocket when you make the decision to begin and maintain a comprehensive physical conditioning program. You don't have to wait until retirement to gain the incredible benefits of being physically active.

Chapter nine gave you an exercise prescription for cardiorespiratory fitness as part of a comprehensive weight-reduction program. Let's review that prescription briefly:

- Type of exercise: Continuous exercise that can be tolerated orthopedically and controlled cardiovascularly (walking, treadmill exercise, cycling, stair climbing, swimming, jogging, etc.).

- Duration: Initially, 30 minutes; eventually 60 minutes or more of continuous exercise per session.

- Intensity: 70 percent to 85 percent of your maximal heart rate, as recorded immediately after exercise.

- Frequency: Continuous exercise on most days, or at least every other day.

- Caloric expenditure: Burn 900 calories per week. After three months of conditioning, burn an additional 100 calories per exercise session until you have used up 2,000 calories.

(You'll find details of the cardiorespiratory exercise prescription and caloric expenditures, along with health benefits, in chapter nine.)

Compare your current exercise program to this prescription. Are you seeing only minimal health improvement or is your program extensive enough to obtain optimal gain?

Make sure your fitness program is providing optimal cardiorespiratory benefits—enhancing the health of your heart and lungs.

Achieving total fitness is more than just cardiorespiratory endurance, however. You also need muscular endurance, muscular strength and flexibility to improve and maintain your physical functionality.

Jogging Toward Total Health

If you walk, jog or cycle, you may have outstanding cardiorespiratory endurance. But are you achieving *total* fitness?

It depends on how comprehensive your conditioning program is. If you're not getting upper body exercise, you may notice changes in the tone, strength and appearance of the muscles in this region of your body. Without some form of resistance training, your upper body muscles are more likely to experience atrophy—a decrease in size and function.

That's not to say your heart, lungs and leg muscles haven't become conditioned. In fact, it would be difficult to determine the age of most conditioned walkers and joggers if you saw them only from the waist to their feet. Looking from the waist up, however, aging becomes easier to spot—especially if the person does not engage in a program of *total* conditioning.

Make your conditioning program complete by including all of these fitness components:

- Cardiorespiratory (heart and lungs) endurance
- Muscular strength
- Muscular endurance
- Flexibility

Regardless of your age right now, don't settle for unproductive senior years. You shouldn't expect to be physically limited when you reach your seventies and eighties. If that happens, it will be your own fault. Research has clearly shown that much of your physical aging will come from the lifestyle decisions you make. If you want to remain functional and truly enjoy your retirement years, then you'll need to exercise most days of the week—and the sooner the better.

Isn't retirement all about being able to do the things you've always dreamed of doing? Well, you can't enjoy your senior years from a hospital or nursing home. Exercise is so essential to your health maintenance that if you choose to be inactive, you'd better hope your parents gave you really good genes to overcome your lack of commitment to exercise.

Developing Muscular Strength and Endurance Through Weightlifting or Resistance Training

The exercise prescription for improving your cardiorespiratory function won't significantly improve other aspects of your fitness. You'll also need resistance training (weight training and resistance training are used interchangeably). This form of conditioning is the most effective way to improve muscular strength and endurance, while increasing muscle mass, bone mass and connective tissue strength.

For many years, resistance training was associated only with bodybuilding and athletics. This form of conditioning intimidated many people. As life expectancy increases and we begin to recognize the importance of maintaining upper body fitness, however, resistance training is earning a more positive image. Seniors in our 60+ program at the Meadow Brook Health Enhancement Institute enthusiastically endorse weight training. It's paying off for them, too; in many cases, they actually see 100 percent improvement in their muscular strength and endurance. And, remember, these are people over age sixty.

Let's make sure you understand each of these terms:

Muscular strength refers to the maximum force that a muscle or group of muscles can generate. You can develop muscular strength by using a resistance that creates maximum or near maximal muscle tension with relatively few repetitions.

Muscular endurance is the ability of a muscle or group of muscles to contract (or work) over a specific period of time until muscular fatigue occurs. This form of conditioning is best achieved by using lighter weights and a greater number of repetitions.

Of course, you need both strength and muscular endurance for everyday life. Muscular strength and endurance is likely to improve if you start your program with ten repetitions of a specific exercise. Most importantly, you have to select the correct resistance or weight. If you can do more than ten repetitions, add more weight; if you can't complete ten repetitions, you're using too much weight. Experiment with different weights if you're just beginning.

After this initial training stage, add sets of a particular exercise to your program. You should see significant improvement in strength and endurance by doing three sets of each exercise each session.

I encourage most people to complete sets of ten, five and three repetitions at each exercise station. As you decrease your repetitions, progressively increase the weight you're using for each set. Once again, it may take some trial and error to adjust weights to match the repetitions you have selected.

Devote twenty to thirty minutes for each resistance training session and consider starting with a three-day-a-week program. This plan should be sufficient to see significant improvement in your muscular strength and endurance. Although you'll see larger gains with more repetitions, additional sets and more frequent training, the difference will be relatively small if you're exercising for health enhancement reasons.

You might also benefit from a personal trainer, who can help you develop a better understanding of the biomechanics of each exercise. Most exercise facilities offer this service; just be sure to check the trainer's education and references. A personal trainer who is inexperienced or lacks adequate education can cause more damage than conditioning benefit.

Holding your breath while completing these exercises can cause an inappropriate increase in blood pressure. So maintain a normal breathing pattern while you perform resistance training. Also, consider getting an exercise partner to provide spotting assistance and motivation.

Finally, select exercises that will improve the muscular strength and endurance of your arms, shoulders, chest, back, abdomen, hips and legs. The illustrations in appendix A offer specific examples of exercises that should be included in your program. All of these exercises are designed for healthy people who don't have orthopedic or cardiovascular limitations.

Developing and Maintaining Flexibility

What is flexibility? And why is it so important?

Flexibility refers to your ability to move a specific joint through a complete range of motion, and it requires a repertoire of exercises to achieve a total body effect. For example, static flexibility exercises—in which you slowly lengthen, or stretch, a muscle and hold it in that position—will improve your range of motion by increasing the elasticity or length of your tendons and muscles.

Body joints that aren't exposed to regular range-of-motion activities lose their flexibility. You'll also lose flexibility if you remain inactive as you age. By including flexibility exercises in your physical conditioning program, you can maintain or improve your range of motion, even while getting older.

Some forms of cardiorespiratory conditioning can improve range of motion for particular joints. For example, the crawl stroke in swimming will improve range of motion of your shoulder joint. On the other hand, joggers and walkers actually can lose range of motion in the lower back, thigh and calf muscles. That's why flexibility exercises are an important element of your comprehensive conditioning program.

Avoid "Ballistic Stretching"

Think back to your physical education class in high school. Your teacher or coach probably taught you to stretch by "bouncing"—reaching toward your toes, for example, and bouncing as you try to stretch further. This technique is referred to as "ballistic stretching."

Well, forget everything you know about it. This type of stretching isn't the most effective way to increase your range of motion and can actually cause small tears in your muscles and tendons. Instead, I recommend a *static stretch*, in which you stretch the muscle and hold it, without bouncing, for ten to thirty seconds. You can significantly increase your flexibility with gentle, static stretches.

Another tip: Avoid any flexibility exercises that are painful.

First, Warm Up Your Muscles

Starting your flexibility exercises as soon as you wake in the morning is a good way to injure yourself. Warm up your muscles first with a slow, three- to five-minute walk. This warm-up will increase muscle temperature enough to make your stretching exercises more comfortable, safe and effective. You'll enjoy stretching much more when your body is properly prepared.

You should also stretch *after* cardiorespiratory exercise such as walking, jogging, aerobics and court sports. Again, perform your flexibility exercises with static stretches, holding each one for fifteen to thirty seconds. Avoid the ballistic movements described earlier.

You have plenty of flexibility exercises to choose from—just look at the sketches in the appendix. Try each one, decide which ones you prefer and put together a stretching program that's right for you. You might also rotate exercises every few months to keep it interesting.

Again, these are intended for healthy individuals who don't have orthopedic or cardiorespiratory limitations.

Talk to Your Doctor

Discuss your comprehensive exercise program with your physician before starting. Your doctor knows your health profile, and can determine whether you need to modify your program to match your physical and clinical capabilities. However, if you simply indicate an *interest* in exercising, your physician may not comment on specific elements of your program. Instead, ask your doctor to react to the prescription I've given you for improving your cardiorespiratory fitness, muscular strength, muscular endurance and flexibility.

Surveys indicate that few physicians give an actual exercise prescription to their patients. By describing your specific plans for exercise, the consultation with your physician is likely to be much more productive.

Why You Need a Stress Test

You may recall that earlier I suggested the best way to create an exercise prescription is to evaluate your work capacity by completing a stress test. This evaluation can provide an objective assessment of your physical capabilities. Instead of telling you simply to be careful and not overdo it, I taught you how to monitor the physiological intensity of your exercise, using your pulse rate. You won't have to guess whether your activity is too intense for your ability to perform physical activity when you monitor your heart rate during exercise.

I should warn you that many physicians believe stress tests are only justified for diagnostic reasons. In my opinion, defining your ability to work so that an accurate exercise prescription can be created is sufficient justification. If your doctor questions your request for a stress test, ask him this question: How will he determine exactly what your exercise program should involve if he doesn't know what you're capable of doing physically? Without the stress test, your doctor simply cannot create an objective exercise prescription. Why should anyone be guessing when they're defining a program of physical activity that is designed to be maintained for the rest of your life?

The American College of Sports Medicine recommends that all men forty-five and older and women fifty-five and older complete a stress test before starting a "vigorous" exercise program. If you're younger, a stress test is recommended before starting an exercise program if you have two or more of the following risk factors (one or more if your HDL cholesterol is 60mg% or above):

- Family history of coronary artery disease

- Cigarette smoking

- High blood pressure

- High cholesterol

- Elevated fasting blood glucose

- Obesity

- Sedentary lifestyle.

If you're between the ages of fifteen and sixty-nine, there's an easy way to determine whether it is safe to begin an exercise program. Try completing this simple questionnaire from the Canadian Society for Exercise Physiology.

❏ Has your doctor ever said you have a heart condition and that you should only perform physical activity recommended by a physician?

❏ Do you feel pain in your chest when you are physically active?

❏ In the past month, have you experienced chest pain when you were not doing physical activity?

❏ Do you lose your balance because of dizziness, or do you ever lose consciousness?

❏ Do you have a bone or joint problem that could be made worse by a change in your physical activity?

❏ Is your doctor currently prescribing drugs (for example, water pills) for your blood pressure or heart condition?

❏ Do you know any reason why you should not be physically active?

It's particularly important to talk with your physician before starting an exercise program if you responded "yes" to any of these questions. If you answered "no" to all of them, you can be reasonably sure it's safe to begin exercising as long as you start slowly and build up gradually.

Exercise Misconceptions

Some providers of exercise equipment and programs have either created or perpetuated misconceptions about exercise, often for financial gain. As you begin your exercise program, you may think about joining an exercise facility or buying home equipment. Keep in mind these common exercise myths:

1. No Pain, No Gain

If your goal is to improve your performance in a sporting event (running a race, swimming competitively, etc.), then you may need high-intensity exercise to reach the highest level of excellence. But for the most part, exercise doesn't have to be difficult to be of significant health benefit.

I can't emphasize enough that you shouldn't feel uncomfortable or experience pain while exercising. If you do, reduce the intensity of your exercise and/or discuss your physical concerns with your personal physician.

2. A Thin Person Is Likely to Be Physically Fit

You can appear to be lean but not have high levels of cardiorespiratory fitness, muscular endurance, muscular strength or flexibility. It's actually difficult to determine someone's health status based on his appearance.

Have you ever heard a person say something like, "It's hard to believe he had a heart attack; he looked so thin and fit." You'd be surprised at the number of patients in our cardiac rehabilitation classes who appear to be thin and fit. As you will see later, appearance has little to do with the development of plaques within arteries that lead to a heart attack. Appearance, then, doesn't really indicate your level of physical fitness or your health status.

3. Women Can Develop Large Muscles If They Lift Weights

Women have limited potential to develop larger muscles from exercise. Muscles increase in size primarily because of the hormone testosterone, and although women do have a certain amount of testosterone, it's typically only one-tenth the amount found in the average male.

Studies of women who lift weights extensively have shown they can achieve significant strength gains with little, if any, change in the size of their muscles. It is, however, possible to improve the shape and tone of your muscles through weightlifting.

4. Exercise Equipment Advertised on TV and in Fitness Magazines Gives Men Muscular Bodies, Just Like the Models

In a weightlifting program designed to improve muscle strength and endurance, like the one outlined in this chapter, even men are unlikely to see a noticeable increase in muscle size. A male's potential for increasing muscle mass is ultimately determined by genetics.

If you're in that small percentage of men capable of creating a bodybuilder's appearance, you'll need to resistance-train more than the three weekly sessions of thirty minutes each I have recommended. So, men, don't be duped into buying a piece of exercise equipment to develop a "bodybuilder's shape" if you inherited a body that makes this goal impossible.

5. Special Foods and Nutritional Supplements Are Beneficial When You Exercise

Even if you're very active, you can easily meet all your nutritional needs by simply increasing your caloric intake to offset your caloric expenditures and by following the nutritional guidelines in chapter seven.

I'm concerned about the proliferation of supplements being sold today, especially protein supplements that are advertised as being essential to build muscle tissue. Research simply doesn't support these claims. When you eat extra protein, your body converts it into fat if your caloric intake is greater than your caloric expenditure.

Follow the nutritional guidelines I've given you and you'll get all the protein, vitamins and minerals you need for any exercise program. The bottom line: It's simply not true that you need special food or nutritional supplements of any kind when you become more physically active.

6. Sports Drinks Are Better Than Water During Exercise

Unless you plan to exercise for more than two hours continuously, sports drinks don't provide physiological or performance benefits. In some cases, sports drinks can actually adversely affect your performance and cause gastrointestinal symptoms.

It may surprise you to learn that the best fluid to drink during most exercise sessions is water. Only during longer duration activities like marathons will you find sports drinks possibly beneficial.

7. Fitness Magazines Provide Reliable Exercise Information

I've spent an incredible number of hours clarifying misconceptions that have been published in national fitness magazines. What really concerns me are the ads that make outrageous claims about the benefits of a specific exercise product or service. In most cases, these claims are rarely scrutinized for accuracy or effectiveness by the publication.

8. Older People Who Are Poorly Conditioned Should Lower Their Exercise Expectations

From the clinical observations I've made in our 60+ program, seniors have incredible potential to improve their overall fitness. Some of our participants do more work at the age of seventy than they did when they were forty. The physical accomplishments of many of our sixty- and seventy-year-olds are truly extraordinary.

In most cases, it's not too late to begin an exercise program that will improve health and functionality. It is *important*, however, that seniors complete a comprehensive physical exam before they begin an exercise program. A stress test should be part of this evaluation, which can ultimately lead to a specific exercise prescription.

9. Toning Tables and Electronic Muscle Stimulators Make You More Fit

Some manufacturers advertise products they claim send low-level electrical impulses to stimulate your muscles in a "passive" approach to becoming fit. Other ads claim you can actually bulk up while watching TV, just by using these muscle stimulators. Mechanical toning tables are advertised that apparently do the work for you. All of this can be yours—for a fee, of course.

My first thought when I heard about these exercise benefit claims was, "Who in the world would ever pay for something like this?" Then one of my graduate students completed a project that required him to visit a facility using these types of equipment and techniques. The establishment promised fitness benefits without the need to sweat or exercise. What really surprised my graduate student was the number of people who were there to pay for the service.

The exercise industry is unregulated. Any entrepreneur can buy equipment, rent space and begin to offer "fitness" services. Electronic muscle stimulators and mechanical tables may have some meaningful purpose in the field of physical therapy, but you won't gain any significant muscular strength and endurance benefits. You still have to do the exercise yourself, so buyer beware.

10. Instructors at Most Exercise Facilities Provide Good Exercise Advice and Guidance

I recommended earlier that you evaluate the credentials of any physical trainer or exercise leader you work with, and I'm emphasizing it again. Instructors at gyms and other exercise facilities perpetuate many of today's fat reduction and fitness myths. Your health is too important to be trusted to an unqualified person.

Here's an example of this problem. A colleague of mine told me he was in perfect orthopedic health until he joined a gym recently and began resistance training under the direction of one of the center's young trainers. Now, after only three months of working out, he has persistent knee symptoms and at times even has trouble climbing stairs. And he's only 37.

When he explained the exercise program that the trainer recommended, I could have predicted the symptoms he developed. The recommended exercise he was given was inappropriate and may have compromised his orthopedic health. (The trainer also urged him to bulk up on protein and fat, by the way.)

Trainers at exercise facilities are not always required to have specific academic training. While some are highly credentialed, most are simply unqualified and uneducated in the areas of nutrition and exercise physiology. Yet people continue to turn to these "experts" for guidance about exercise, fitness and even nutritional supplements. Because the industry is unregulated, consumer misinformation about health is rampant.

Make sure you check the academic training of any personal trainer or exercise leader you work with. In most cases, their training should be appropriate if they have a degree in exercise physiology or a closely related field. Also, check references. In addition, the American College of Sports Medicine certifies individuals in exercise leadership positions.

12

What About Dietary Supplements?

In This Chapter:
- ✔ Who's regulating the supplements you take?
- ✔ Seven vitamin and diet supplement claims to watch out for
- ✔ What research says about twenty-two popular supplements
- ✔ The best "natural supplements" you can choose

As director of the primary prevention program at a major university in the Midwest, I am constantly responding to the outrageous health claims made about dietary supplements. They prevent colds. They cure colds. They prevent osteoporosis, arthritis, heart disease and cancer. They elevate your mood and reduce your body fat. They even enhance your weight training.

Do you know *for sure* that the supplements you take do what they promise—or that they're even safe? Or do you blindly believe the advertising hype because you *want* to believe it?

Well, if you take supplements, you're not alone. Surveys suggest that more than half of your neighbors take at least one dietary supplement. So it's no surprise that sales of supplements are approaching $16 billion a year in the United States alone. This is big business, and it's not going away—unless we demand to see the evidence associated with nutritional supplement claims. Short of a more educated population, it's unlikely this trend toward greater use of dietary supplements will decline in the near future. Americans are pushovers for products that promise enhanced health the easy way …by simply taking a pill.

It's time for a reality check.

Currently, dietary supplements are unregulated. In 1994, the federal government approved the Dietary Supplement Health and Education Act (DSHEA), which stripped control and regulation of these products from the Food and Drug Administration (FDA). The dietary supplement industry was instrumental in promoting this deregulating legislation.

The Act allows manufacturers to make health claims for their products without evidence of benefit. The result is that you, not the government, have the responsibility for evaluating the safety of dietary supplements and the truthfulness of their claims.

Before DSHEA, dietary supplements were products made primarily of vitamins, minerals and other nutrients. This legislation broadened the definition of a dietary supplement to include vitamins, minerals, herbs, botanicals, amino acids and metabolites. As long as manufacturers sell their products as dietary supplements, they don't have to provide evidence that their products are effective and they can make health claims that escape scrutiny.

Once a dietary supplement appears on the market, the burden of proof that a product is unsafe falls on the FDA. Unfortunately, someone has to bring health consequences to the attention of the FDA before action can be considered.

Manufacturers of dietary supplements rely on claims of impressive health benefits to sell their products. Some don't bother to provide research support, while others cite studies that seem to endorse their products. Look closer and you discover that the studies typically lack research fundamentals.

Another marketing ploy is to suggest that dietary supplements are "natural" and therefore a more acceptable alternative to prescription medications. Well, mushrooms are natural, but you can also die if you eat the wrong type.

There is now evidence that the adverse health consequences of taking dietary supplements are increasing. Unregulated herbs have been associated with serious illnesses and even death. A recent survey revealed dangerous contaminants and poor quality control in supplement ingredients. In California, nearly one-third of 216 imported Asian herbals were either spiked with drugs not listed on the label or contained lead, arsenic or mercury. [1]

Stephen Barrett, M.D., a board member of the National Council Against Health Fraud, has identified typical claims made by dietary supplement manufacturers and health practitioners that can indicate fraud:

- Be skeptical of claims that taking dietary supplements can cure most diseases. While many diseases seen in America are related to our diet, don't assume that dietary supplements can replace a healthy diet.

- Watch out for anecdotes and testimonials. One of my favorites involves the claim that vitamin C can prevent the common cold. People will frequently say they experienced fewer colds when they started to take vitamin C. Well, we develop immunities as we get older and become less susceptible to infectious problems simply as a matter of aging. Double-blind studies have consistently failed to demonstrate that vitamin C makes you less susceptible to the common cold.

- Be skeptical of "pseudomedical" jargon (words that are unfamiliar or don't seem to make sense). Have you seen products that claim to "detoxify" your body, balance your body's chemistry, bring your body into harmony with nature or correct a supposed weakness of a particular system or organ? These claims are impossible to measure and evaluate.

- Look out for conspiracy claims. I've seen claims by practitioners and supplement manufacturers that pharmaceutical companies and traditional medicine are conspiring to suppress medical information to ensure profitability. They say the medical establishment knows if people don't get sick, they won't need doctors or medication. To suggest that anyone would encourage or allow illness simply to advance profits is irresponsible.

- Don't be seduced by "secret cures," "miracle cures" or "new discoveries." Researchers do not suppress medical findings. If a medical "breakthrough" is found in this era of instantaneous media communication, you'll know about it.

- Be aware of the potentially toxic effects of herbal agents. Herbs contain thousands of chemicals; the health consequences of consuming them remain under investigation. Future research may identify some herbs as beneficial, but it will also find others to be toxic. Are you willing to jeopardize your health under these circumstances?

- Be skeptical of dietary supplements that claim to prevent a wide range of chronic degenerative diseases. Unfortunately, a dietary supplement "cure all" is fiction.

Vulnerability can often increase a person's susceptibility to dietary claims. Unfortunately, traditional medicine doesn't have the answer to all our health problems. Be guided by medical research that has made our health care system the envy of the world.

Common Dietary Supplements

It may help you to know the current research on some of the most common dietary supplements. Here's a brief summary, along with my recommendations:

Beta Carotene

Claim: Prevents cancer and heart disease. Also promoted as an antioxidant.

Facts: The most recent clinical trials involving smokers failed to demonstrate cancer prevention benefit; in fact, cancer death rates were actually higher in groups taking beta carotene as a supplement. Beta carotene was widely recommended before these recent trials, but is rarely recommended as a dietary supplement by responsible organizations today.

Not recommended as a dietary supplement.

Calcium

Claim: Prevents osteoporosis.

Facts: Interestingly, the nations that consume the most calcium tend to have the highest incidence of osteoporosis. This observation is linked to the amount of animal protein you consume. Excess protein intake results in calcium loss. Some research suggests that when you eat a lot of protein, you may need more calcium. In this case, a calcium supplement may be beneficial.

Recommendation depends on your diet; discuss with your physician before taking. Plant sources of calcium are highly preferable.

Coenzyme Q-10

Claim: Another supplement for whatever ails you.

Facts: Recommended by some cardiologists, but where is the evidence it's effective?

Not recommended as a dietary supplement.

Creatine

Claim: Improves human performance and lean body mass.

Facts: Creatine is an amino acid (building block of protein). Studies currently fail to consistently demonstrate benefits. It's unlikely to provide an advantage for people who are exercising for health enhancement purposes.

Not recommended as a dietary supplement.

DHEA

Claim: Promoted as an anti-aging hormone, among other health claims.

Facts: DHEA is a human hormone, yet it's allowed to be sold as a dietary supplement. I don't get it! Some have challenged its labeling accuracy for this reason. Others have expressed concerns about possible links to prostate and endometrial cancer. Even if you wanted DHEA, you may not be getting it based on a review of the products being sold. I don't recommend playing around with hormones. The only thing it's sure to do is lighten your wallet.

Not recommended as a dietary supplement.

Echinacea

Claim: Promoted as a cold remedy.

Facts: Used extensively in Europe for colds and influenza and recently introduced in the United States. For the most part, research has shown no evidence of its benefits. Potential toxic effects are unknown.

Not recommended as a dietary supplement.

Ephedra

Claim: A major player in the weight-control business.

Facts: The active ingredient in ephedra is ephedrine, an ingredient found in allergy and decongestant medications. Ephedrine stimulates the cardiovascular system, making it a significant concern for diabetics and heart patients. Reported side effects in healthy people include insomnia, headaches, seizures, heart arrhythmias, strokes, heart attacks and even death. Taking supplements is absolutely the wrong approach to weight control. The use of ephedra has the potential to seriously compromise your health.

Not recommended as a dietary supplement.

Folic Acid

Claim: Used to prevent heart disease, cancer and birth defects.

Facts: Research on folic acid and heart disease appears promising. The benefits to pregnant women are well established (400 micrograms above dietary sources is generally recommended). For everyone else, the full benefit of taking folic acid to supplement a well-balanced diet remains to be determined.

Recommended for pregnant women or those anticipating pregnancy, but discuss first with your personal physician. Research is too preliminary to recommend to the general population.

Garlic

Claim: Promoted as a cardiovascular enhancer. Advertisements claim garlic can reduce your cholesterol.

Facts: Clinical trials have failed to provide sufficient evidence that it is beneficial as a supplement.

Not recommended as a dietary supplement.

Ginseng

Claim: A benefit for numerous health problems.

Facts: Frequently used to increase energy levels, but evidence is lacking that it provides any health benefit. Save your money.

Not recommended as a dietary supplement.

Glucosamine and Chondroitin

Claim: Advertised as arthritis remedies.

Facts: Potential toxic effects are unknown, and inadequate research has been reported to date on their benefit. Other arthritis-treating options are available that clearly provide advantages.

Not recommended as a dietary supplement.

Lysine

Claim: Advertised for the prevention and cure of cold sores.

Facts: The amount of lysine needed to provide any benefit would expose you to potential side effects. If you're concerned about cold sores, talk with your physician about effective prescription options.

Not recommended as a dietary supplement.

Melatonin

Claim: Primarily promoted to enhance sleep and combat travel lag in different time zones.

Facts: You run the risk of numerous physiological consequences taking this hormone. (That's right, melatonin is a human hormone—not a dietary supplement. How in the world can the supplement industry possibly call a human hormone a dietary supplement and get away with it? In France and Britain, melatonin has been banned.) Current research suggests it has little, if any, impact on sleep.

Not recommended as a dietary supplement.

Saw Palmetto

Claim: Taken by men to improve prostate symptoms.

Facts: Research on its benefit has been inconsistent to date. I would recommend saw palmetto only if you have first consulted with your physician.

Not recommended as a dietary supplement.

Selenium

Claim: Prevents heart disease and cancer.

Facts: Unfortunately, some physicians are promoting this dietary supplement, causing some people to assume more is better. Yet selenium is toxic in high concentrations. As for its benefits, research support is lacking.

Not recommended as a dietary supplement.

St. John's Wort

Claim: Mood elevator. Some people use it as an antidepressant.

Facts: Prescribed frequently in Europe as an antidepressant. Clinical trials in Europe support its effectiveness in favorably altering mood. It may benefit mild forms of depression and should be taken only in consultation with a physician. Never take it with other antidepressants. If you believe St. John's wort would help you, talk with your physician first. If you have symptoms of depression, more effective prescription medications that have been scrutinized through clinical trials are available.

Not recommended as a dietary supplement; take only if directed by your physician.

Vitamin B12

Claim: Recommended for seniors to treat possible B12 deficiencies.

Facts: Found only in animal products unless a food product is fortified. Solid research supports its benefit to seniors who have atrophic gastritis, which affects 10-30 percent of Americans over the age of 60.

Recommended as a dietary supplement for vegetarians and for seniors in a multipurpose form.

Vitamin C

Claim: Promoted most heavily for the prevention of the common cold. Sold also as an antioxidant.

Facts: Clinical trials have failed to support the benefits of this vitamin in preventing infectious problems. At levels above 1,000 milligrams per day, it is associated with an increased risk of kidney stones and diarrhea. A recent study is particularly concerning. After one year, subjects taking vitamin C ended up with thicker artery walls when compared to those not taking supplements. The more vitamin C that subjects took, the greater the arterial thickening. At 480 milligrams per day, artery thickening was almost three times greater. You need vitamin C, but get it from your diet.

Not recommended as a dietary supplement.

Vitamin D

Claim: Also recommended for seniors.

Facts: Found only in animal products unless food is fortified. You can get all the vitamin D your body needs naturally, through proper exposure to the sun.

Recommended as a dietary supplement for vegetarians.

Recommended as a dietary supplement for people with inadequate sun exposure. Take only in multipurpose form, such as the One-A-Day or Centrum brands.

Vitamin E

Claim: The last of the big three antioxidants. Promoted for the prevention of many chronic degenerative diseases, especially heart disease.

Facts: In the largest clinical trial to date, patients at high risk for cardiovascular events were treated with vitamin E for nearly five years but saw no positive benefits on their cardiovascular outcomes. The benefit of vitamin E supplements remains to be established.

Not recommended as a dietary supplement.

Zinc

Claim: Reduces symptoms and duration of a cold. Also taken to enhance vision and to reduce urinary problems in men.

Facts: Research on the ability of zinc lozenges to influence the length or severity of cold symptoms is inconclusive. Research on its benefit associated with vision is unimpressive. Several well-respected clinical groups do not recommend zinc supplements for urinary symptoms in men.

Not recommended as a dietary supplement.

So there you have it. There just isn't a lot of rigorous research to support using dietary supplements. Worse yet, many of them can actually bring on serious health consequences. It appears that dietary supplements are necessary only for the adequate intake of folic acid in expectant women and possibly vitamins D and B12 for seniors and vegetarians.

Don't confuse this discussion on vitamin and mineral supplements with the benefits of eating a plant-based diet. Numerous studies have shown that a diet rich in fruits, vegetables and grains can have protective benefits against the major causes of death in the United States. Plants are amazingly capable of taking thousands of chemicals and arranging them in a way that creates this incredible prevention benefit. Almost every time we try to extract out a specific chemical from a plant and provide it as a supplement, we end up with supplements that have no benefit or become toxic in high concentrations. We just can't seem to duplicate what's been done naturally in plants.

Which Supplements Get My Approval?

OK, this book is supposed to emphasize Good News. So is there any good news in all this? Are there other supplements I can recommend?

You bet! In fact, aside from the few above, there are several I can advocate wholeheartedly. The absolute best dietary supplements you can choose are strawberries, carrots, peaches, a cup of whole grains or other plant selections. You'll never go wrong with these delicious "natural supplements."

If you really understand the disease prevention power that lies within the chemistry of fruits, vegetables and grains, you might finally decide to replace the morning vitamin pill you're now taking with something more palatable such as a ripe, juicy strawberry.

13

How to Live to Be 100 (and Why You Should Want To): Ten Steps to a Longer, Better Life

In This Chapter:
- ✔ Develop a physical morality
- ✔ What seventy-five-year-old Americans can—and can't—do
- ✔ Ten steps to reach 100
- ✔ The importance of spirituality

Many people can live to be 100 years old. That's the good news. It's possible you could be healthy and energetic enough to actually enjoy life at age 100. That's the *better* news.

I've heard an argument against longevity that goes something like this: "Why would I want to live to be 100? I'll be old, feeble and probably sick. After all, my grandparents had a terrible quality of life in their senior years."

But what if you could live to be 100 and still be healthy? What if—thanks to your healthy lifestyle choices—you could reach the century mark mentally alert, physically fit and spiritually sound? And what if your friends followed the same lifestyle program and also were able to enjoy their senior years?

Believe me, it *can* be done. The lifestyle principles I've shared with you in this book have the potential to provide 100 years of high-quality living.

What a Difference a Century Makes

We have a family friend named Ed who, until recently, lived here in the Detroit area. He stood about 6 feet, with a muscular frame and weighed about 220 pounds. A widower, he lived alone and kept up his historic brick house nearly single-handedly. His children visited from Chicago about once a year.

A few years ago, we held his birthday party at my house. He drove himself, as he always did, and bounded into the house full of energy. His handshakes were deadly; he could almost fracture the bones in my hand with his powerful greeting.

We spent the afternoon talking about family, current events and the latest books he was reading; he's an insatiable reader and a fantastic conversationalist. He also challenged me to a wrestling match on the living room floor. (He was dead serious, and I have no question he would have taken me!)

Not bad for someone who's a century old.

That's right, it was the 100th birthday party for this absolutely robust gentleman. In just a few years from now, you may be just like

Ed—able to pass that magical age of 100 with enthusiasm and good health while making a contribution to society. Still characterized by a zest for living and a hunger for knowledge. A remarkable symbol of a healthy body and sound mind. What a goal to establish!

Entering the new millennium, many articles were written about the how far we have come in the last century. We've seen incredible societal advancements including the development of telephones, electricity, automobiles, tractors, television, radio and computers. The most impressive of all, however, may be the thirty-year increase in life expectancy Americans have experienced during that same time period.

In 1900, life expectancy in the United States was forty-seven years. The major causes of death at that time were primarily infectious and included influenza (flu), pneumonia and tuberculosis.

Since then, thanks to medical research, these causes of death have been either eliminated or significantly reduced. We now have a life expectancy of approximately seventy-six years—that's nearly three decades added to our lives.

Today, the major causes of death are chronic degenerative diseases (heart disease, cancer, stroke and diabetes). Research has unequivocally linked these diseases to the way we live. That means in the future, medical technology may no longer drive increases in life expectancy. Instead, changes you make in your lifestyle will have the greatest impact on achieving an expanded life span.

My friend Ed escaped the major causes of death from the last century. I believe his lifestyle significantly contributed to his 100 years of good health.

Develop 'Physical Morality'

Likewise, I'm firmly convinced that, in the near future, the average American who follows the ten steps outlined in this chapter will live to be 100 years of age. This prediction is very realistic when you consider the following:

- The current life expectancy of seventy-six years is for a newborn male or female. The older you are, the longer your life expectancy becomes. Therefore, life expectancy for you may well be eighty years of age and above.

- If a couple lives to be age sixty-five, life expectancy for at least one of the pair is ninety-three years.

- Americans age sixty-five and older now outnumber teenagers.

- In the history of the world, it is estimated that more than half the people who have ever lived to age sixty-five are alive today.

It's not a stretch for the average American to live to be one hundred. Living to one hundred becomes an even greater probability when you live a lifestyle that's consistent with the ten steps that follow.

What will happen if Americans continue to experience an increase in life expectancy? How functional will you be when you reach the age of seventy-five? Will you play golf every day—or shuffleboard? Will you walk on the beach with your spouse or walk only with assistance? Will you enjoy playing with your grandchildren or sit passively watching them grow? To a large degree, it depends on the lifestyle choices you make.

Already, the fastest-growing segment of our population is above the age of 100. So you have to wonder whether the senior population will become a burden to the rest of society. At first glance, a report by the National Institute on Aging appears discouraging. According to the report, among Americans beyond the age of seventy-five:

- 40 percent can't walk two blocks

- 32 percent can't climb 10 steps

- 22 percent can't lift 10 pounds

- 7 percent can't walk across a small room

- 50 percent who fracture a hip never walk independently again; many of these people die of the complications.

I'm sure you know senior citizens with a poor quality of life. I often hear people say, "I don't want to live to be that old and end up being a burden and dependent on other people." This is the typical perception we have of aging: We inevitably become weak and helpless.

Is reduced functionality and devastating physical aging inevitable? For most of us, the answer is absolutely *no. The New England Journal of Medicine* recently addressed a report on aging, health risks and cumulative disability. Researchers demonstrated that disability is strongly linked to specific risk factors that are modifiable by committing to a healthy lifestyle.

How important are genetics in determining your quality and length of life? Well, current research summarized by the Mayo Clinic suggests that only one-third of our physical and half of our mental fitness later in life is genetically controlled. The potential to live a long, high-quality life is, to a large extent, determined by your motivation to maintain what I call a *physical morality*.

My friend Ed had an impressive physical morality. Are you willing to maintain the lifestyle discipline that's necessary to achieve your health and life expectancy goals? Unfortunately, Americans find it too easy to abuse their bodies and thus substantially reduce their life expectancy and quality of life.

But you can drastically influence the probability of living to 100 and being just like Ed.

Ten Steps to Achieving 100 Years of Quality Life

As we begin to identify these ten steps, remember your two objectives:

- increase your life expectancy (live longer)

- improve and maintain your quality of life (*enjoy* living longer).

Some of the steps will add years to your life, while others will improve your feeling of well-being. We've discussed five of the steps in detail in previous chapters and will only mention them briefly here.

Ready?

1. Maintain a Comprehensive Exercise Program

Throughout this book, I've emphasized the benefits of physical activity because it is critically important if you hope to be functional as your life expectancy increases.

I want you to be able to fish a mountain stream, cycle for an hour, climb a mountain or play baseball with your grandchildren on your eightieth birthday. Believe me, these are realistic goals if you maintain a program that emphasizes cardiorespiratory fitness, muscular strength, muscular endurance and flexibility.

How do I know? At Oakland University's Meadow Brook Health Enhancement Institute, we have outstanding role models in our 60+ programs who have demonstrated that it can be done. They are living models of fitness and the enjoyment of life at any age.

Exercise profoundly influences life expectancy as well as your feeling of well-being. That's why I've identified physical activity as the *single most important lifestyle factor* in your quest to achieve a long and functional life.

Across the country, clinicians are using exercise to treat anxiety and depression. For most people, rainy days and Mondays are never as bad when the day starts with exercise. And when you exercise with a friend or a group, it can be an excellent social activity.

It's also one of the most effective stress management interventions we can choose. This is especially meaningful given the impact stress has on our emotional and psychological health. Researchers have even demonstrated that some people experience euphoria—associated with increased levels of endorphins—when they participate in continuous exercise for long periods of time.

Humans were meant to be active. When you choose to be inactive, or when you're unable to exercise, your quality of life is likely to be substantially reduced.

2. Avoid Tobacco Products

Many preventive medicine specialists believe smoking is the single most preventable cause of premature death in the United States.

More than 440,000 Americans die each year from causes related to cigarette smoking. In the United States, one in every five deaths is believed to be smoking related. Researchers have identified smoking as the major cause of lung, larynx, oral and esophageal cancers. Reports have also concluded that cigarette smoking significantly increases death rates for cancers of the bladder, kidney, pancreas and cervix in women. Still other studies have linked smoking with cancers of the stomach, liver, prostate, colon and rectum.

Your risk of developing these cancers depends on:

- the number of cigarettes you smoke each day

- the age you began smoking

- how many years you've smoked.

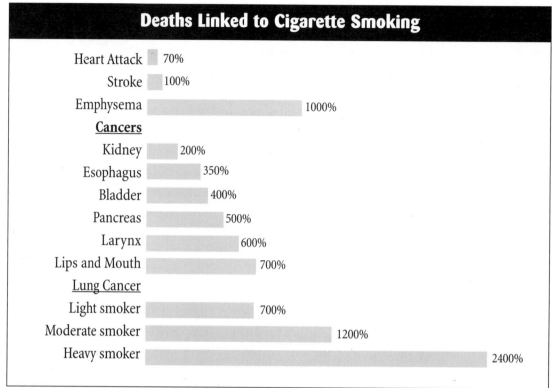

If you smoke, your chances of succumbing to one or more of these major diseases (above) increase, as shown, when compared to a non-smoker.

To appreciate the magnitude of risk associated with tobacco use, realize that lung cancer is 2,000 percent higher in men and 1,200 percent higher in female smokers than it is in non-smokers.

There's more. Smoking is also related to a greater risk of heart disease, stroke, emphysema and other respiratory diseases. Smokers are twelve times as likely to suffer from emphysema and three times as likely to die from heart disease.

The British Medical Journal recently calculated the impact of cigarette smoking on life expectancy. In this study, every cigarette reduced the smoker's life expectancy by eleven minutes. The researchers found that the average smoker lost a total of 6.5 years of life, compliments of cigarettes. (The calculation was based on an average number of cigarettes smoked annually from the median starting age of seventeen until death at the average age of seventy-one.)[1] *Obviously, if you want to live longer, you need to avoid tobacco products.*

Stop-smoking campaigns light up airwaves while smokers just keep lighting up

Isn't it interesting that the trend toward a decline in smoking would be reversed at a time when our society and the government have begun the most intensive antismoking campaign our country has ever seen?

Education is the key to reducing tobacco use as well as promoting good health behavior. Regulating behavior in an attempt to improve the health status of any group of people is typically met with resistance and less than optimal success.

(Remember the early battles over seatbelts and motorcycle helmets.)

Surveys indicate that smokers know the health consequences of using tobacco products. However, most believe these health statistics just don't apply to them. Do you know a smoker who is in denial?

Once a tobacco user decides to quit, however, behavioral modification and pharmacological interventions are available that can significantly increase the chances of success. Ultimately, the success of any smoking cessation program is determined by how motivated the smoker is to quit.

Fortunately in the United States, the percentage of smokers has decreased from more than 40 percent of the population to 23 percent in recent years. This decline reached a plateau in the 1990s, however. We now have evidence that for the first time in years, the number of high school students who smoke has started to rise.[2] It is safe to predict that cigarette smoking among adult Americans will increase as well, since more than 80 percent of adult tobacco users started smoking cigarettes before age eighteen.

3. Maintain an Optimal Lipid Profile (Blood Cholesterol, HDLs, LDLs, Triglycerides and Cholesterol/HDL Ratio)

The number-one cause of death in America for both men and women is coronary artery disease. Through our clinical work at the Meadow Brook Health Enhancement Institute, we have identified a health and lifestyle profile that if achieved will make coronary artery disease unlikely.

As a researcher, I would never suggest to you that anything is absolute. However, we have tested tens of thousands of people in our Primary Prevention Program and as of this date, *we are not aware of even one person who achieved this profile who died of a heart attack, due to coronary artery disease.*

One other point: I have trained more than five hundred physicians in preventive medicine and I've challenged all of them to identify one patient with this profile who developed coronary artery disease. They have yet to bring a case study to my attention.

Here is the health and lifestyle profile that dramatically lowers your chances of a heart attack:

- Achieve a total cholesterol of less than 150mg% or a cholesterol/HDL ratio less than 3.4

- Avoid tobacco products

- Maintain a blood pressure of 120/80 (less if you're healthy and your blood pressure isn't being influenced by medication)

- Avoid diabetes (see earlier chapter on how to achieve this goal)

- Maintain a cardiorespiratory exercise program consistent with the prescription provided in chapter nine.

In your attempts to prevent a heart attack, the most important element of the health and lifestyle profile above involves optimizing your lipid profile (blood cholesterol and associated measurements). Several researchers believe that if your blood cholesterol is low enough, coronary artery disease is not likely to occur even when other risk factors are present. In nations that have an average cholesterol level of 150mg%, heart disease is virtually unknown as a public health issue and ischemic strokes are less likely to occur.

So, how likely is it that you can achieve a blood and cholesterol of 150mg% or a cholesterol/HDL ratio of 3.4 or less? Well, the aver-

Whom do you blame for your poor health habits?

Have you ever heard a person justify their poor health behavior by pointing to a ninety-five-year-old person who smokes cigarettes? Why stop smoking if someone else has survived?

On an individual basis, the influence of poor health behavior varies considerably. We can, however, conclude that for any person who smokes cigarettes for an extended period of time, they will in fact experience a reduction in life expectancy. The ninety-five-year-old smoker will also die prematurely. No matter the age of death, life expectancy would likely have been extended as a result of maintaining a lifestyle consistent with disease prevention.

If you smoke and choose to quit, the good news is that you greatly reduce the risk of the diseases mentioned before. As an example, death due to heart disease decreases by 50 percent in one year when compared to a person who continues to smoke. While people who smoke for many years never reach the same risk category nonsmokers enjoy, after ten to fifteen years of avoiding tobacco products, your health risk can be fairly close to that of a nonsmoker.

age vegetarian maintaining a low-fat diet has an average cholesterol level of 150mg%. Also, there are other lifestyle choices you can make to optimize your blood lipid profile.

For example, restricting fat intake to no more than 25 grams per day is of primary importance. Of the fat you eat, limit hydrogenated and saturated fats. In addition, eat at least 25 grams of fiber per day. These lifestyle strategies can also be helpful:

- Minimize your intake of refined carbohydrates

- Achieve your recommended weight based on body fat measurements

- Maintain a cardiorespiratory exercise program (again, see chapter nine)

- Avoid tobacco products.

If you're unable to achieve these optimal blood lipid values for genetic reasons, medication can be prescribed that will dramatically reduce your cholesterol. Clinical trials involving the use of these medications have demonstrated a 30-50 percent reduction in all-cause mortality.

So, is there anyone who can't achieve this profile? Probably, but not many. I've estimated that if every American chose an optimal lifestyle and, if necessary, began medication, less than one half of one percent of all Americans would *not* be able to achieve the desired lipid levels. In other words, the number-one cause of death in America—heart attacks—could be reduced to an insignificant cause of death. Our nation's life expectancy would literally catapult.

So, how do the results of your last blood studies compare to the definition of what world research suggests is optimal? If you have a family history of coronary artery disease, why wouldn't you work with your physician to achieve the health and lifestyle profile I have defined above? Imagine the impact on life expectancy in America if we established this cholesterol standard for our nation.

4. Maintain Optimal Nutrition

Earlier, I presented a review of worldwide research that demonstrated the relationship between nutrition and good health. In chapter seven, I presented *The Good News* Diet, a nutritional plan that not only helps you reduce and maintain your body fat content, but also helps prevent many health problems.

Here again, based on current research, are the guidelines you should follow to ensure you have the best opportunity to increase your life expectancy:

- Limit fat consumption to no more than 25 grams per day

- Consume at least 25 grams of fiber per day

- Include food groups and recommended servings from *The Good News* Food Pyramid in chapter seven

- Avoid animal products

- Avoid refined carbohydrates; when eating foods individually, choose those with low glycemic index values

- Minimize use of alcohol and caffeine.

5. Achieve an Optimal Body Fat Percentage

As indicated in chapter nine, you should base your recommended weight on the amount of body fat you have, not what a standard weight chart suggests. Too much body fat can increase your risk for significant health problems:

- Cancer

- Coronary artery disease

- Diabetes

- Gall bladder disease

- Hypertension

- Stroke.

Most Americans can achieve a recommended body fat content by implementing this comprehensive program:

- Participate in continuous (cardiorespiratory) exercise on most days of the week

- Reduce calories by limiting fat consumption to 25 grams per day and eating at least 25 grams of fiber each day

- Avoid alcohol, or at least reduce caloric intake from alcohol

- Know the behavioral factors that influence your eating decisions (know *why* you eat and begin avoiding those eating cues).

6. Minimize Alcohol Consumption

It's unfortunate that many people, even some physicians, assume that alcohol provides health benefits that outweigh health risks. While some evidence suggests alcohol can help reduce your risk of developing coronary artery disease, the net effect on your health and quality of life doesn't justify it. Here are potential health consequences associated with alcohol consumption.[3]

- Alcohol can increase your risk of lung, esophageal, gastric, pancreatic and urinary tract cancers

- Long-term drinking (three or more drinks a day) increases your risk of liver disease, high blood pressure, hemorrhagic stroke as well as damage to the brain and pancreas

- Alcohol increases your risk of osteoporosis, car accidents, workplace injuries, homicide and suicide

- Alcohol is a significant source of calories—a major concern for a nation that is experiencing an obesity epidemic

- Alcohol use brings increased risk of alcoholism and social drinking problems.

While some studies suggest alcohol can lower your risk for heart attacks, you can get similar risk reduction benefits from medications that improve your lipid profile. And prescribed medications don't have the health and social risks associated with alcohol.

When you evaluate the benefits and risks of drinking alcohol, the optimal decision appears to be abstinence. But if you choose to drink alcohol, I encourage you to abstain at least five days a week. Also, restrict your quantity to no more than three ounces of pure alcohol per week—the equivalent of six 12-ounce beers, 28-30 ounces of wine, or 3-4 mixed drinks (1.5 ounces of liquor per mixed drink).

Medicine's traditional definition of alcohol moderation—1-2 drinks per day—is simply irresponsible and inconsistent with increasing your life expectancy and maintaining a high quality of life.

7. Learn to Manage Stress Effectively

I don't believe in theories that suggest the physiology of stress causes, in general, chronic degenerative diseases. Yes, there's a clinical relationship between stress and heart disease, liver disease, cancer, diabetes and other health problems. But my own clinical observations suggest the reason is more related to how stress influences our health behavior. People who are under stress frequently choose to live a lifestyle that's conducive to poor health. They're more likely to smoke, eat on the run, drink too much alcohol, exercise less and, in general, disregard the principles of health enhancement.

I know many high-level executives who are under incredible amounts of stress yet experience few, if any, health consequences. Why are they different? They're able to manage stress effectively by developing a well defined "physical morality." When health is not a priority in your life, you become more willing to sacrifice your physical well-being to achieve other goals, such as financial or career success. If you successfully apply the lifestyle principles found in this book, the chances that stress will reduce your life expectancy are very low.

While stress may not physiologically shorten your life span, it is the single most important factor related to the feeling of well-being of most Americans. If you manage stress well, you'll have a higher level of well-being. If not, life can be one trial after another, regardless of your success in other aspects of life.

The most common symptoms of stress, as reported by patients in our Primary Prevention Program, include:

- Overt anxiety

- Development of phobias

- Constipation

- Diarrhea

- Hyperventilation

- Chest pain

- Heart palpitations

- Insomnia

- Headaches

- Hypertension

- Dizziness

- Backache

- Stomach or intestinal pain

- Chronic fatigue

- Chronic irritability

- Nervousness

- Depression

- Muscle tension

- Restlessness

- Irritable bowel (gas, cramps, stomach bloating).

So how do you deal with the crises in your life? Do you have a personal plan to manage stress? Try these strategies; they've been particularly effective in helping people manage stress more effectively in our program:

Avoid nicotine, caffeine and alcohol

These socially accepted drugs influence adrenal function (a gland at the top of your kidney that releases adrenaline). Many of the aforementioned stress symptoms are the result of having too much adrenaline in your bloodstream. Prescription drugs, over-the-counter medications and sugar-binging can also adversely affect your ability to physiologically manage stress.

I've worked with many people whose depression, anxiety or panic attacks were induced by nicotine, caffeine or alcohol. To compensate for a schedule that is overly demanding, people too often turn to these mood-altering drugs. Your body is capable of being exposed to incredible levels of stress without becoming symptomatic. Unfortunately, too often we compromise our body's ability to manage stress through chemical abuse.

The best possible approach to enhance your ability manage stress is to decaffeinate your drinks and eat less chocolate. Learn the side effects of all your prescription drugs and over-the-counter medications. Make it your goal to achieve a physiological equilibrium in which you don't experience mood swings induced by chemicals.

Get active on most days

Most people who exercise report an enhanced relaxation state after completing the activity. That's one reason this intervention is being used across the nation in the treatment of anxiety and depression. Even corporations are now beginning to provide exercise opportunities for their employees because they see the emotional and psychological benefits of physical activity.

It's been my experience that most types of exercise can create a relaxation response. However, cardiorespiratory exercise performed continuously for at least forty minutes has been particularly effective in reducing anxiety levels.

Always remember, humans were born to be physically active. When you're not, you frequently pay an emotional price. With technology ever increasing, you'll find greater opportunities to be physically *inactive*. If you'll implement my prescription for exercise, your feeling of well-being and ability to manage stress can be profoundly enhanced.

Participate in stress management educational and behavioral modification programs

Many communities provide classes, seminars and programs that emphasize time management skills, relaxation strategies and other behavioral tools for managing stress.

At Meadow Brook Health Enhancement Institute, we've established Wellness Coaching sessions that are directed by a behavioral psychologist. We review occupational and family factors that influence anxiety levels and help you develop a plan to manage stress through behavior modification. These behavioral skills are integrated into a comprehensive program that includes exercise and the avoidance of mood-altering drugs.

Too many stress management programs have focused almost exclusively on the psychology of stress management. If you're currently not exercising or increasing adrenaline levels through artificial means (caffeine and other drugs), I hope you will consider the three interventions I've outlined above. This plan can create a sense of well-being that you probably haven't experienced in many years.

8. Minimize Stimulants

You know my concerns about stimulants, especially caffeine, our favorite "upper" in this country. I have yet to find research that conclusively links caffeine to any chronic degenerative disease; even so, the impact of stimulants on your quality of life can be substantial. If you eat a lot of chocolate or drink caffeinated beverages, determine whether you have one or more of the following symptoms:

- Nervousness
- Irritability
- Headaches
- Rapid breathing
- Tremulousness/shakiness
- Insomnia
- Restlessness
- Rapid heart rate
- Irregular heartbeat
- Nausea
- Diarrhea
- Heartburn
- Irritable bowel.

Did you notice that many of the symptoms associated with caffeine are also linked to stress? You're anxious and stressed, so you drink a cup of coffee or cola, which in turn increases your heart rate and makes you more restless and unable to sleep. It doesn't make sense for you to consume a stimulant like caffeine if you are experiencing increased anxiety.

Chances are, you're unaware of how much caffeine you consume in products such as those listed below:

Caffeine Content of Selected Products	
Average cup of coffee	135 mg/cup
Average cup of tea	50 mg/cup
Colas	37-45 mg/12 oz
Sunkist orange soda	41 mg/12 oz
Excedrin	130 mg/2 tablets
Starbucks coffee ice cream	40-60 mg/cup
Dannon coffee yogurt	45 mg/cup

9. Maintain Spirituality

Our medical history questionnaire at the Meadow Brook Health Enhancement Institute asks clients to prioritize the following:

- Ego

- Family

- Health

- Money

- Occupation

- Power

- Spirituality.

Take a moment to prioritize these for yourself. What does your list look like? Is your behavior consistent with your priorities?

It has been my clinical experience that people who list spirituality, family and health as their top priorities in life tend to deal with life crises more effectively. They typically also have a better quality of life than those who list power, money and occupation as their top priorities. Having a purpose in life that supercedes monetary and occupational priorities can provide a sense of contribution and accomplishment that is essential to your well-being.

I've met with people who are atheists, yet indicated in their medical history that their number-one priority in life is spirituality. While God is part of my own personal spirituality, others base their spirituality on other paradigms. One patient, for example, identified spirituality as her most important priority, but did not believe in God. When I asked her to explain, she said it was her belief that she is part of a network of people around the earth who are dependent on one another. Even if she became disabled, as long as she was able to help other people, she felt her life would be meaningful and fulfilled. I found her definition of spirituality qualified as a life-enhancing aspect of the wellness program.

Centenarians frequently identify spirituality as one of the factors they associate with their longevity. Research also suggests that people who have made spirituality a high priority tend to have better outcomes when they become sick.

10. Complete a Comprehensive Physical Examination Every Year

Many U.S. doctors today recommend and perform physical exams only for diagnostic purposes. Many tests and procedures that I believe are important in a comprehensive physical exam are oftentimes not performed. Also, annual exams unfortunately are not always recommended for certain age groups.

I believe you should interact with your personal physician at least once a year, no matter what your age. Your annual physical exam should serve as a barometer of health and lifestyle change, helping you monitor your health enhancement progress and identify health and lifestyle areas requiring improvement.

Make it your personal goal to minimize the risk factors you now know are linked to the major causes of death. When you request an exam, ask your physician to perform the tests that will help you identify health trends so you can achieve the best possible health profile (see the following checklist). This approach and philosophy is, of course, consistent with preventive medicine.

It is important to be aware that physicians today are not financially rewarded for spending time with you to explain results or establish personal health goals. Because of our third-party system of payment, physicians are basically rewarded for doing procedures. I encourage you to find a physician who has a particular interest in preventive medicine and is willing to spend time with you.

And if you have to pay something beyond what your insurance

will cover, recognize the benefits of investing in your health. Don't take the position that everything in health care must be provided by third-party reimbursement. (You'll pay $7 for a movie, $20 for dinner or $40 for a day at the ballpark; how much are you willing to pay for a lifetime of good health?) If good health is one of your highest priorities in life, then be willing to make an investment even if your insurance program won't pay for some preventive medicine procedures.

One other important point: Make sure you get the results of all studies completed during your physical examination. Take on this responsibility by requesting the results as you start the evaluation; don't wait for your physician to send the results. Many times when I ask patients for the results of their last physical examinations, they tell me they assume the results were normal because they never heard back from the doctor's office. Much of the progress we're making toward preventing heart disease, cancer and diabetes is occurring because people are making changes in their lifestyles. But to make those changes, you need to take responsibility for getting—and understanding—your test results.

Your physical exam should include the following:

❏ Eyes, thyroid, lymphatic system, ears, lungs, cardiovascular system, hernias, spleen, genitals, pelvic exam for women, digital rectal exam, skin, and neurological and musculoskeletal findings

❏ Cancer screenings for women should include breast exams, digital rectal exams, hemoccults, mammography (based on your age and symptoms), sigmoidoscopy/colonoscopy (based on your age and symptoms) and skin exam

❏ Cancer screenings for men should include digital rectal exam, hemoccults, PSA, sigmoidoscopy/colonoscopy (based on your age and symptoms), skin exam and testicular exam

❏ An appropriate assessment of your body composition

❏ Stress test (determination of your functional work capacity).

Again, your physician should present the results of all of these evaluation components to you with conclusions and recommendations. Make follow-up appointments to evaluate your progress toward reducing the specific risk factors that have been identified in the exam. Create your own health database. This will permit you to monitor your personal physiological trends and your overall progress toward adding years of functional living to your life.

Here's the Good News: These Ten Steps Are Achievable

There you have it, ten specific steps toward a longer, functional life. I hope you agree that most of these health and lifestyle recommendations are achievable. In fact, I'll bet you have four or five of them in place already. Take the time to develop a strategy for implementing the others.

Implement these ten steps and I'll see you at your 100th birthday party.

IV

APPENDICES

Stretches and Exercises

As emphasized earlier in the book, a comprehensive program of physical conditioning should include flexibility exercises, resistance training (weight lifting), as well as cardiorespiratory exercise. With all forms of conditioning, make sure you follow a reasonable progression of activities. If you lack flexibility, muscular strength or muscular endurance, don't expect optimal results in a short period of time. Deconditioning occurs over a long period of time. So don't expect significant improvement in your flexibility, strength and muscular endurance after only a few exercise sessions.

With the following flexibility exercises always warm up prior to stretching. Perform the movement without bouncing. Movements should be controlled while holding each stretch for ten to thirty seconds. Maintain only stretch tensions that feel comfortable.

Your breathing should be slow, deep and rhythmical. Don't be overly concerned with how far you can stretch initially. As you continue your flexibility exercises, your range of motion will automatically improve. Perform three to five repetitions of each flexibility exercise each session.

Resistance Training (weight lifting)

As you develop your resistance training program, remember to emphasize safety. I encourage you to obtain good instruction in the proper use of this type of equipment. If you plan to use free weights, a spotter or exercise partner is an absolute prerequisite to ensure your safety. Be sure to also breathe appropriately during the exercise. Many people make the mistake of holding their breath while initially using resistance equipment. Failure to breathe regularly during this form of exercise can influence pressure in the chest cavity, ultimately reducing blood flow to your heart. Follow the exercise prescription described in chapter nine when you implement your resistance training program.

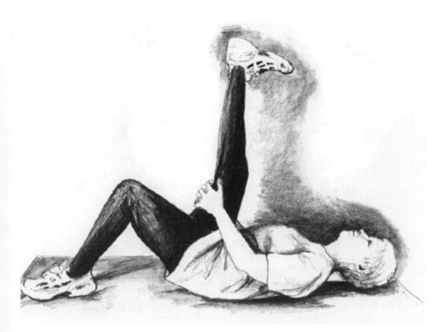

Supine

Lie on your back with one knee bent so that your foot is set firmly against the floor. Gently extend your other leg toward your head. Grasp your thigh with both hands to control the intensity of the stretch. Repeat this same stretch with your other leg.

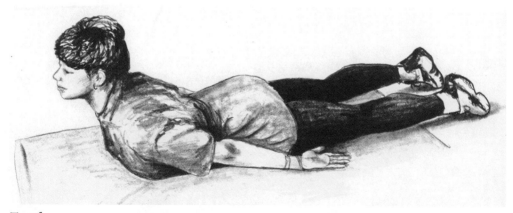

Trunk

Lie face down with both of your arms at your sides. Gently lift your head, neck and chest. Keep your feet in contact with the floor to minimize the risk of straining your back.

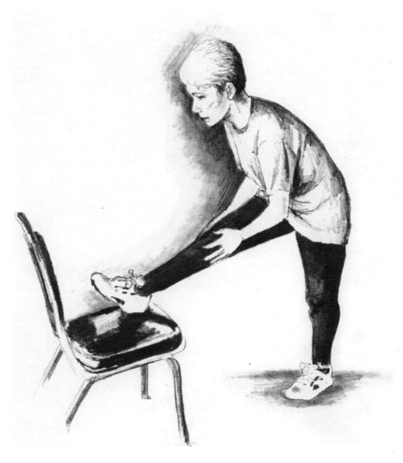

Hamstring

Rest your foot on a chair or elevated object at a comfortable height. The supporting leg should be nearly straight with your foot pointed forward. Slowly bend forward from your hip. Repeat this stretch with your opposite leg.

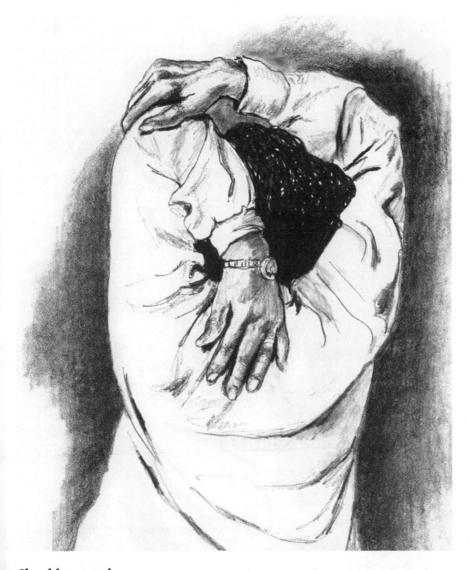

Shoulder stretch

Extend one arm above your head. Bending at the elbow, drop your lower arm behind your head. Use your opposite hand to exert gentle pressure on your elbow. Repeat this stretch with your other arm.

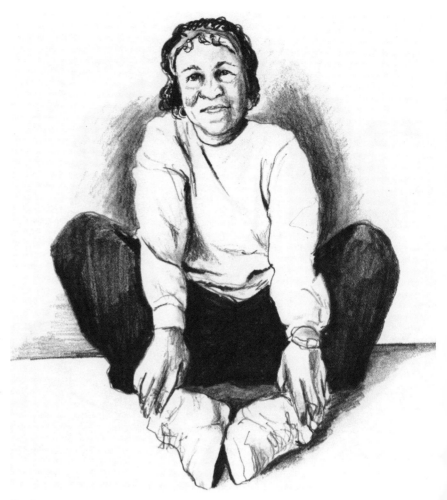

Groin
Position your legs so that the soles of your feet can meet each other. Place your hands on your feet or ankles. Lean forward from your hips to stretch. Avoid bending from your shoulders.

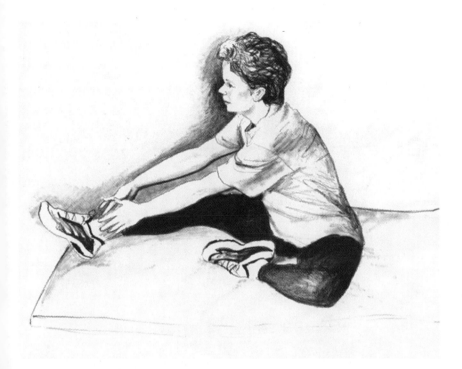

Hurdle

With one leg straightened, rest the sole of your opposite foot against your inner thigh. Lean forward from your hip to stretch your hamstring. Do not lock the straightened knee. Repeat this stretch with your opposite leg.

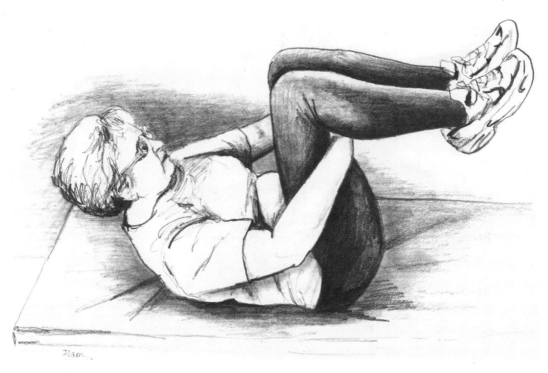

Lower back
Lie on your back with both knees bent. Grasp both legs behind your knees and pull them toward your chest. Lift your head.

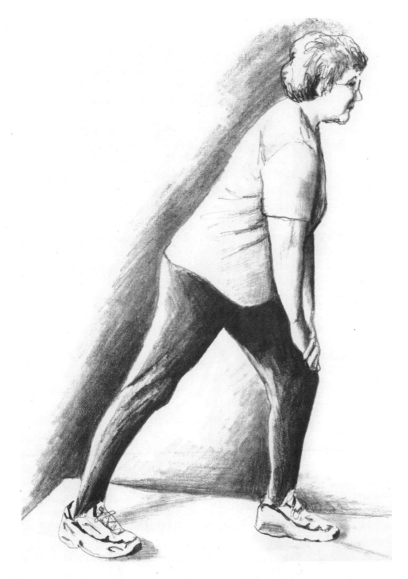

Calf

Bending one leg, place your foot in front of you. Your other leg should remain straight and behind you. Rest both arms on your forward thigh, supporting your upper body. Keep the heel of the straight leg on the ground with your toes pointing forward. Repeat this stretch with your opposite leg.

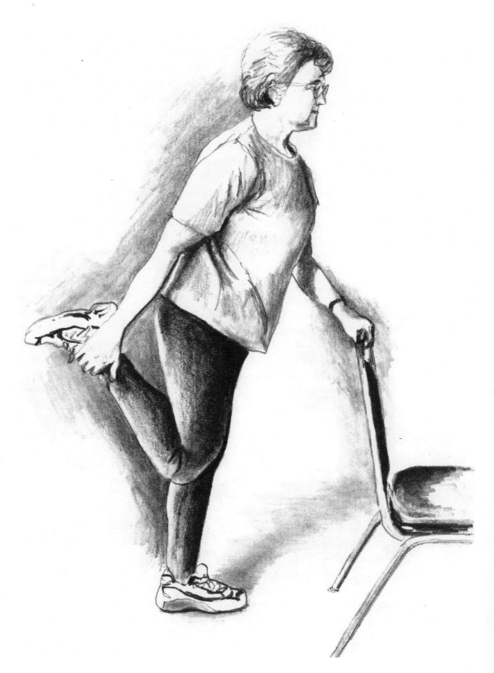

Quadriceps

Standing on one leg, bend the knee of the opposite leg and hold your foot with the same-sided hand. Gently pull your foot toward your buttocks. Do not lock the knee of your supporting leg. Repeat this stretch with your other leg.

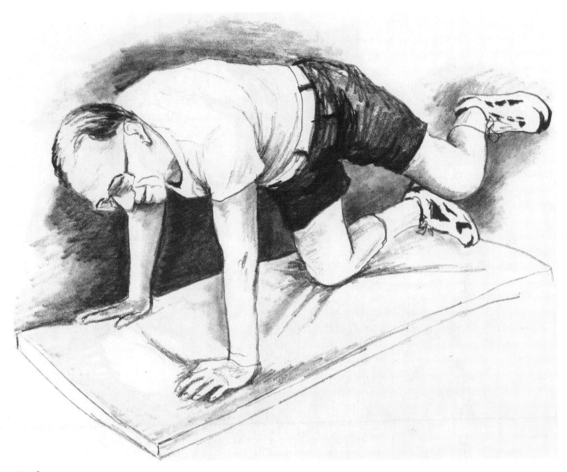

Hydrant
On your hands and knees, evenly distribute your body weight. Your hands should be shoulder width apart, while your knees should be hip width apart. Keep one knee bent while lifting one leg to the height of your hip. Return to your starting position. Continue lifting and returning until you feel fatigue. Repeat this exercise with your other leg.

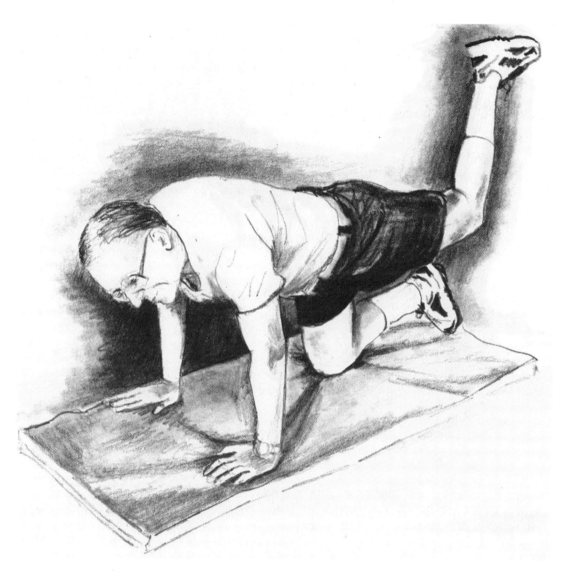

Donkey

On your hands and knees, distribute your weight evenly. Straighten one leg and bend at the knee so that your lower leg is perpendicular to your upper leg. Maintaining this position, lift and lower your leg (as if you were attempting to balance a plate on your foot). Continue lifting and lowering until you feel fatigue. Repeat this exercise with your other leg.

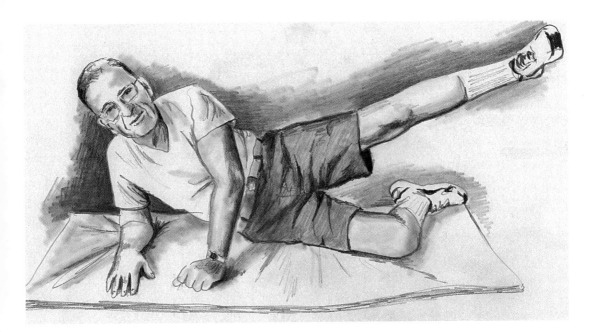

Outer leg

Lie on your side, using both arms for support. Bend your lower leg at the knee. Keep your upper leg straight as you raise and lower it. Continue lifting and lowering your leg until you feel fatigue. Repeat this exercise with your opposite leg.

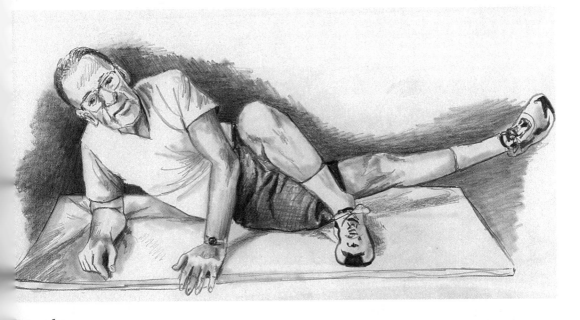

Inner leg

Lie on your side, using both arms for support. Cross your upper leg in front of your body. Keeping your lower leg straight, raise and lower it until you feel fatigue. Repeat the exercise on your opposite side.

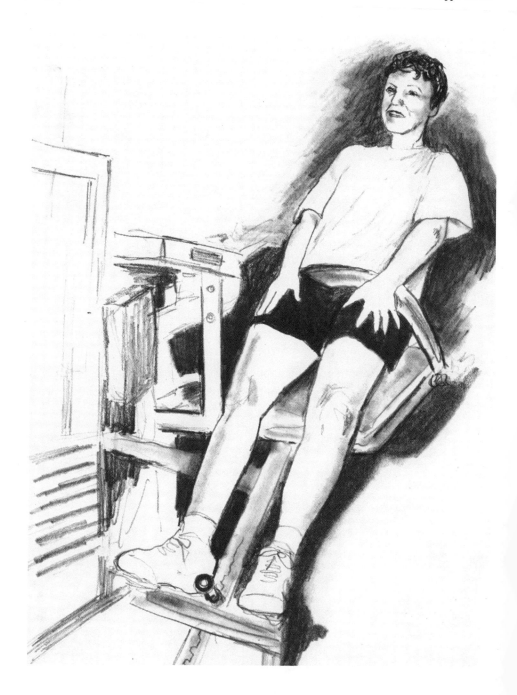

Back

Adjust the foot plate so that your knees are bent and your hips are aligned with the axis of the machine. Secure the seat belt and place your hands on your thighs. As you extend and bend your back, lift and lower with steady control.

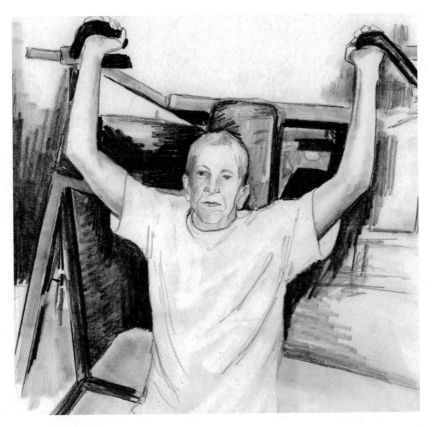

Shoulder

Adjust your seat so that the handles are level with your shoulders. Select a grip, then slowly lift and lower yourself, being careful to control your weight. Avoid locking your elbows as you reach the maximum extension of your arms.

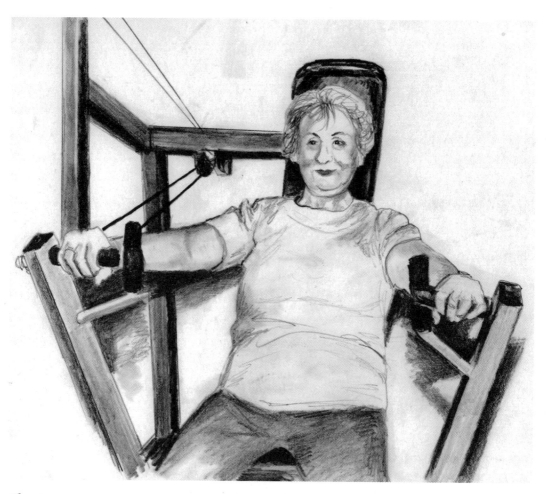

Chest

Adjust the seat height so that the handles are even with your sternum. Use the foot pedal to raise the handles and position your arms. Select your grip. Steadily lift and lower the weight. Avoid locking your elbows at your maximum arm extension.

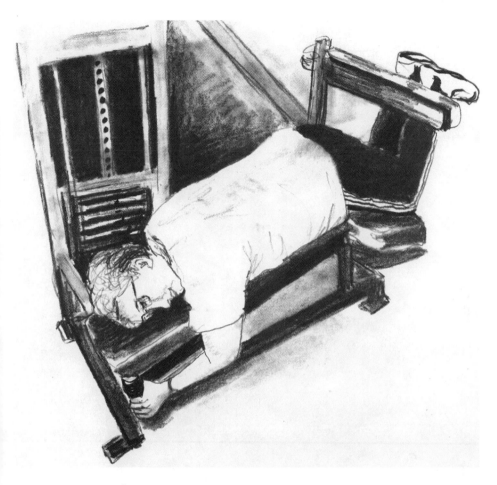

Leg curl

Adjust the leg pad so that it rests above your Achilles tendon. Position your body so that your knees are off the surface of the body pad. Lightly grip the handles. Raise and lower the weight with steady control.

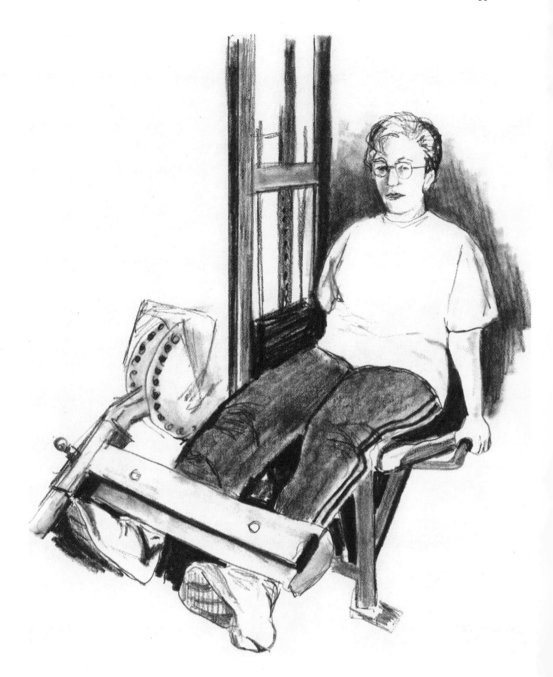

Leg extension
Adjust the leg pad so that it rests above your ankle. Adjust the back pad so that your knee is positioned at the edge of the seat. Lift the weight until your leg is straight and slowly return it to the starting position. Lift and lower the weight with steady control.

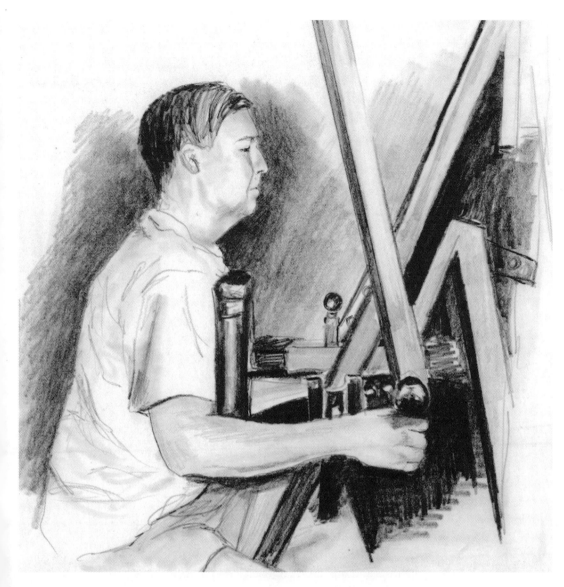

Rowing

Adjust your seat height so that the arms of the machine are parallel to the floor as you grasp the handles. Position the chest pad so that your arms are fully extended as you grasp the handles. Select your desired grip and lift and lower the weight with steady control.

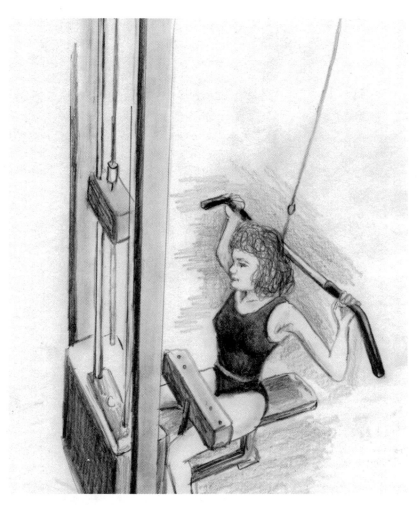

Lateral pull

Sit so that your lower legs are vertical to the floor. Your knees should be at 90-degree angles. Adjust your thigh pad to touch your legs. Grasp the handles and pull down. At the lowest point, the bar can be either in front of or in back of your head. Lift and lower the weight with steady control.

7-Day Food Diary

TIME	MINUTES SPENT EATING	DEGREE OF HUNGER - SCALE FROM 1-5 (1-not hungry) (5-very hungry)	ACTIVITY WHILE EATING	LOCATION WHILE EATING	DESCRIBE FOOD, TYPE & QUANTITY (BRAND NAMES WHERE POSSIBLE) PLEASE BE SPECIFIC (one per line)	AMOUNT	FAT GRAMS / FIBER GRAMS

Make copies of this food journal and use it for seven days to become aware of your food intake patterns.

Delicious Good News Recipes

Appetizers

Sauces

Soups and Chilis

*Recipes are adapted from American Institute for Cancer Research

APPETIZERS

LITE HUMMUS SPREAD

One 15-oz can garbanzo beans, drained; reserve 6 tablespoons of
   the liquid
1 tablespoon sesame tahini
2 tablespoons lemon juice
1-2 cloves of garlic
Paprika
Fresh ground black pepper
Salt to taste

Serves:	4
Calories:	160
Fat:	3.7 g
Saturated Fat:	0.1 g
Fiber:	4.9 g

Blend the beans, reserved liquid, tahini, lemon juice and garlic together in
a blender or food processor until smooth. Pour the mixture into a bowl.
Sprinkle with paprika, black pepper, and, if desired, salt.

MARINATED MUSHROOMS

¼ cup balsamic vinegar
1 tablespoon lemon juice
1 teaspoon dried oregano
½ teaspoon sea salt (can use regular salt)
1 teaspoon pepper
¾ lb button mushrooms
½ cup onion, sliced
½ cup green peppers, chopped
½ cup sweet red pepper, chopped

Serves:	4
Calories:	52
Fat:	0.4 g
Saturated Fat:	0.1 g
Fiber:	2.4 g

In a large bowl, whisk together vinegar, lemon juice, oregano, salt, pepper
and 2 teaspoons of water. Next, remove and discard stems on mushrooms
and cut large mushrooms in half. Add mushrooms, onions and peppers to
marinade and stir, coating them well. Refrigerate overnight or for 8 hours,
stirring every few hours.

BLUE CHEESE SPREAD

Serves: 10
Calories: 43
Fat: 1.6 g
Saturated Fat: 1.1 g
Fiber: 0.1 g

Vegetable cooking spray
1 cup fat-free cottage cheese
2 oz crumbled blue cheese
½ cup nonfat plain yogurt
1 green onion, finely minced
1 medium clove garlic, minced
1 tablespoon freshly squeezed lemon juice
1 tablespoon fresh dill, finely chopped
1 teaspoon Worcestershire sauce
1 tablespoon gelatin
2 tablespoons cold water
1 head red leaf lettuce

Lightly spray a 10-inch tart pan with removable bottom. In the bowl of your food processor or blender, combine cottage cheese and blue cheese and puree until smooth; add yogurt. Add the onion, garlic, lemon juice, dill and Worcestershire sauce, pulse to combine. Dissolve gelatin in water and stir in mixture. Pour blue cheese mixture into pan. Cover with plastic wrap and chill until mixture is set. Line a plate with red leaf lettuce and turn dip onto plate.

NEPTUNE SPREAD

Serves: 10
Calories: 74
Fat: 0.5 g
Saturated Fat: 0.1 g
Fiber: 0 g

12 oz nonfat cottage cheese
3 tablespoons fat-free cream cheese
1 cup fat-free mayonnaise
¼ teaspoon lemon pepper or ½ teaspoon white pepper
2 tablespoons lemon juice
7½-oz can king crabmeat, drained
4½-oz can cocktail shrimp, drained

In a blender combine nonfat cottage cheese, cream cheese, mayonnaise, pepper and lemon juice. Remove from blender and mix in seafood. Cover and chill. Serve with whole grain or nonfat saltine crackers.

MEXICAN LAYERED BEAN DIP

1 pkg seasoning taco mix
Two 15-oz cans of fat-free refried beans
16 oz fat-free sour cream
6 oz taco sauce
2 cups fat-free cheddar cheese
1 cup scallions

Serves:	12
Calories:	146
Fat:	0 g
Saturated Fat:	0 g
Fiber:	4 g

Mix half of the seasoning mix with beans. Mix remaining seasoning mix with sour cream. In a rectangular glass dish, layer bean mixture, taco sauce, sour cream mixture and shredded cheese. Top with onions and serve with baked tortilla chips.

ROASTED EGGPLANT AND ONION PATÉ

1 lb eggplant
1 large clove garlic, sliced
½ large onion
2 sprigs fresh oregano
¼ cup plain fat-free yogurt
2 teaspoons lemon juice
1 teaspoon chopped fresh marjoram
1 teaspoon chopped fresh oregano
1 teaspoon salt
½ teaspoon black pepper

Serves:	12
Calories:	16
Fat:	0 g
Saturated Fat:	0 g
Fiber:	1 g

Cut slits in the eggplant and stick the garlic slices into the slits. Remove the skin from onion. Wrap the eggplant, onion, and oregano sprigs tightly in a large piece of foil and bake at 350 degrees until the eggplant is completely soft all over, 1-1½ hours. Turn the eggplant halfway during cooking time. Open the package and let it sit for 10 minutes. Discard the oregano and any liquid. When the eggplant is cool enough to handle, scrape the flesh and add this to garlic and onion into the bowl of a food processor. Discard the skin of the eggplant. Add the yogurt, lemon juice, marjoram and salt and pepper. Process until smooth and serve at room temperature.

KING CRAB SPREAD

Serves: 8
Calories: 65
Fat: 0.5 g
Saturated Fat: 0 g
Fiber: 0 g

Two 7.5-oz cans crabmeat, drained well
½ cup fat-free mayonnaise
3 tablespoons chopped parsley
2 tablespoons chopped chives
½ teaspoon Worcestershire sauce
¾ teaspoon lemon juice
3 hard-cooked egg whites, chopped finely
1 cup diced, peeled and seeded cucumber

Remove any cartilage from crabmeat and flake. In a medium bowl, combine mayonnaise, parsley, chives, Worcestershire, and lemon juice. Mix well. Cover and chill for one hour. Serve with whole grain crackers or with lettuce on whole grain bread. Line plates with leaf lettuce and serve as a salad.

DILLY CUCUMBER SPREAD

Serves: 12
Calories: 38
Fat: 0.5 g
Saturated Fat: 0.3 g
Fiber: 0.1 g

2 (8-oz) pkg softened fat-free cream cheese
2 teaspoons lemon juice
1 tablespoon minced onion
2 teaspoons dill weed
¼ teaspoon prepared horseradish
Dash of hot pepper sauce
¾ cup finely diced peeled and seeded cucumber

In a mixing bowl, beat cream cheese until smooth. Add lemon juice, onion, dill, horseradish, and hot pepper sauce. Fold in cucumber. Cover and chill for at least an hour. Serve with crackers or raw vegetables.

BROILED CHEESE BREAD

Per slice:
Calories: 109
Fat: 0.8 g
Saturated Fat: 0.2 g
Fiber: 1.4 g

1 slice of French bread per person
2 tablespoons creamy pesto sauce/dip (see recipe in the sauce section)

Place two tablespoons of dip on each slice of bread, place on baking tray and broil until golden brown. Great with spaghetti or Italian dishes.

TASTY AND TANGY SWEET AND SOUR MEATBALLS

1 lb ground turkey breast (no skin or dark meat)
¼ cup minced onion
2 tablespoons minced parsley
2 tablespoons mustard
1 garlic clove, finely minced
1 tablespoon Worcestershire sauce
2 teaspoons oregano flakes
1 egg white, beaten
¼ cup bread crumbs

Sauce:

8-oz can tomato sauce
½ cup water
2 tablespoons soy sauce
2 tablespoons lemon juice
1 tablespoon sugar

Serves:	**12**
Calories:	**50**
Fat:	**0.7 g**
Saturated Fat:	**0.2 g**
Fiber:	**0.2 g**

Combine all ingredients for meatballs. Shape into 1-inch balls (about 30-36 meatballs). Brown these in a skillet sprayed with vegetable oil. Turn to brown evenly. In a separate bowl combine all sauce ingredients. Pour this mixture over cooked meatballs. Heat thoroughly and serve. Note: For a thicker sauce, dissolve three teaspoons cornstarch in cold water and add once sauce is hot. Stir until thickened. Variation: Omit sauce and use meatballs in spaghetti sauce or shape as burgers.

SALSA DIP

8-oz block of fat-free cream cheese
One 16-oz jar of salsa
4 green onions, chopped
½ green bell pepper, chopped
8 oz fat-free cheddar cheese

Serves:	**6**
Calories:	**123**
Fat:	**0.8 g**
Saturated Fat:	**0.4 g**
Fiber:	**1.6 g**

Spread cream cheese in 8-inch x 8-inch container. Spread salsa on top of cream cheese. Sprinkle diced green onions and green peppers on top of salsa. Top with cheddar cheese. Serve cold or with tortilla chips or rolled in lawash bread.

PARTY CHEESE BALL

Serves: 8
Calories: 63
Fat: 0.2 g
Saturated Fat: 0.1 g
Fiber: 0 g

2 cups (8-oz) fat-free shredded cheese
¼ cup fat-free mayonnaise
1½ teaspoon Worcestershire sauce
3-oz block of fat-free cream cheese, softened
½ teaspoon onion powder
½ teaspoon celery powder
¾ teaspoon garlic powder

Mix all ingredients well. (Easiest to mix with your hands.) Cover with plastic wrap and chill cheese mix until firm. Once chilled, shape into a ball. Cover again and chill until firm (approximately two hours). For variety, roll into crumbled low-fat cheese flavored crackers or Grape Nuts cereal.

GUACAMOLE GONE SKINNY

Serves: 8
Calories: 33
Fat: 0.2 g
Saturated Fat: 0 g
Fiber: 2.2 g

10-oz bag of frozen peas
½ jalapeno pepper, minced
1 clove garlic, minced
1½ teaspoons lemon juice
½ teaspoon cumin
1 teaspoon salt
¾ cup chopped and seeded tomato
¼ cup finely chopped onion

Cook peas according to directions on package. Drain very well to decrease liquid (or pat dry). Put jalapeno, garlic, and lemon juice in food processor and blend. Add cumin and salt and pulse until blended. Add peas and puree. Remove the pea puree and stir in the tomato and onion. Chill for one hour or until cool and serve. Great with baked tortillas, pita, on fajitas or as a sandwich spread.

SAUCES

ROASTED RED PEPPER AND FETA CHEESE SAUCE

15-oz jar of roasted red pepper (in water)
1 cup white wine
1 cup vegetable broth
3 cloves garlic
1 teaspoon sweet basil
½ teaspoon hot pepper flakes
2 oz reduced-fat feta cheese, crumbled

Serves: 4
Calories: 110
Fat: 1.8 g
Saturated Fat: 1 g
Fiber: 0 g

Put jar of peppers in blender and puree. Combine wine and broth in frying pan and add garlic, basil, and hot pepper flakes. Simmer until reduced in half (approximately 15 minutes). Add pepper, puree, and stir until combined. Add feta cheese and heat for 2 minutes. Stir until combined. Great over pasta, rice, or meat.

TERIYAKI SAUCE/MARINADE

½ cup brown sugar
⅓ cup soy sauce (low sodium)
1 cup warm water
1-1½ teaspoons freshly grated ginger
½-¾ teaspoon garlic powder
3 teaspoons cornstarch

Serves: 4
Calories: 125
Fat: 0 g
Saturated Fat: 0 g
Fiber: 0 g

Stir brown sugar, soy sauce, water, ginger, and garlic powder together until sugar dissolves; blend. Heat on medium high until bubbles. Dissolve cornstarch in cold water and add to mixture. Continue heating until thick. Note: This sauce can be made directly in your stir-fry. If using as a marinade sauce, cool completely before adding to food. If meat is being used, do not reserve the marinade used. Suggestion: Use half of the sauce for marinating food and the other half with serving.

SPAGHETTI SAUCE

Serves: 4
Calories: 118
Fat: 1.2 g
Saturated Fat: 0 g
Fiber: 5.4 g

48 oz stewed tomatoes
1 tablespoon sugar
1½ tablespoons fresh chopped oregano
2 teaspoons fresh chopped basil
1 clove garlic, minced
¾ cup sliced mushrooms

Put cans of tomatoes into food processor or blender and blend. Put in a pot and add remaining ingredients. Bring to a boil. Let simmer until thick (about 15 minutes). For variation, add fat-free Parmesan on top or add ground "meatless burger."

HOT VEGETABLE SAUCE

Serves: 6
Calories: 122
Fat: 0.5 g
Saturated Fat: 0.1 g
Fiber: 8.1 g

5½ cup vegetable medley
1 cup vegetable broth
1 tablespoon instant minced onion
2 tablespoons tomato paste
1 teaspoon dried basil leaves
1½ teaspoons garlic powder
½ teaspoon black pepper
2 tablespoons cornstarch

In a large saucepan, combine vegetable medley, broth, the minced onion, tomato paste, basil, garlic powder and black pepper. Bring to a boil and cook until vegetables are soft. Place vegetable mixture in blender or food processor and process until blended. Mixture will still be lumpy. Return to pan and bring to a boil. Dissolve cornstarch in ¼ cup water and add to mixture. Stir until sauce is thickened. Serve over pasta, rice or baked potato.

CREAMY PESTO SAUCE/DIP

Serves: 4
Calories: 81
Fat: 0 g
Saturated Fat: 0 g
Fiber: 1.3 g

16 oz fat-free cottage cheese
¼ cup fresh basil, chopped
2 tablespoons fresh oregano, chopped
1 teaspoon garlic powder

In a food processor or blender add all ingredients and blend until smooth. Uses: Toss with hot pasta or use as a vegetable dip.

SOUPS AND CHILIS

STRAWBERRY SOUP IN MELON BOWLS

2 pints of fresh strawberries, washed and hulled
1 cup orange juice
½ teaspoon cornstarch
¼ teaspoon cinnamon
Dash of ground cloves
1 tablespoon lemon juice
2 tablespoons + 2 teaspoons sugar
1 cup skim milk
2 cantaloupes

Serves:	4
Calories:	187
Fat:	0.7 g
Saturated Fat:	0.1 g
Fiber:	4.8 g

Puree the strawberries with the orange juice in a blender or food processor and pour into a 4-quart saucepan. Put a few spoonfuls of the puree into a small cup and stir in the cornstarch until well blended. Return the mixture to the saucepan, and add the cinnamon and cloves. Stirring frequently, heat the puree over a medium heat until the mixture comes to a boil. Cook for one minute and remove from the heat, stirring in the lemon juice and sugar. When the mixture has cooled, pour the milk into a large bowl and gradually add the strawberry mixture to it, stirring constantly. The soup should be covered and chilled for three hours. Cut the cantaloupes into halves, scoop out the seeds and turn them upside down to drain. To serve, fill each melon with chilled soup.

SAVORY SALMON CHOWDER

Serves: 4
Calories: 353
Fat: 4.8 g
Saturated Fat: 1.3 g
Fiber: 4.8 g

¾ cup chopped onion
½ cup chopped celery
1 clove garlic, minced
3 cups frozen hash brown potatoes (no fat added)
1 cup diced carrots
2 cups vegetable broth
1-2 tablespoons of water
1 teaspoon dill weed
7½-oz can pink salmon
12-oz can evaporated skim milk
8¾-oz can cream style corn
Pepper, to taste

In a large nonstick saucepan coated with vegetable spray, cook onion, celery and garlic, stirring often until vegetables are tender. Add some water if vegetables start to stick. Add potatoes, carrots, broth, water, and dill weed; bring to a boil. Reduce heat, cover and simmer for thirty minutes or until vegetables are tender. Drain and flake salmon, reserve liquid. Add salmon, reserved liquid, evaporated milk, corn, and pepper to taste. Cook over low heat just until heated through. Serve.

CRIMINI MUSHROOM CHOWDER

Serves: 4
Calories: 173
Fat: 2.4 g
Saturated Fat: 0.8 g
Fiber: 3 g

Two 11-oz cans low-fat tomato soup
½ cup skim milk
¾ cup water
2 teaspoons instant vegetable granules
½ lb crimini mushrooms, sliced
2-3 green onions with stems, cut ¼-inch slice
1 clove garlic, minced
2 teaspoons seafood seasoning
4 tablespoons fresh chopped parsley

Heat soup, skim milk, water and vegetable granules to just near boiling point. Sauté mushrooms in skillet sprayed with vegetable oil. Add onion and garlic. Add one tablespoon water or vegetable broth during sauté. Add seafood seasoning, mushrooms, onions and garlic to the soup; stir gently. Simmer twenty minutes, stirring constantly. Stir in parsley one minute before serving.

INDIAN PUMPKIN SOUP

4 cups pumpkin flesh
Three 14.5-oz cans fat-free vegetable broth
2 baking apples, peeled, cored and chopped
1 carrot, chopped
¼ cup chopped onion
2 teaspoons grated gingerroot
1 teaspoon curry powder
½ teaspoon ground cumin
¼ teaspoon ground cinnamon
2 tablespoons sugar
1 cup croutons

Serves:	8
Calories:	93
Fat:	1.2 g
Saturated Fat:	0.1 g
Fiber:	3 g

In a large pot, combine the four cups of pumpkin flesh, broth, apples, carrot, onion, gingerroot, curry powder, cumin, and cinnamon and sugar. Bring to a boil, reducing heat. Cover, simmer for 10-12 minutes or until the vegetables are tender. Cool slightly. Blend or process mixture, a third at a time, in a blender or food processor until smooth. Return pumpkin mixture to pot and simmer for twenty minutes. Serve with croutons as garnish.

SPINACH, CORN AND SHRIMP SOUP

4 cups frozen sweet corn
Vegetable cooking spray
2 cloves garlic, minced
1 small onion, chopped
12 medium shrimp deveined
8 oz evaporated skim milk
1 cup water
1 cup vegetable broth
1 pkg spinach leaves
Salt to taste

Serves:	6
Calories:	188
Fat:	1.7 g
Saturated Fat:	0.3 g
Fiber:	7.6 g

Cook corn according to directions. Blenderize two cups of corn. Set aside. Spray pan with vegetable cooking spray and sauté garlic and onions until onions are tender. Add shrimp and cook until pink. Add blenderized corn and the rest of the corn kernels. Add milk, water and broth. Bring to a boil and simmer for five minutes. Add spinach and cook until wilted. Serve.

LENTIL SOUP WITH HERBS AND LEMON

Serves: 4
Calories: 209
Fat: 2.0 g
Saturated Fat: 0.1 g
Fiber: 15.9 g

1 cup lentils, soaked overnight in 1 cup water
6 cups vegetable broth, reserve ¼ cup
1 yellow onion, thinly sliced
1 teaspoon dried tarragon
½ teaspoon dried oregano
Salt and pepper to taste
1 tablespoon lemon juice
4 thin slices of lemon

Bring the lentils to a boil in the broth. Reduce the heat and simmer until tender, approximately fifteen minutes (if you have not pre-soaked the lentils, increase your cooking time by about fifteen minutes more). While the lentils are cooking, sauté the onions in the reserved ¼ cup of broth. Remove from heat and set aside. When the lentils are tender, add the onions, herbs, salt, and pepper. Cook for two minutes. Stir in the lemon juice and garnish with lemon slices.

CREAMY ASPARAGUS AND POTATO SOUP

Serves: 6
Calories: 214
Fat: 2.0 g
Saturated Fat: 0.3 g
Fiber: 3.8 g

Vegetable cooking spray
3 cups defrosted hash brown potatoes (no fat added)
1 teaspoon fresh garlic, minced
½ cup celery, cut in small pieces
1 cup fresh green beans, chopped
3 cups asparagus, cut in small pieces (discard the tough ends)
2 tablespoons flour
3 cans (15-oz cans) vegetable broth
2 teaspoons dill weed
1 teaspoon salt
1 teaspoon pepper
1 can evaporated skim milk
½ cup fat-free sour cream

In a large pot sprayed with vegetable spray, cook potatoes for four minutes. Add garlic, celery, green beans, and asparagus and cook for five more minutes. Add flour and stir to coat vegetables. Add broth and spices, bring to a boil, and then simmer for twenty minutes. Stir in milk and sour cream. Serve.

MOM'S GAZPACHO SOUP

4 cups tomato juice
2 cups vegetable broth
1 medium onion, chopped
2 cups fresh tomatoes, diced
1 cup green pepper, diced
1 tablespoon garlic powder
1 tablespoon dried parsley
1 large cucumber, diced
1 cup scallions, diced
Juice of 1 lemon
Juice of 1 lime
2 tablespoons Worcestershire sauce
2 tablespoons wine vinegar
1 teaspoon tarragon
1 teaspoon basil
¾ teaspoon black pepper

Serves:	6
Calories:	87
Fat:	0.8 g
Saturated Fat:	0.1 g
Fiber:	3.2 g

Combine all ingredients. Refrigerate at least two hours. Overnight is best because spices have a chance to blend. Serve cold. Add pepper sauce as desired.

CARROT SOUP

6 cups of vegetable broth
1½ lb of carrots peeled and sliced into 1-inch pieces
1 medium onion
Pam cooking spray
½ cup skim milk or buttermilk
1½ tablespoons fresh thyme
½ teaspoon nutmeg
½ teaspoon salt
½ teaspoon white pepper

Serves:	4
Calories:	121
Fat:	2.1 g
Saturated Fat:	0.1 g
Fiber:	5.9 g

Bring broth to a boil. Add carrots and simmer twenty minutes. Cool slightly and puree in food processor. Spray pan with vegetable spray. Sauté onion. Add carrot puree to onions. Add milk and spices. Simmer five minutes. Soup is great hot or cold.

WHITE CHILI

Serves: 10
Calories: 249
Fat: 2.6 g
Saturated Fat: 0.6 g
Fiber: 7.4 g

Two 14.5-oz cans vegetable broth
1 large onion, chopped
2 rounded teaspoons minced garlic
4-oz can green chilies with liquid
48-oz jar Great Northern beans with liquid
2 teaspoons ground cumin
1 teaspoon oregano
3-4 dashes pepper sauce
⅛ teaspoon cayenne pepper
*4 boneless, skinless chicken breasts, poached or grilled and
  cubed*

In a large saucepan pour just a bit of the broth (enough to cover bottom) and set the rest aside. Add onion and minced garlic. Simmer and stir until onion is wilted and hot. Add chilies and stir well. Add the beans, including the liquid, then mix in the cumin, oregano, pepper sauce, cayenne pepper, broth, and add chicken pieces. Combine and simmer, cover, and stir occasionally, for a minimum of thirty minutes. It will continue to thicken.

VEGETARIAN SOUTH OF THE BORDER CHILI

1 yellow onion, chopped
1 green pepper, chopped
1 yellow pepper, chopped
1½ cups carrots, sliced
2 cloves garlic, minced
2 teaspoons paprika
¼ teaspoon cayenne pepper
2 tablespoons chili pepper
1 tablespoon ground cumin
1½ teaspoons dried oregano
1½ teaspoons dried basil
Two 16-oz cans tomatoes
1 small jalapeno pepper, minced (remove seeds)
15-oz can light kidney beans
15-oz can black beans
¼ cup plain non-fat yogurt or fat-free sour cream
1 cup coarsely crushed baked tortilla chips

Serves:	8
Calories:	167
Fat:	1.2 g
Saturated Fat:	0.1 g
Fiber:	10 g

Coat large skillet with vegetable cooking spray. Add onions, peppers, carrots, and spices. Sauté five to ten minutes. Add canned tomatoes, jalapeno pepper and beans. Simmer for fifteen to twenty minutes or longer. Add water if needed. Top with yogurt or sour cream and baked chips.

TURKEY BLACK BEAN CHILI

Serves: 6
Calories: 208
Fat: 3.0 g
Saturated Fat: 0.8 g
Fiber: 5.8 g

1 lb ground turkey breast (no skin or dark meat)
1 cup coarsely chopped onions
1 sweet red pepper, coarsely chopped
1 jalapeno chili pepper, seeded and finely chopped
2 cloves garlic, minced
1 can (28-oz) salt-free tomatoes, coarsely chopped (save juice)
1 can (16-oz) black beans, rinsed and drained
1 tablespoon chili powder
2 teaspoons ground cumin
1 teaspoon ground coriander
½ teaspoon dried oregano
½ teaspoon dried marjoram
¼ teaspoon crushed red pepper
½ teaspoon ground cinnamon
¾ cup coarsely chopped and loosely packed fresh cilantro

Spray a large saucepan with vegetable cooking spray. Cook the turkey, onions, sweet peppers, jalapeno peppers and garlic over medium heat or until the turkey is no longer pink and the vegetables are tender. Stir in tomatoes, juices, beans, and all spices except cilantro. Bring to a gentle boil, then reduce heat. Cover and simmer for five minutes. Stir in cilantro and serve.

SALADS AND SIDE DISHES

ZESTY CUCUMBER SALAD

4 cucumbers, peeled, seeds removed and sliced thinly
2 tablespoons salt
2 tablespoons vinegar, white or rice vinegar
2 teaspoons prepared horseradish
2 tablespoons fresh dill, minced
1 teaspoon pepper
½ cup green onions, sliced

Serves	4
Calories	50
Fat	0.9 g
Saturated fat	0.4 g
Fiber	2.9 g

Place cucumbers in a colander and salt them. Let drain for thirty to forty-five minutes (this will get rid of excess water). Rinse cucumbers thoroughly; pat dry. In a bowl mix vinegar, horseradish, dill and pepper. Add cucumbers and onion and toss to well coat. Chill for forty-five minutes; stir occasionally to coat cucumbers.

APPLE-GLAZED PEAS AND CARROTS

10-oz pkg frozen peas and carrots
1 cup frozen small whole onions, or 1 cup coarsely chopped onion
1½ cups water
¼ cup apple juice concentrate
¼ teaspoon ground cinnamon
⅛ teaspoon ground nutmeg

Serves	4
Calories	79
Fat	0.3 g
Saturated fat	0.1 g
Fiber	4.7 g

In two-quart casserole, combine peas and carrots, onions and water. Cover. Microwave on high for seven to ten minutes, or until vegetables are hot, stirring once. Add apple juice concentrate, cinnamon and nutmeg. Toss to coat. Serve.

COLESLAW

Serves: 8
Calories: 65
Fat: 0.3 g
Saturated Fat: 0 g
Fiber: 2.5 g

2 tablespoons honey
3 tablespoons white vinegar
¼ cup non-fat plain yogurt
¼ cup fat-free mayonnaise
¼ teaspoon celery seed
1 teaspoon salt
1 teaspoon pepper
4 cups shredded cabbage
2 large carrots, grated
2 medium apples, grated
½ cup red onion, chopped

For dressing, mix honey, vinegar, yogurt, mayonnaise, celery seed, salt and pepper together. In another bowl combine cabbage, carrots, apples and onion. Pour dressing over cabbage mixture and mix well. Chill. Serve.

CARROT AND APPLE SUNSHINE

Serves: 6
Calories: 48
Fat: 0.5 g
Saturated Fat: 0.9 g
Fiber: 2.0 g

⅓ cup water
1 lb baby carrots, cut in thick "pennies"
1 medium apple, unpeeled, sliced thin
⅓ cup orange juice
½ teaspoon salt

Bring water to a boil. Add carrots, cover and cook three minutes. Drain. Arrange apple slices over carrots. Then add orange juice and salt, cover and bring to a boil. Boil for another three minutes or until liquid is almost gone. Remove from heat and let stand two minutes. Serve.

HERBED LIMA BEAN SALAD

16-oz pkg frozen baby lima beans, thawed
½ cup finely diced fresh tomato
½ cup finely diced celery
2 tablespoons red wine vinegar
1 teaspoon freshly chopped parsley
½ teaspoon freshly minced garlic
1 teaspoon dried thyme
1 teaspoon dried sage
½ teaspoon salt
¼ teaspoon pepper

Serves:	4
Calories:	123
Fat:	0.5 g
Saturated Fat:	0.1 g
Fiber:	7.3 g

Microwave lima beans for 3 minutes and then rinse under cold water. Combine the lima beans, tomato and celery. Pour vinegar over bean mixture and toss. Add parsley, garlic, thyme, sage, salt and pepper. Toss again.

CREAMY BROCCOLI SALAD WITH DRIED CHERRIES

1 cup fat-free mayonnaise
¼ cup fat-free parmesan cheese
2 tablespoons sugar
2 tablespoons cider vinegar
1 teaspoon cinnamon
8 cups broccoli, in bite size pieces
1 red onion, chopped
1 cup dried cherries (or raisins)

Serves:	8
Calories:	132
Fat:	0.4 g
Saturated Fat:	0.1 g
Fiber:	3.9 g

In a small bowl, stir together mayonnaise, parmesan cheese, sugar, vinegar and cinnamon. In a large bowl combine broccoli, onion and cherries. Toss dressing mixture with broccoli mixture. Chill and serve.

PINEAPPLE SLAW

Serves: 6
Calories: 107
Fat: 0.5 g
Saturated Fat: 0.1 g
Fiber: 3.1 g

½ cup low-fat yogurt, peach flavored
½ teaspoon cinnamon
20-oz can crushed pineapple, drained (reserve 1 tablespoon juice)
4 cups coleslaw mix
½ cup raisins

Stir yogurt, cinnamon and reserved juice in a bowl until blended. Combine pineapple, coleslaw and raisins in a bowl; set aside. Pour yogurt dressing over coleslaw mixture; toss to evenly coat. Cover; refrigerate one hour to allow flavors to blend.

BEAN SALAD WITH DIJON MARINADE

Serves: 8
Calories: 87
Fat: 1.3 g
Saturated Fat: 0.1 g
Fiber: 4.7 g

2 cups frozen green beans
1 cup cooked kidney beans
1 cup cooked chickpeas
1 large tomato, seeded and diced
3 tablespoons Dijon mustard
2 tablespoons water
1 tablespoon fresh basil, chopped
1 tablespoon honey
¼ teaspoon black pepper
¼ cup snipped chives

Cook the green beans until crisp-tender. Rinse under cold water. Drain well. In a bowl combine beans, chickpeas and tomato. In bowl, whisk mustard, water, basil, honey and pepper. Pour this over the salad and garnish with chives. Chill for thirty minutes and serve.

BAKED POTATOES WITH HERBED CHEESE TOPPING

4 large baking potatoes
1⅓ cups fat-free cottage cheese
¼ cup minced green onion
½ cup cilantro
2 tablespoons lemon juice
1 teaspoon salt
1 teaspoon pepper

Serves:	4
Calories:	281
Fat:	0.3 g
Saturated Fat:	0.1 g
Fiber:	5.5 g

Prick potatoes and microwave on high for 6 to 8 minutes per potato, turning occasionally. Test with fork for doneness and continue to cook if needed. In a medium bowl combine cottage cheese, green onion, cilantro, lemon juice, salt and pepper. Stir to blend. To serve, cut an "X" in the top of each potato, gently squeeze open and fluff the interior with a fork. Caution—potatoes are very hot. Take ¼ of the mixture and top potato. Mix slightly and serve while hot.

FRUIT PASTA SALAD WITH CURRY CITRUS DRESSING

8 oz uncooked elbow macaroni
½ cup plan fat-free yogurt
3 tablespoons orange juice
1½ teaspoons curry powder
1½ teaspoons lemon juice
1 teaspoon sugar
1 can pineapple chunks, drained
2 cups seedless green grapes, halved
1 cup sliced celery
½ cup chopped red onion

Serves:	8
Calories:	170
Fat:	0.9 g
Saturated Fat:	0.2 g
Fiber:	2.1 g

Cook macaroni as directed on package. Drain and rinse with cold water. Combine yogurt, orange juice, curry, lemon juice and sugar. In large bowl combine drained pasta, pineapple, grapes, celery and onion. Pour dressing over pasta mixture and mix well. Chill for thirty minutes and serve.

ASIAN CHICKEN SALAD

Serves: 6
Calories: 229
Fat: 1.8 g
Saturated Fat: 0.5 g
Fiber: 5.6 g

3 cups cooked whole-wheat pasta
8 oz skinless chicken breast
1 teaspoon garlic powder
2 tablespoons honey
1 tablespoon water
2 tablespoons sugar
6 tablespoons soy sauce, divided
4 teaspoons fresh grated ginger, divided
4 tablespoons vinegar
1 teaspoon pepper
1 teaspoon Chinese 5 spice
6 cups shredded cabbage or coleslaw mix
4 green onions

Cook pasta according to package directions, drain and keep warm. Cut chicken into small chunks. Combine in a bowl garlic powder, honey, water, sugar, two tablespoons soy sauce and one teaspoon ginger. Mix well. Coat chicken with this sauce. Spray skillet with cooking spray, cook chicken on medium heat, stirring constantly to prevent burning. Cook three to five minutes, check to make sure no longer pink. Make dressing by combining vinegar, pepper, remaining soy sauce and ginger and Chinese 5 spice. Combine chicken, cabbage, onion and noodles. Drizzle dressing over salad. Serve warm.

GARLICKY FAVA BEANS

Serves: 6
Calories: 97
Fat: 0.4 g
Saturated Fat: 0.1 g
Fiber: 5.2 g

10-oz jar fava beans (or lima beans), drained and rinsed
½ cup fat-free Italian dressing
1 clove garlic, chopped
1 medium onion, chopped
2 teaspoons fresh rosemary, chopped
1 teaspoon fresh oregano, chopped
2 medium tomatoes, seeded and chopped
¼ cup fresh savory, chervil OR parsley, chopped

In a large bowl, combine beans, dressing, garlic, onion, rosemary, oregano and tomatoes. Let stand at room temperature for twenty minutes. Stir in savory (or chervil or parsley) and serve.

PEA DELIGHT

16-oz pkg frozen peas
2 cups cooked rice
½ cup mushrooms, sliced
½ cup chopped onions
8-oz jar fat-free chicken or turkey gravy

Serves:	6
Calories:	156
Fat:	0.5 g
Saturated Fat:	0.1 g
Fiber:	4.6 g

Cook peas and rice according to package directions. In a skillet sprayed with cooking spray, sauté mushrooms and onions. Add gravy, peas and rice, mix well. Heat on low for 5 minutes and serve.

BLACK-EYED PEAS WITH GARLIC AND KALE

1½ lb kale, washed and drained
Vegetable cooking spray
1 tablespoon chopped fresh garlic, or more to taste
Pinch of dried red pepper
2 cups canned or cooked black-eyed peas
1 tablespoon cider vinegar, to taste

Serves:	6
Calories:	125
Fat:	1.1 g
Saturated Fat:	0.2 g
Fiber:	6.0 g

Pull the kale leaves from the tough stems. Discard the stems and chop the leaves into 1-inch pieces. Place about two inches of water in a large pot and heat to boiling. Add the kale, cover and cook until tender, stirring occasionally, fifteen to twenty minutes. Drain. Reserve the water for soup, if desired. Coat a non-stick skillet with vegetable cooking spray; add garlic. Cook the garlic over low heat, stirring, until it begins to sizzle, about two minutes. Add the peas and red pepper and cook until blended, stirring, about three minutes. Add the kale and stir to blend over low heat. Add the cider vinegar just before serving. Serve hot or at room temperature.

SEASONED RED POTATOES

Serves: 4
Calories: 70
Fat: 2.9 g
Saturated Fat: 0.5 g
Fiber: 1.6 g

1 lb small red potatoes
½ cup water
¼ teaspoon salt
3 teaspoons melted margarine (or 3 teaspoons butter-flavored
*   sprinkles in 3 teaspoons water)*
1 tablespoon chopped chives
½ teaspoon dill weed
pepper

Peel a thin strip around center of each potato, or cut into quarters. Place in pan with water and salt. Cover and bring to a boil. Reduce heat and simmer twenty minutes until tender.

Just before potatoes are done, melt margarine. Add chives and dill. Pour over cooked potatoes and toss gently. Season with pepper to taste.

GARLIC GREENS

Serves: 4
Calories: 62
Fat: 0.7 g
Saturated Fat: 0.1 g
Fiber: 5.7 g

Vegetable cooking spray
1 small leek, white part only, sliced, ¾ cup
3 scallions, chopped
2 large cloves garlic, minced
3 cups chopped kale
3 cups chopped mustard greens
2 cups collards, cut in ½ inch ribbons
3 cups fresh spinach or 10-oz pkg frozen, defrosted
1 cup fat free chicken or vegetable broth
salt and freshly ground pepper to taste

Coat heavy skillet with vegetable cooking spray and heat over medium heat. Add the leek, scallions and garlic. Sauté until leeks are limp, about four minutes.

Add the kale, mustard greens, and collards, stirring until they are wilted. Mix in the spinach. Add broth and simmer until the greens are tender, about fifteen minutes, stirring occasionally. Season to taste with salt and pepper. Serve.

QUINOA TABBOULEH

2 cups cooked quinoa (about ¾ cups dry)
½ cup green bell pepper, cut into ½ inch cubes
½ cup chopped tomato, seeded and cut into ½ inch cubes
⅓ cup chopped radish, cut into ½ inch cubes
2 scallions, chopped
2 tablespoons chopped mint
2 tablespoons chopped parsley
Juice of ½ lime
1 tablespoon water
Salt and pepper to taste

Serves:	4
Calories:	137
Fat:	2.0 g
Saturated Fat:	0.2 g
Fiber:	3.0 g

In a large bowl, combine the quinoa with the green pepper, tomato, radishes, scallions, mint, and parsley. Coat quinoa mixture well with vegetable cooking spray. Add the lime juice and water and toss to combine. Season to taste with salt and freshly ground pepper.

QUICK KASHA PILAF

1 small carrot, sliced
1 small onion, cut in 8 pieces
½ celery rib, sliced
2¼ cups vegetable broth, divided
½ cup whole buckwheat groats
Salt and pepper to taste

Serves:	4
Calories:	96
Fat:	1.2 g
Saturated Fat:	0.1 g
Fiber:	3.0 g

In a food processor, pulse the carrot, onion, and celery until they are finely chopped.

In a large, heavy saucepan heat ¼ cup of broth over medium high heat. Stir in chopped vegetables. Sauté until they are soft, about four minutes, stirring occasionally.

Mix the buckwheat into the vegetables, stirring until it is slightly darker in color, one to two minutes. Pour in the remaining broth. Cover the pot tightly. When the liquid boils, reduce the heat and simmer ten minutes. Turn off the heat and let the pilaf sit five minutes.

Fluff pilaf with a fork, add salt and pepper as desired, and serve.

RED BEANS AND RICE SALAD

Serves: 4
Calories: 276
Fat: 1.6 g
Saturated Fat: 0.3 g
Fiber: 10.1 g

2 cups cooked brown rice, such as basmati or Texmati
15-oz can red kidney beans, drained and rinsed
¾ cup finely chopped green bell pepper
½ cup fresh mango, cut in ½ inch cubes
½ cup finely chopped red onion
½ cup salsa
salt and freshly ground pepper to taste
2 tablespoons chopped cilantro

In a large bowl, use a fork to combine the rice, beans, pepper, mango and onion. Drain the salsa well and mix it into the salad. Season to taste with salt and freshly ground pepper.

Just before serving, sprinkle with the cilantro.

FRENCH FRIES

Serves: 2
Calories: 220
Fat: 0.2 g
Saturated Fat: 0.1 g
Fiber: 4.8 g

2 large baking potatoes
Vegetable cooking spray

Clean potatoes. Cut each potato in half lengthwise, then each of these halves into six wedges. Spray generously with cooking spray. Add seasonings (i.e., garlic powder, onion powder, salt). Cover with paper towel and microwave on full power for seven minutes, or until potatoes are tender. Rotate dish halfway to help evenly cook.

Variation: Try using sweet potatoes for a nice change.

FRENCH FRIES ITALIAN STYLE

Serves: 2
Calories: 248
Fat: 0.3 g
Saturated Fat: 0.1 g
Fiber: 5.0 g

Follow French fries recipe above
¼ cup fat-free Parmesan cheese
1 teaspoon garlic powder, ½ teaspoon oregano.

Mix ingredients together and sprinkle over fries.

ENTREÉS

TUNA KABOBS WITH A TWIST

⅓ cup fresh lime juice (about 2 limes)
1 tablespoon reduced sodium soy sauce
1 garlic clove, minced
2 tablespoons chopped Thai or Italian basil leaves
¼-½ teaspoon red pepper flakes
¼ teaspoon freshly ground pepper
Vegetable cooking spray
¼ cup vegetable broth

Kabobs:
1 lb fresh tuna cut in 12 chunks
6-inch cucumber, peeled
8 large cherry tomatoes
1 medium red onion halved vertically, and cut in ½-inch
crescents

Serves:	4
Calories:	157
Fat:	1.4 g
Saturated Fat:	0.3 g
Fiber:	1.5 g

Preheat a gas grill or broiler.

In a glass or other non-metal bowl, combine the lime juice, soy sauce, garlic, basil, pepper flakes, pepper, and broth. Coat tuna chunks with a vegetable cooking spray.

Halve the cucumber lengthwise, scoop out the seeds and cut each half crosswise into eight crescents.

Assemble the kabobs using four 10-inch skewers, metal or well-soaked bamboo. Slip a cucumber piece almost to the bottom of a skewer. Add a tuna chunk. Slip on a two to three layer onion crescent, followed by a tomato. Repeat with more cucumber, fish, onion and tomato. Finish the kabob with a final cucumber crescent, turned toward the onion. In the same way make up three more skewers.

Broil the kabobs three minutes. Turn and cook until the fish is firm to the touch and the vegetables are browned, another two to three minutes. Do not overcook or the tuna will be dry. Serve either hot or at room temperature.

SWEET AND SOUR CHICKEN ON RICE

Serves:	**4**
Calories:	**392**
Fat:	**3.5 g**
Saturated Fat:	**0.9 g**
Fiber:	**3.1 g**

½ cup pineapple juice drained from pineapple chunks
1 tablespoon cornstarch
3 tablespoons vinegar
2 tablespoons honey
1½ teaspoons soy sauce, low sodium
⅔ cup rice
Vegetable cooking spray
1 garlic clove
1 carrot
1 green pepper
3 green onions
2 skinless boneless chicken breasts cut into chunks
2½ cups pineapple chunks
1 cup seedless red grapes, halved
½ teaspoon cayenne pepper sauce

Mix pineapple juice, cornstarch, vinegar, honey and soy sauce and set aside. Prepare rice as directed on package; omit the salt and butter. Spray large skillet or wok with cooking spray, heat on high. Stir-fry garlic fifteen seconds. Add carrots and stir-fry two minutes. Add green pepper and green onions; and stir-fry for approximately 1 minute or until vegetables are crisp-tender. Remove vegetables from skillet. Spray skillet again and stir-fry chicken for three minutes or until no longer pink. Push chicken to one side of the skillet and stir in vinegar mixture. Cook and stir two more minutes. Stir in vegetables, add pineapple and grapes. Stir, cover and let cook for two minutes or until hot. Add cayenne pepper sauce. Serve with rice.

QUICK ITALIAN SCALLOPS

Three 15-oz cans stewed tomatoes
1 lb angel hair pasta
1 lb small bay scallops
1 teaspoon garlic salt
3 tablespoons grated romano cheese
1 teaspoon basil
1 teaspoon oregano

Serves:	6
Calories:	435
Fat:	4.3 g
Saturated Fat:	0.6 g
Fiber:	3.5 g

Heat tomatoes on low and cut up large pieces. Cook pasta. Sauté scallops five minutes (with garlic salt) and then mix with tomatoes. Drain pasta. Put on plates. Ladle on tomato and scallop mixture. Sprinkle with romano cheese, basil, and oregano; serve.

CHICKEN AND SWISS CHEESE ROLL-UPS

6 boneless, skinless chicken breasts
6 slices fat-free Swiss cheese
½ cup diced celery
½ cup carrots
½ cup onion, chopped
2 cups cubed whole wheat bread
1 can low-fat cream of chicken soup
¾ cup white wine
½ cup fat-free parmesan cheese
Paprika

Serves:	6
Calories:	329
Fat:	6.0 g
Saturated Fat:	1.7 g
Fiber:	1.6 g

Pound chicken breasts between wax paper, lay half slice of fat-free Swiss cheese on top of each. Place two tablespoons vegetables and two tablespoons bread crumbs on top of the cheese. Roll each and lay seam-down in baking dish (secure with toothpicks).

Mix soup and wine together. Pour sauce over chicken. Bake at 350 degrees for twenty-five to forty minutes depending of the thickness of the chicken. Check chicken; when no longer pink, top chicken mixture with cheese and paprika and bake for five minutes.

BAKED HADDOCK GREEK STYLE

Serves: 4
Calories: 182
Fat: 4.1 g
Saturated Fat: 2.2 g
Fiber: 1.3 g

1 pound fresh or frozen haddock fillets
Vegetble cooking spray
1-4 green onions with tops, chopped
1 rib celery, finely chopped
1-2 cloves garlic, minced
¼ cup dry white wine
2 medium fresh tomatoes, peeled and chopped
2 parsley sprigs, chopped
5 fresh basil leaves minced (or ½ teaspoon dried)
2 tablespoons lemon juice
⅛ teaspoon white pepper
4 oz reduced-fat feta cheese
Parsley sprigs (optional garnish)
Lemon wedges (optional garnish)

Allow haddock fillets to stand at room temperature thirty to sixty minutes (if frozen). Preheat oven to 425 degrees. Coat generously a large skillet with cooking spray. Prepare sauce: sauté green onions, celery and garlic for three minutes. Add wine, chopped tomatoes, parsley, and basil. Simmer uncovered over medium heat, stirring occasionally until thickened (about twenty minutes).

With sharp knife, cut fish into eight portions of equal thickness, cutting on a slant. Place into a baking pan just large enough to fit portions. Cover with mixture of lemon juice and pepper. Bake fish fifteen minutes uncovered.

Remove pan from oven and drain excess juices. Fish may be left in pan or transferred to an ovenproof platter if desired. Spoon hot sauce over fish and top with cheese. Reduce oven to 350 degrees and bake five to eight minutes longer, or until fish becomes opaque and cheese has heated.

To serve: garnish with parsley sprigs and wedges of lemon.

SPICY GRILLED SHRIMP OVER RICE

18 oz shrimp (about 18 to 20 large) peeled and deveined
1½ tablespoons fresh lime juice
3 garlic cloves, crushed through a press
1½ teaspoons fresh thyme leaves (or ¾ teaspoon dried)
⅓-½ teaspoon crushed red pepper (or to taste)
Cilantro sprigs

Rice:

1 teaspoon ground tumeric
¼ teaspoon ground cumin
2⅔ cups water
1⅓ cups long grain rice, preferable basmati
½ teaspoon salt

Serves:	4
Calories:	344
Fat:	3.7 g
Saturated Fat:	0.4 g
Fiber:	2.8 g

Toss shrimp with lime juice, garlic, thyme, and red pepper. Cover and marinate at least one hour. When ready to cook, start with the rice. Place tumeric and cumin in a skillet and heat over low heat, just until fragrant (about thirty seconds). Add water, rice and salt. Heat to boiling, then cover and cook over low heat until water is absorbed and rice is tender (about fifteen minutes). Prepare shrimp when rice is almost done; either grill, broil or cook quickly in a preheated nonstick skillet until lightly browned on both sides. Don't overcook. Spoon rice onto a platter and top with shrimp. Garnish with cilantro and serve.

FRUITED CHICKEN OVER WILD RICE

⅓ cup low sodium soy sauce
1 cup fat-free Kraft Catalina Salad Dressing
½ cup chopped onion
½ cup raisins
1 cup crushed pineapple with juice
4 cups cooked wild rice
2 cups grilled chicken breast, cubed

Serves:	4
Calories:	458
Fat:	2.9 g
Saturated Fat:	0.7 g
Fiber:	5.8 g

In a mixing bowl, combine soy sauce, dressing, onion, raisins, and pineapple. Set aside. Add rice to a 2-quart baking dish. Arrange chicken chunks on top. Pour dressing on top of chicken rice mixture. Cover and cook in the microwave for six minutes or until hot. Serve warm.

CASSOULET

Serves:	6
Calories:	311
Fat:	4.1 g
Saturated Fat:	1.3 g
Fiber:	6.4 g

1 medium onion, peeled and chopped
1½ cups 1-inch chopped carrots
1 stalk celery
2 bay leaves
2 cloves garlic, crushed and minced
½ cup defatted chicken broth
2½ cups cooked white beans, drained
1½ lb boneless-skinless turkey breast, in strips
1 medium tomato, seeded and chopped
1 teaspoon dried thyme
½ teaspoon pepper sauce
¼ cup chopped fresh parsley
½ teaspoon salt

Sauté onions, carrots, celery, bay leaves, and garlic in broth for five minutes. Add beans, turkey, tomato, thyme, and pepper sauce. Bring to a low boil for about five minutes or until turkey is opaque and cooked through. Discard bay leaf. Sprinkle with parsley and salt.

CHICKEN WITH CINNAMON-RAISIN SAUCE

Vegetable cooking spray
½ cup chopped onion
¾ teaspoon cinnamon
⅛ teaspoon fresh ground pepper
3 cloves garlic, minced
4 boneless, skinless chicken breast halves
2 tablespoons water
¾ cup orange juice
¼ cup raisins
Fresh orange slices (optional)

Serves:	4
Calories:	210
Fat:	3.1 g
Saturated Fat:	0.9 g
Fiber:	1.1 g

Coat large skillet with vegetable cooking spray and heat. Add onion, cinnamon, pepper and garlic. Cook over medium-high heat for three to four minutes, stirring frequently to prevent sticking. Add chicken and cook about five minutes on each side (add more water if needed). Add two tablespoons water, orange juice and raisins; cover and simmer over low heat about ten minutes more. When chicken is done (juices run clear when pierced with a fork), serve chicken with some of the onion-raisin mixture spooned on top. Garnish with orange slices if desired.

Variation: Grill chicken first and add to sauce.

POACHED FISH WITH TOMATOES

Serves: **4**
Calories: **145**
Fat: **2.3 g**
Saturated Fat: **0.3 g**
Fiber: **1.8 g**

Vegetable cooking spray
¾ cup scallions, coarsely chopped
2-4 cloves garlic, minced
2 cups fish or vegetable stock, or water
2 tablespoons lemon juice
2 cups chopped tomatoes
2 teaspoons red wine vinegar
1 bay leaf
2 whole cloves
Dash hot pepper
Pepper to taste
1½ lbs fresh or frozen sole

Coat skillet with vegetable cooking spray. Sauté scallions until very lightly browned. Add garlic and cook for thirty seconds. Add all remaining ingredients except fish. Bring to a boil, then reduce heat, cover and cook for five minutes. Remove cover and cook about twenty minutes more, until sauce begins to thicken. Add fish and cook ten minutes per inch of thickness of fish (measured at thickest point). To test that fish is done, see that it flakes easily with a fork and that it is opaque throughout. Do not overcook.

Remove bay leaf and cloves; serve promptly.

CHICKEN MARSALA

Vegetable cooking spray
¾ lb boneless chicken breast cut into 1-inch cubes
2 cups sliced mushrooms
4 medium onions cut into large chunks
1 cup marsala wine
16-oz can of fat-free chicken broth, divided
2 tablespoons cornstarch
½ teaspoon salt
Dash of pepper
2 cloves garlic, chopped
⅛ teaspoon cayenne pepper
4 dashes cayenne pepper sauce
4 cups cooked brown rice
Chopped parsley (optional)

Serves:	**4**
Calories:	**463**
Fat:	**5.4 g**
Saturated Fat:	**1.2 g**
Fiber:	**5.9 g**

Coat skillet with vegetable cooking spray; brown chicken. Move chicken to side of skillet. Add mushrooms and onions and cook until onions are tender. Add wine, bring to a boil.

Mix two cups chicken broth, cornstarch, salt, pepper, garlic and cayenne pepper sauce, in a small pan. Stir into skillet, bring to boil, reduce heat, cover and simmer ten minutes. Add chicken mixture.

Spoon rice into a baking dish and top with chicken mixture.

Bake fifteen minutes at 300 degrees. Sprinkle with parsley and serve.

FILLET OF SOLE FLORENTINE

Serves: 4
Calories: 131
Fat: 1.3 g
Saturated Fat: 0.3 g
Fiber: 2.2 g

2 cups chopped fresh spinach
¼ cup dry bread crumbs
1 tablespoon minced shallots
½ teaspoon fresh thyme leaves, or ¼ teaspoon dry thyme
½ teaspoon minced fresh rosemary, or ¼ teaspoon dry, crushed
3 or 4 gratings fresh nutmeg, or pinch of ground nutmeg
¼ teaspoon salt
¼ teaspoon freshly ground pepper
1 lb fillet of sole, in 4 pieces
½ cup defatted chicken broth
1 teaspoon cider vinegar
1 teaspoon sugar
Paprika for garnish

Preheat oven to 350 degrees.

In a large bowl, combine the spinach, bread crumbs, shallots, thyme, rosemary, nutmeg, salt and pepper. Arrange the spinach mixture to cover the bottom of an 8-inch square pan or other shallow baking dish just large enough to hold the fish in one layer. Arrange the fillets in a single layer over the spinach, overlapping them as little as possible.

In a small saucepan, combine the broth, vinegar and sugar, and bring to a boil. Pour the hot liquid over the fish. Dust the fillets lightly with paprika.

Bake until the fish is opaque all the way through and flakes easily. Serve immediately.

PARMESAN BARLEY RISOTTO WITH CHICKEN

1 lb chicken breast-skinless and boneless
Vegetable cooking spray
¾ cup diced carrot
1 thyme sprig
1 cup diced celery
¾ cup thinly sliced leek
½ cup finely chopped onion
¼ teaspoon salt
½ teaspoon pepper
1¾ cup uncooked pearl barley
4 cups chicken broth, fat-free
⅓ cup chopped fresh flat leaf parsley
½ cup fat-free parmesan cheese

Serves:	6
Calories:	383
Fat:	3.1 g
Saturated Fat:	0.8 g
Fiber:	10.4 g

Cut chicken into strips, set aside. Coat generously a dutch oven with vegetable cooking spray, and heat. Add carrots and thyme; sauté one minute. Add celery, leek and onion; sauté one minute. Add salt, pepper and chicken; sauté five minutes. Add barley; sauté one minute.

Add broth, bring to a boil. Cover, reduce heat and simmer thirty-five minutes. Remove from heat; discard thyme sprig. Stir in parsley and cheese.

PASTA WITH TUNA SAUCE

Serves: 2
Calories: 537
Fat: 4.5 g
Saturated Fat: 1.0 g
Fiber: 6.7 g

Vegetable cooking spray
1 clove garlic, minced
6½-oz can water-packed white tuna, drained
1¾ cups tomato puree
1 tablespoon fresh parsley, minced (or 1½ teaspoons dried)
½ to 1 teaspoon oregano
1 or 2 pinches cayenne pepper
5-6 oz dry pasta
1½ tablespoons fat-free grated parmesan

Coat skillet with vegetable cooking spray. Add garlic and sauté, stirring constantly until just golden. Add remaining ingredients except pasta and cheese. Simmer uncovered for about fifteen minutes. Add water if sauce gets too thick.

Meanwhile, cook pasta in boiling water until tender but still firm. Drain. Serve immediately, topped with sauce and cheese.

VEGETARIAN ENTREÉS

PORTABELLO FAJITAS

4 large portabello mushrooms
2 tablespoons fresh lime juice
2 cloves garlic, crushed, divided
½ cup nonfat plain yogurt
½ cup packed cilantro leaves
4 large (10 inch) whole wheat flour tortillas
Vegetable cooking spray
2 red, green, or yellow bell peppers, thinly sliced
1 medium onion, sliced
1 large tomato, diced

Serves:	4
Calories:	209
Fat:	1.7 g
Saturated Fat:	0.8 g
Fiber:	5.8 g

Wash and remove stems from mushrooms. Cut into strips. Preheat oven to 350 degrees. Combine the lime juice and 1 clove garlic in a bowl. Add the mushroom strips, turn to coat and marinate for 15 minutes. Process the yogurt and cilantro and 1 garlic clove in a food processor until smooth; transfer to a small bowl and refrigerate until ready to use.

Wrap the flour tortillas in foil and place in the oven until warm, about 10 minutes.

Coat skillet generously with cooking spray and heat. Add the mushrooms, peppers, and onions in batches and cook until they are lightly browned.

Place warm tortillas on plate and add ¼ of the mushroom mixture and ¼ cup of tomatoes. Drizzle sauce on top. Fold and serve.

SPINACH AND ARTICHOKE STUFFED PASTA SHELLS

Serves: 6
Calories: 261
Fat: 1.5 g
Saturated Fat: 0.2 g
Fiber: 5.4 g

10-oz pkg frozen spinach
1 cup frozen artichoke hearts
12 jumbo pasta shells
1 cup fat-free ricotta cheese
5 tablespoons chopped fresh basil, divided
1 tablespoon chopped parsley
¼ teaspoon salt
2 tablespoons lemon juice
⅓ cup fat-free sour cream
28-oz can stewed tomatoes
2 tablespoons cornstarch

Cook spinach (thawed) and artichoke hearts (thawed) according to package directions, drain well. Chop artichoke hearts, and set aside. Cook pasta shells according to package directions, omitting salt and fat; drain and set aside. In food processor bowl, add spinach, ricotta cheese, two tablespoons basil, parsley, salt and lemon juice. Process thirty seconds or until smooth. Transfer to bowl, stir in chopped artichokes and sour cream. In a saucepan combine tomatoes (undrained, chopped), cornstarch, and 3 tablespoons basil, stir well. Cook over medium heat until thickened, stirring frequently. Spoon one cup tomato mixture in bottom of 11-inch x 7-inch x 1½-inch baking dish coated with cooking spray. Spoon spinach mixture evenly into shells. Arrange shells in baking dish. Pour remaining tomato mixture over shells. Bake uncovered at 350 degrees for thirty minutes or until bubbly.

COUSCOUS CASSEROLE

1½ cups water
1 cup dry couscous
15-oz can black beans, rinsed and drained
8-oz can corn kernels, vacuum packed
8-oz can water chestnuts, drained and chopped
7-oz jar roasted bell pepper packed in water, drained and cut
½ cup minced green onion
2 tablespoons minced green chile
1 cup fat-free ricotta cheese
2 tablespoons balsamic vinegar
1½ teaspoon sesame oil
1½ teaspoon ground cumin

Serves:	6
Calories:	300
Fat:	2.7 g
Saturated Fat:	0.4 g
Fiber:	7.6 g

In a saucepan, bring water to a boil. Remove from heat. Add couscous; stir well. Cover and let stand approximately five minutes or until all water is absorbed. Add black beans and next five ingredients.

Combine ricotta cheese, vinegar, oil, and cumin; stir into mixture. Spoon mixture into 11-inch x 7-inch x 2-inch baking dish coated with vegetable cooking spray.

Bake uncovered at 350 degrees for twenty-five to thirty minutes.

BLACK BEANS AND RICE

Vegetable cooking spray
2 sweet red peppers, finely chopped
1 large onion, finely chopped
1 stalk celery, finely chopped
2 cloves garlic, minced
¼ teaspoon dried thyme
2 cups cooked black beans
2 tablespoons cider vinegar
3 cups hot cooked rice
1 cup non-fat yogurt

Serves:	4
Calories:	323
Fat:	1.0 g
Saturated Fat:	0.3 g
Fiber:	10.2 g

Spray a large non-stick frying pan with vegetable cooking spray. Add the peppers, onions, celery, garlic and thyme. Sauté over medium heat until the vegetables are tender, about ten minutes.

Add the beans and vinegar. Cook until the beans are hot, about three minutes. To serve, divide the rice among shallow bowls. Top with the beans and yogurt.

MUSHROOM RISOTTO

Serves: **4**
Calories: **426**
Fat: **3.5 g**
Saturated Fat: 0.4 g
Fiber: **3.4 g**

3 cups vegetable broth
Vegetable cooking spray
½ cup onions, chopped
1 clove garlic, minced
½ cup coarsely chopped sweet red pepper
6 cups sliced mushrooms (1 lb)
1½ cups dry arborio rice
1 cup dry white wine
salt and pepper
½ cup scallions chopped fresh parsley
2 tablespoons fat free parmesan cheese

In a saucepan bring broth to a low simmer.

Meanwhile, coat a wide shallow saucepan with vegetable cooking spray and heat. Add onions, garlic, red pepper and mushrooms, stirring for about 10 minutes or until tender and most of the liquid released by the mushrooms has evaporated.

Add rice, stirring to coat. Stir in about half of the wine or additional broth; cook, stirring often, until liquid is absorbed, about two minutes. Add remaining liquid and cook, stirring often, until absorbed.

Add hot broth ¼ cup at a time, stirring after each addition, until all of the stock is absorbed and rice has swelled to double its size and is tender but still a little firm, about twenty minutes. Add additional broth or water if necessary to make risotto creamy and moist. Season with salt and pepper to taste. Serve and then sprinkle with scallions, parsley and parmesan cheese.

JERKED VEGGIE BURGERS

1 medium onion, finely chopped
1 small green bell pepper, seeded and cut in ½-inch pieces
½ cup finely chopped scallions, both white and green parts
2 garlic cloves, finely chopped
1 teaspoon grated fresh ginger
¼ teaspoon freshly grated nutmeg
2 slices toasted whole wheat bread, cut in 1-inch pieces
2 cups cooked or one 15-oz can black beans, rinsed and
    drained (if canned)
1 cup cooked long grain white rice
½ habanero pepper or 1 teaspoon hot pepper sauce
Salt
Freshly ground pepper
1 large egg white
Mustard, iceberg lettuce and sliced tomato, for garnish

Serves:	8
Calories:	131
Fat:	1.2 g
Saturated Fat:	0.2 g
Fiber:	5.6 g

Sauté onion, pepper, and scallions until very soft, about five minutes, but do not let them color. Mix in the spices. Reduce the bread to crumbs using a blender or food processor. Add the beans, cooked vegetables, rice and chili pepper or hot sauce. Pulse until the mixture is coarsely chopped. Do not overprocess or the burgers will be mushy. Season the burger mixture with salt and pepper to taste. Add the egg white and pulse to blend. Form the mixture into eight patties. They can be individually wrapped in plastic wrap and frozen or refrigerated up to twenty-four hours before cooking. Defrost frozen burgers in the refrigerator. Brush a grill with oil and preheat. You can also use a skillet over medium-high heat. Cook the burgers until they are browned. If grilling, cook about one and one-half minutes; in pan, cook until the burgers are browned and crisp on the bottom, about three minutes. Carefully turn to brown other side, for about two minutes or less, if grilling.

Serve the cooked burgers on a toasted whole wheat grain bun whose insides have been spread with mustard. Top the burger with lettuce and tomato slice, then serve. These are great reheated.

TEXAS BBQ PASTA

Serves: 6
Calories: 292
Fat: 2.4 g
Saturated Fat: 0.3 g
Fiber: 4.1 g

8 oz macaroni pasta, cooked
1 onion, chopped
1 chopped green bell pepper
1 tablespoon chili powder
1 tablespoon dried oregano
¼ teaspoons salt
2 garlic cloves or 1 teaspoon minced garlic
8-oz can tomato sauce
1 cup barbecue sauce
2½ cups of canned corn

Cook macaroni according to package directions until al dente. Drain.

Meanwhile, in a large non-stick skillet sprayed with non-fat cooking spray, cook onion, bell pepper, chili powder, oregano, salt, garlic, tomato sauce, barbecue sauce and corn. Bring mixture to boil. Reduce heat to medium and simmer until slightly thickened, about three to four minutes, stirring occasionally.

In a large serving bowl, combine the mixture with the pasta. Serve immediately.

WARM ITALIAN SALAD SANDWICHES

Serves: 4
Calories: 240
Fat: 4.8 g
Saturated Fat: 1.2 g
Fiber: 5.6 g

3 medium tomatoes cut into thin wedges
1 small red onion, thinly sliced
1 roasted red pepper, cut into thin strips
10 pitted black olives, sliced
½ cup fat-free Italian dressing
4 whole grain rolls or 8 Italian bread slices
¼ cup shredded reduced-fat mozzarella
¼ cup shredded fresh basil

Preheat broiler. In a medium bowl, combine tomatoes, onion, red peppers, and olives. Add dressing; toss well to coat. Let stand for twenty minutes. Spoon tomato mixture evenly onto rolls. Place sandwiches on a baking sheet. Sprinkle with mozzarella. Broil, 4 inches from the heat, until cheese melts and edges of rolls are golden. Sprinkle with basil, and serve immediately.

WHOLE WHEAT PASTA WITH FRESH TOMATO AND BASIL

3½ lb fresh tomatoes (about 13 medium size)
1 cup vegetable broth
2 medium onions, chopped
1 teaspoon minced garlic
½ cup fresh basil, chopped
¼ teaspoon hot red pepper flakes, crushed
1 teaspoon salt
1 lb whole wheat pasta

Serves:	**4**
Calories:	**508**
Fat:	**3.3 g**
Saturated Fat:	**0.5 g**
Fiber:	**14.6 g**

Peel, seed and dice tomatoes.

In a large nonstick skillet, heat broth over moderately high heat until boiling. Add onions and garlic. Cook, stirring, until softened, three to five minutes. Stir in tomatoes, basil, hot red pepper flakes, and salt. Simmer, stirring occasionally, until sauce thickens, ten to fifteen minutes.

Cook pasta according to package directions, until al dente. Drain and transfer to a large warm bowl. Add sauce and toss well.

Serve immediately

Serving size: 2 cups pasta, 1 cup sauce

RICE AND BARLEY PILAF

¾ cup pearl barley
¾ cup brown rice
5½ cups vegetable broth, divided
¾ cup red onion, chopped
1 cup fresh parsley, chopped
1½ teaspoon salt
1 teaspoon pepper

Serves:	**4**
Calories:	**303**
Fat:	**3.0 g**
Saturated Fat:	**0.3 g**
Fiber:	**8.1 g**

Combine barley and rice in pot, add five cups of vegetable broth. Bring to a boil and simmer for thirty minutes, or until water is absorbed and grains are tender. Add remaining broth, onion, parsley, salt and pepper. Cook for three more minutes on medium heat. Fluff with a fork and serve.

PENNE BOLOGNESE—VEGETARIAN STYLE

Serves: 4
Calories: 399
Fat: 2.0 g
Saturated Fat: 0.4 g
Fiber: 7.3 g

Vegetable cooking spray
1 cup onion, finely diced
1 carrot, finely diced
1 cup celery, finely diced or thinly sliced
1 cup canned whole tomatoes, coarsely chopped
*1 sun-dried tomato (not oil-packed) halved, soaked in hot
    water until soft, coarsely chopped*
½ cup dry white wine
1 cup vegetable broth
1 cup evaporated skim milk
½ teaspoon nutmeg
1 cup thawed frozen peas
¼ cup water
8 oz penne pasta cooked (hot)
4 tablespoons grated fat-free parmesan cheese

Coat medium nonstick saucepan with vegetable cooking spray, and heat. Add onions, carrots and celery and cook, stirring constantly until onions are translucent, about eight minutes. Add canned and sun-dried tomatoes and wine.

Cook, stirring constantly, until liquid has evaporated, about five minutes. Add broth, milk and nutmeg, and bring to a simmer. Reduce heat to low and cool, stirring occasionally, until vegetables are soft, fifteen to twenty minutes, adding quarter cup water if liquid evaporates too quickly. Add peas and quarter cup water; simmer, stirring occasionally, until peas are cooked through, about five minutes. Toss with hot cooked pasta, cooked according to package directions.

Arrange in serving bowls, and sprinkle each with 1 teaspoon parmesan cheese. Serve immediately.

THREE PEPPER TOFU STIR-FRY

1 lb reduced/low-fat firm tofu (not silken) cubed
Vegetable cooking spray
½ purple onion, sliced
½ yellow bell pepper, chopped
½ green bell pepper, chopped
1 red bell pepper, chopped
1 green onion, sliced
1 stalk celery, sliced
1 tablespoon reduced sodium soy sauce
1 teaspoon cornstarch or arrowroot
1 teaspoon sesame seeds
¼ cup chopped cilantro

Serves:	4
Calories:	179
Fat:	5.8 g
Saturated Fat:	0.9 g
Fiber:	2.4 g

Marinade:

½ cup pineapple juice
1 tablespoon packed light brown sugar
2 tablespoons reduced sodium soy sauce
¼ teaspoon toasted sesame oil
1 tablespoon hoisin sauce
½ teaspoon ground ginger
½ teaspoon garlic granules or garlic powder

Mix together the marinade ingredients and marinate the tofu for one hour or as long as overnight. Coat pan generously with vegetable cooking spray and heat. Add tofu and cook, turning gently with a spatula every few minutes to evenly brown all sides. Reserve the marinade in a bowl for later use. When the tofu has browned, transfer it to a bowl. Over sink, recoat pan with cooking spray. Stir all of the vegetables and the soy sauce together until the peppers are crisp-tender. Add the cornstarch to the leftover marinade. Mix until dissolved. Add this to the vegetables. Quickly add back the tofu and stir gently until the marinade has turned clear and thick (this happens quickly). Transfer to a serving dish and garnish with sesame seeds and cilantro. Serve over rice or pasta.

VEGETABLE RICE ITALIANO

Serves: 4
Calories: 420
Fat: 1.6 g
Saturated Fat: 0.3 g
Fiber: 18.4 g

6-oz box long grain wild rice
2 teaspoons instant low-sodium bouillon
Vegetable cooking spray
1 medium onion, chopped
½ lb carrots, chopped (about 1½ cup)
1 teaspoon dried rosemary or oregano
⅓ cup quick-cooking brown rice
16-oz can tomatoes with no added salt
9-oz pkg of frozen artichoke hearts
1 cup frozen peas, thawed
15.5-oz can kidney beans, drained and rinsed

In a 4-quart saucepan or Dutch oven over high heat, bring to a boil the long grain and wild rice combination, using water according to package instructions, and bouillon. Do not add seasoning packet if one is enclosed in package of rice. Reduce heat to low and simmer, covered.

Meanwhile, coat a saucepan with vegetable cooking spray. Add onion, carrots and rosemary. Sauté until onion is softened and carrots are crisp-tender. Set aside.

When long grain and wild rice mixture has about ten minutes cooking time left, add quick-cooking brown rice, tomatoes (with their juice) and artichoke hearts.

When rice is tender and liquid absorbed, stir in peas, kidney beans and cooked carrot-onion mixture. Heat throughly and serve.

MACARONI SPINACH CASSEROLE

1½ cups dry macaroni	
1 lb pkg frozen chopped spinach	
½ cup fat-free ricotta cheese	
¼ cup fat-free parmesan cheese	
¼ cup low-fat mozzarella cheese	
1 tablespoon garlic powder	
Vegetable cooking spray	
15-oz can kidney beans, rinsed and drained	
28-oz jar low-fat spaghetti sauce	

Serves:	4
Calories:	400
Fat:	4.4 g
Saturated Fat:	3.1 g
Fiber:	15.6 g

Cook macaroni according to package directions. Drain and place in medium mixing bowl. Mix spinach, cheeses, garlic, and beans together. Toss with pasta. Spray an 8-inch x 8-inch glass casserole dish with vegetable oil cooking spray. Place one third of spaghetti sauce in bottom of casserole dish. Layer half of pasta mixture on top; follow with another third of sauce then the rest of the pasta mixture and last third of sauce; top with grated cheese. Cover and bake in microwave oven until heated through, about fifteen to twenty minutes.

TACO SALAD

½ cup fat-free Thousand Island dressing	
½ cup taco sauce	
½ packet of taco seasoning	
15-oz can of kidney beans, drained	
15.25-oz can corn, drained	
8 cups of lettuce torn in bite-size pieces	
4 oz baked seasoned tortilla chips	
2 cups fat-free cheddar cheese	

Serves:	4
Calories:	465
Fat:	2.7 g
Saturated Fat:	0.3 g
Fiber:	14.5 g

Mix dressing, taco sauce and seasoning in large sauté pan or wok. Once bubbling, add kidney beans and corn. Heat on low for five minutes. Turn heat off. Add lettuce and tortilla chips. Toss well. Sprinkle with cheese and serve.

MEDITERRANEAN BARLEY

Serves: 4
Calories: 199
Fat: 1.4 g
Saturated Fat: 0.1 g
Fiber: 8.2 g
g

1 cup pearl barley
3 cups reduced fat/sodium chicken or vegetable broth
1 large clove garlic, minced
Vegetable cooking spray
¼ cup chopped fresh parsley
4 tablespoons fresh lemon juice
2 tablespoons vegetable broth
1 tablespoon fresh grated lemon peel
¼ teaspoon salt
⅛ teaspoon coarse ground black pepper
⅛ teaspoon fennel seed

Rinse the barley and place in a medium saucepan with broth. Cover and simmer, stirring occasionally, over medium heat until barley is tender, about thirty-five minutes. Add garlic; cook for five minutes. Transfer the barley mixture to a fine sieve; drain well. Transfer mixture to a bowl. Lightly coat with cooking spray. Cover and chill completely. To serve, add parsley, lemon juice, broth, lemon peel, salt, pepper and fennel seed; toss well to combine.

WEST COAST PASTA SALAD

Serves: 4
Calories: 333
Fat: 2.0 g
Saturated Fat: 0.3 g
Fiber: 6.7 g
g

8 oz dry shaped pasta
Vegetable cooking spray
16 oz frozen mixed vegetables (broccoli, cauliflower and carrots)
⅔ cup fat-free Italian salad dressing
2 tablespoons balsamic vinegar
¼ cup fat-free Parmesan cheese
½ teaspoon garlic powder
¼ cup sliced black olives

Cook pasta according to package directions. Rinse under cold water. Drain well. Spray pasta with a light coating of cooking spray. Cook vegetables according to directions. Rinse under cold water. Combine all ingredients in large serving bowl. Toss well and chill. Serve.

SUN-DRIED TOMATOES AND SHIITAKE MUSHROOMS ORZO

1 cup dried shiitake mushrooms, soaked and diced
1 cup sun-dried tomatoes packed in water, diced
Vegetable cooking spray
1 clove garlic, crushed
2 cups orzo (rice-type semolina pasta)
2 cups water, soaking liquid from mushrooms
2 cups vegetable broth
1½ teaspoon oregano
½ cup fresh basil, minced

Serves:	4
Calories:	373
Fat:	2.6 g
Saturated Fat:	0.1 g
Fiber:	6.2 g

Soak mushrooms in two to three cups of very hot water until soft (thirty minutes to two hours). Save liquid. Once tender, dice or cut into pieces with scissors. Dice or cut tomatoes in the same manner. In a large pot (6-quart dutch oven) sprayed with vegetable cooking spray, add garlic and orzo until it crackles and is slightly golden brown. Stir frequently so as not to burn. Add soaking liquid, two cups vegetable broth, tomatoes, mushrooms, oregano and bring to a boil. Reduce heat, cover and simmer until tender but not mushy (about fifteen to twenty minutes). Stir and check tenderness occasionally. Cooking time may vary depending on desired consistency of orzo.

Mix in minced basil before serving.

WHOLE WHEAT SPINACH PASTA WITH HONEY MUSTARD DRESSING

1 lb whole wheat spinach noodles
Vegetable cooking spray
1 red onion, sliced
8-oz pkg mushrooms, sliced
2½ cups fat-free honey mustard dressing

Serves:	6
Calories:	438
Fat:	1.8 g
Saturated Fat:	0.3 g
Fiber:	10.2 g

Cook pasta according to directions. Spray skillet with vegetable cooking oil and sauté onions and mushrooms; add salad dressing and heat until warm. Pour dressing mixture over cooked pasta, add more salad dressing if needed until moist. Serve.

VEGETABLE FRIED RICE

Serves: 4
Calories: 318
Fat: 3.9 g
Saturated Fat: 0.8 g
Fiber: 7.8 g

Vegetable cooking spray
2 green onions, sliced in 1-inch pieces
2 cloves garlic, minced
2 stalks celery, sliced thinly on a diagonal
2 carrots, sliced thinly on a diagonal
2 cups broccoli florets, in bite-size pieces
½ yellow or red pepper, chopped
1 tablespoon reduced sodium soy sauce
1 egg, lightly beaten
4 cups cooked long grain brown rice
2 tablespoons finely diced scallions

Seasoning sauce:
3 tablespoons reduced-sodium soy sauce
1 tablespoon mirin or white wine
¼ teaspoon ground ginger
½ teaspoon toasted sesame oil
Fresh ground black pepper

Coat wok well with vegetable cooking spray. Stir-fry the onions, garlic and celery for one minute. Add the remaining vegetables and one tablespoon soy sauce. Stir-fry five minutes or until the vegetables are crisp-tender. Transfer to a bowl. Add the egg and fry it, breaking it into small pieces as it cooks. When the egg is done, return the vegetables to the wok. Add the rice, breaking it up and dispensing it evenly in the pan. Stir in the seasoning sauce, mixing well. Adjust the seasonings to taste. Transfer to a serving dish and garnish with scallions, if desired.

DESERTS, BAKED GOODS AND SMOOTHIES

APPLE STREUSEL MUFFINS

¾ cup white sugar
½ cup unsweetened applesauce
3 egg whites, beaten
1½ teaspoons pure vanilla
2½ cups peeled, diced tart green apples
1 cup all purpose flour
½ cup whole wheat flour
1½ teaspoons baking soda
½ teaspoon salt
½ teaspoon cinnamon
¾ cup golden raisins

Serves:	12
Calories:	175
Fat:	0.3 g
Saturated Fat:	0 g
Fiber:	2.4 g

Streusel topping:

¼ cup brown sugar
2 tablespoons all-purpose flour
½ teaspoon cinnamon
2 teaspoons applesauce

Preheat oven to 350 degrees. In a bowl combine white sugar, applesauce, egg whites and vanilla. Add apples. In another bowl sift together flours, baking soda, ½ teaspoon cinnamon, and salt. Add dry ingredients to apple mixture. Stir in raisins. Spoon mixture into muffin pan lined with paper cups.

Streusel Topping: In a small bowl, combine ¼ cup brown sugar, 2 tablespoons all-purpose flour and ½ teaspoon cinnamon. Stir in 2 teaspoons applesauce with fork or crumb mixture.

BLUEBERRY-RHUBARB COBBLER

Serves: 8
Calories: 171
Fat: 0.9 g
Saturated Fat: 0.1 g
Fiber: 1.8 g

1 cup light buttermilk baking mix
⅓ cup skim milk
¼ cup sugar
2 tablespoons plus 1 teaspoon cornstarch
2 tablespoons orange juice
2 cups frozen blueberries
2 cups frozen rhubarb, no sugar
½ cup sugar
½ teaspoon ground ginger

Preheat oven. Combine buttermilk mix, milk, and sugar until moist and set aside. Dissolve cornstarch in orange juice and set aside. In a large saucepan combine fruit, sugar, ginger and orange juice mixture. Heat on medium heat until it thickens (10-15 minutes). Pour mixture into a 1½-quart baking dish. Drop spoonfuls of baking mix mixture on fruit mixture. Bake for 27-32 minutes or until golden brown. Serve warm with fat-free ice cream or yogurt if desired.

COFFEE SOUFFLÉ

Serves: 6
Calories: 167
Fat: 2.7 g
Saturated Fat: 2.7 g
Fiber: 0 g

2 envelopes unflavored gelatin
¾ cup sugar, divided into ½ and ¼ cups
3 cups boiling fresh brewed decaffeinated coffee
2 egg whites
2 cups fat-free whipped topping

Place gelatin and ½ cup sugar in a mixing bowl. Pour hot coffee over this. Stir to dissolve sugar and gelatin. Chill mixture until slightly firm. In a separate bowl, add remaining sugar (¼ cup) and egg whites and beat with mixer on high until soft peaks form. Spoon soufflé in bowls and top with a dollop of whipped topping.

POACHED PEARS WITH CHOCOLATE SAUCE

2½ cups water
½ cup granulated sugar
Grated rind and juice of 1 lemon
1 cinnamon stick
4 pears
4 tablespoons fat-free chocolate syrup

Serves:	8
Calories:	126
Fat:	0.4 g
Saturated Fat:	0.1 g
Fiber:	2.5 g

In large saucepan combine water, sugar, lemon rind, lemon juice, and cinnamon stick. Bring to a boil, stirring until sugar is dissolved.

Peel, halve and core pears. Add pears to boiling syrup. (Pears should be covered in liquid; if not, double the amount of poaching liquid or poach in batches.) Reduce heat to medium-low and simmer gently for 15-20 minutes or until pears are almost tender (time will vary depending on ripeness and type of pear; remember, pears will continue to cook while cooling). Remove from heat and let cool in liquid.

Drain pears thoroughly and pat dry on paper towels. Arrange pear halves on individual plates. Drizzle with chocolate syrup. Serve at room temperature.

BEST BROWNIES

Vegetable cooking spray
3 egg whites, beaten until frothy
¾ cup sugar
½ cup applesauce, unsweetened
1½ teaspoons vanilla
½ cup flour sifted
½ cup cocoa
¼ teaspoon salt
3 tablespoons Grape Nuts cereal

Serves:	8
Calories:	140
Fat:	0.6 g
Saturated Fat:	0.3 g
Fiber:	2 g

Preheat oven to 350 degrees. Spray 8-inch square pan with vegetable spray. In large bowl, whisk together egg whites, sugar, applesauce, and vanilla. In a medium bowl, combine flour, cocoa, and salt. Stir flour mixture into applesauce mixture. Pour brownie mix into pan and bake for 15 minutes. Remove pan from oven and sprinkle with Grape Nuts. Return to oven and continue to bake until a toothpick inserted comes out clean (about 10 minutes). Cool and cut into squares.

LEMON TORTE WITH FRESH RASPBERRIES

Serves: 12
Calories: 72
Fat: 0.2 g
Saturated Fat: 0 g
Fiber: 1.4 g

4-oz pkg low-calorie lemon flavored gelatin
½ cup boiling water
3 oz lemonade concentrate
Vegetable cooking spray
12-oz can of evaporated skim milk
2 cups cubed angel food cake
2 cups fresh raspberries; keep chilled

In a large bowl, dissolve lemon gelatin in the boiling water. Stir in thawed lemonade concentrate and evaporated skim milk. Cover and chill in the refrigerator for 1½ hours or until the mixture mounds when spooned. With an electric mixer on medium high speed, beat chilled lemon mixture until fluffy. Spray the bottom only of an 8-inch springform pan with cooking spray; set aside. Arrange angel food cake cubes in the bottom of the springform pan. Pour gelatin mixture over cake cubes. Cover with plastic wrap and chill until firm (about 4½ hours). Arrange raspberries on top and serve.

BANANA SPLIT CAKE

Serves: 12
Calories: 221
Fat: 4.4 g
Saturated Fat: 2.5 g
Fiber: 2.5 g

16 graham cracker sheets, finely crushed
1 large box sugar-free vanilla pudding mix
3 cups skim milk (used to make the pudding)
4 small bananas sliced
8 oz fat-free whipped topping
2 cups fresh strawberries
Two 8-oz cans crushed pineapple, no sugar added
¼ cup fat-free chocolate syrup

Spread crushed graham crackers evenly on a 13-inch x 9-inch pan. Mix pudding according to package directions. Pour over crumbs and chill. Layer bananas over pudding. Cover banana layer with whipped topping. Cover with strawberries. Cover strawberries with pineapple. Drizzle chocolate syrup on top. Refrigerate until serving time.

GRANNY'S APPLE CAKE

1¼ cup whole wheat flour
1¼ cup unbleached flour
¾ cup packed brown sugar
2 teaspoons baking soda
2½ teaspoons ground cinnamon
¾ cup and 2 tablespoons light maple syrup
4 egg whites, beaten lightly
2 teaspoons vanilla extract
4 cups chopped Granny Smith apples (about 5 medium sized)
½ cup raisins

Serves:	12
Calories:	215
Fat:	0.5 g
Saturated Fat:	0.1 g
Fiber:	3.3 g

In a mixing bowl combine the flours, sugar, baking soda, and cinnamon and stir to mix well. Add ¾ cup maple syrup, egg whites, and vanilla extract and stir to mix well. Fold in the flour mixture in thirds. Stir in apples and raisins. Coat 9-inch x 13-inch pan with nonstick cooking spray. Spread batter evenly in pan and bake at 350 degrees for forty to fifty minutes or just until a wooden toothpick inserted in the center of the cake comes out clean. Cool cake for at least twenty minutes. Cut into squares. Drizzle with the remaining syrup.

OATMEAL COOKIES WITH A TOUCH OF CHOCOLATE

1 cup all purpose flour
¾ cup whole wheat flour
½ cup cocoa
½ teaspoon salt
2½ teaspoons baking powder
1½ cup packed brown sugar
¾ cup applesauce
2 teaspoons vanilla
½ cup skim milk
1½ cups quick cooking oatmeal

Serves:	30
Calories:	91
Fat:	0.5 g
Saturated Fat:	0.1 g
Fiber:	1.3 g

Heat oven to 350 degrees. Sift the flours, cocoa, salt, and baking powder together and set aside. Combine sugar, applesauce, vanilla, and milk together in a bowl. Blend in flour mixture ⅓ at a time. Stir in the oatmeal. With a spoon, drop cookie mix onto an ungreased baking sheet. Bake for eight to nine minutes.

CHOCOLATE ÉCLAIR DESSERT

Serves: 20
Calories: 206
Fat: 4.3 g
Saturated Fat: 2.3 g
Fiber: 1.2 g

3 small pkg sugar-free vanilla pudding (instant)
4 cups skim milk plus 1-2 tablespoons
8-oz fat-free dairy whip
1 box low-fat graham crackers
1 can low fat chocolate frosting (1½ cups)
2 tablespoons skim milk

Mix four cups of milk with pudding mix. Fold in dairy whip. Line bottom of a 9-inch x 13-inch pan with a layer of graham crackers, then pudding. Top with final layer of graham crackers. Mix one to two tablespoons of milk with can of frosting, spread evenly over top. Refrigerate for at least eight hours.

LEMON-GLAZED CRANBERRY ROLLS

Serves: 12
Calories: 116
Fat: 0.9 g
Saturated Fat: 0.2 g
Fiber: 1.6 g

Vegetable cooking spray
10-oz can of refrigerated pizza crust
½ cup orange marmalade
⅔ cup dried cranberries soaked in ½ cup water
½ cup powdered sugar
2 teaspoons lemon juice
1 teaspoon hot water

Preheat oven to 375 degrees. Coat muffin pan with vegetable spray. Unroll refrigerated crust dough, pat into a 12-inch rectangle. Spread marmalade over dough, leaving a ½-inch border. Drain cranberries. Sprinkle cranberries over marmalade, pressing gently into dough. Beginning with the long side, roll dough in a jellyroll like fashion. Pinch the sides to seal (do not seal the ends of the roll.) Cut roll into twelve 1-inch slices. Place slices into muffin tins, bake for fifteen minutes or until golden. Cool for five minutes and remove the rolls from the pan on a wire rack. Combine sugar, lemon juice and water; mix completely. Place rolls on a plate and drizzle with glaze.

BANANA BREAD

4 egg whites
1 cup mashed banana
½ cup buttermilk
⅓ cup applesauce
2 teaspoons vanilla
1 cup flour
1 cup whole wheat flour
1 cup packed brown sugar
1 teaspoon cinnamon
¼ teaspoon baking soda
1 tablespoon baking powder
½ cup raisins, soaked in ¼ cup water

Serves:	12
Calories:	181
Fat:	0.4 g
Saturated Fat:	0.1 g
Fiber:	2.1 g

Preheat oven to 350 degrees. In a large bowl beat egg whites until foamy. Add banana, buttermilk, applesauce and vanilla. In another large bowl, combine dry ingredients. Stir dry ingredients into wet mixture. Drain raisins and add them to the mixture. Pour into a lightly greased bread loaf pan. Bake for forty-five to fifty-five minutes or until golden. Cool and cut into twelve slices. Keep bread covered to prevent drying out.

BLACKSTRAP MOLASSES BARS

½ teaspoon salt
½ teaspoon ground cinnamon
½ teaspoon ground cloves
½ teaspoon baking soda
¾ cup whole wheat flour
¼ cup Blackstrap molasses
¼ cup light molasses
1⅔ cup hot water
½ cup raisins

Serves:	8
Calories:	167
Fat:	0.6 g
Saturated Fat:	0.1 g
Fiber:	3.7 g

Preheat oven to 350 degrees. Stir dry ingredients together and set aside. Combine the molasses, hot water, and raisins. Bring to a boil, cover and cool to room temperature. Stir flour mixture into cooled molasses mixture until smooth. Spray an 8-inch x 8-inch baking pan and pour mixture into a pan. Spread evenly. Bake for forty-five minutes. When cooled, cut into squares.

PUMPKIN PRALINE CHEESECAKE

Serves: 8
Calories: 221
Fat: 2.2 g
Saturated Fat: 0.4 g
Fiber: 3.5 g

Vegetable cooking spray
1½ cups wheat germ
¼ cup packed brown sugar
3 tablespoon applesauce
1 egg white, beaten
16-oz nonfat cottage cheese
½ cup canned pumpkin
½ cup packed brown sugar
½ teaspoon vanilla
½ teaspoon cinnamon
Dash cloves
Dash nutmeg
2 egg whites
2 tablespoons fat-free caramel topping
Grape Nuts cereal (optional)

Preheat oven to 350 degrees. Lightly spray 9-inch pie plate with nonstick cooking spray. For crust, combine wheat germ and brown sugar. Add applesauce and egg white; mix well. Press mixture onto bottom and sides of pie plate. Bake eight to ten minutes. Remove from oven. For filling, blend cottage cheese in blender or food processor until smooth. Add pumpkin, brown sugar, vanilla, and spices; blend well. Add egg whites; blend just until all ingredients are combined. Pour into crust. Bake forty to forty-five minutes or until center is almost set. Cool completely. Refrigerate three hours or overnight. Just before serving, sprinkle with Grape Nuts cereal on top of cheesecake (optional) and drizzle with caramel.

GINGERED PEACH SMOOTHIE

2 medium peaches, frozen
8-oz fat-free vanilla yogurt
¾ cup skim milk
2 tablespoons honey
1½ teaspoons ground ginger
4-6 large ice cubes

Serves:	**4**
Calories:	**124**
Fat:	**0.9 g**
Saturated Fat:	**0.6 g**
Fiber:	**1.1 g**

Cut peaches into cubes. Discard pits. In a blender combine fruit, yogurt, milk, honey, and ginger. Blend until smooth. With blender on, add ice cubes one at a time (through opening in lid). Blend until smooth.

BANANA SPLIT SUPREME FRUIT SMOOTHIE

1 cup ripe large banana, frozen
½ cup ripe strawberries, frozen
¾ cup skim milk
1 cup fat-free vanilla ice cream
¼ cup fat-free chocolate syrup
4-6 large ice cubes

Serves:	**4**
Calories:	**150**
Fat:	**0.5 g**
Saturated Fat:	**0.3 g**
Fiber:	**1.6 g**

Peel banana and cut into chunks. Wash strawberries and remove stems. Cut strawberries in half. In a blender combine fruit, milk, ice cream and chocolate syrup. Blend until smooth. With blender on, add ice cubes one at a time (through opening in lid). Blend until smooth.

Suggestion: Top with toasted wheat germ or Grape Nuts cereal.

BERRY SURPRIZE FRUIT SMOOTHIE

Serves: 4
Calories: 111
Fat: 1.1 g
Saturated Fat: 0.4 g
Fiber: 2.2 g

1½ cups mixed berries (strawberries, blueberries, raspberries, etc.), frozen
¾ cups skim milk
8 oz fat-free vanilla or berry flavored yogurt
2 tablespoons powdered sugar
4-6 large ice cubes

Wash berries and cut any large ones in half. In a blender, combine fruit, milk, yogurt and sugar. Blend until smooth. Add ice cubes one at a time (through an opening in the lid). Blend until smooth.

Variation: Use low-fat soymilk instead of skim milk, and soft silken tofu instead of yogurt.

28-Day Menu Plan

Breakfast
Calories–344   *Fat –1.1*   *Saturated Fat –0.0*   *Dietary Fiber –10.3*

Calories	1820
Fat	11.3
Saturated Fat	2.0
Dietary Fiber	51.8

Scrambled eggs
   ¼ cups egg substitute
   2 slices whole grain toast
   1 tablespoon jelly

Lunch
Calories–692   *Fat –5.2*   *Saturated Fat –1.0*   *Dietary Fiber –16.1*

Veggie burger
   1 low-fat veggie patty
   1 whole grain bun
   Lettuce, tomato, onion, mustard, ketchup
1 serving Italian Fries*
2 cups tossed salad of spring greens
   1½ tablespoons fat-free dressing

Dinner
Calories –784   *Fat –5.0*   *Saturated Fat –1.0*   *Dietary Fiber –25.4*

Spaghetti
   2 cups whole wheat pasta
   1 cup Spaghetti Sauce*
1 serving Black Eyed Peas Barley with Kale*
1 serving Broiled Cheese Bread*
8 oz skim milk or equivalent

Calories	1742
Fat	13.2
Saturated Fat	2.3
Dietary Fiber	46.8

Breakfast
Calories –583   *Fat –1.8*   *Saturated Fat –0.5*   *Dietary Fiber –7.9*

2 slices Banana Bread*
1 cup fat-free, low-sugar Yogurt
¼ cup Grape Nuts cereal

Indicates the recipe is provided in the previous section.

Lunch
Calories –453   *Fat –6.3*   *Saturated Fat –0.5*   *Dietary Fiber –23.5*

Rolled Hummus Lawash
    1 serving (¼ cup) Lite Hummus*
    1 whole wheat lawash bread
    ¼ cup thinly sliced cucumber
    ¼ cup thinly sliced tomato
    2 leaves lettuce
1 serving Quinoa Tabbouleh*
1 cup cantaloupe or melon

Dinner
Calories –706   *Fat –5.1*   *Saturated Fat –1.3*   *Dietary Fiber –15.4*

1 serving Portabello Fajitas*
1 cup brown rice mixed with ½ cup salsa
½ cup mixed vegetables
1 serving Peach Gingered Smoothie*

Day 3

Calories	**1632**
Fat	**13.5**
Saturated Fat	**2.8**
Dietary Fiber	**54.5**

Breakfast
Calories –429   *Fat –3.2*   *Saturated Fat –0.3*   *Dietary Fiber –15.3*

1½ cup Raisin Bran
1 cup skim milk or equivalent
1 cup strawberries

Lunch
Calories –537   *Fat –6.7*   *Saturated Fat –1.5*   *Dietary Fiber –17.1*

1 serving Warm Italian Sandwich*
1 serving Red beans and Rice Salad*
½ cup steamed asparagus

Dinner
Calories –666   *Fat –3.6*   *Saturated Fat –1.0*   *Dietary Fiber –22.1*

1 serving Parmesan barley Risotto with Chicken*
Salad
    1½ cup spinach
    ½ cup tomatoes
    2 tablespoons onions
    2 tablespoons fat-free French dressing, warmed
1 serving Poached Pears with Chocolate Sauce*

Day 4

Breakfast
Calories –428   *Fat –4.3*   *Saturated Fat –1.0*   *Dietary Fiber –6.5*

Calories	1631
Fat	17.1
Saturated Fat	3.5
Dietary Fiber	32.3

1 pkg instant flavored oatmeal
½ cup skim milk or equivalent
1 slice whole grain bread
1½ teaspoons jelly
6 oz orange juice with calcium

Lunch
Calories –498   *Fat –6.4*   *Saturated Fat –1.0*   *Dietary Fiber –9.6*

Peanut butter and Jelly sandwich
    2 tablespoons Peanut Wonder Spread
    1 tablespoon jelly
    2 slices whole grain bread
8 oz skim milk or equivalent
1 apple
1 cup carrot sticks

Dinner
Calories –705   *Fat –6.4*   *Saturated Fat –1.5*   *Dietary Fiber –16.2*

1 serving Taco Salad*
1 serving Peach Gingered Smoothie*
4 Ginger Snaps

Day 5

Breakfast
Calories –483   *Fat –6.1*   *Saturated Fat –1.1*   *Dietary Fiber –7.4*

Calories	1741
Fat	18.8
Saturated Fat	5.3
Dietary Fiber	50.1

2 slices of whole grain bread
2 tablespoons Peanut Wonder Spread
1 banana
Sugar-free hot cocoa with
8 oz skim milk or equivalent

Lunch
Calories –542   *Fat –6.4*   *Saturated Fat –0.5*   *Dietary Fiber –16.6*

¼ cup Lite Hummus*
1 piece whole wheat pita
1 cup carrots
1 cup cucumber
1 serving Creamy Pesto Sauce Dip*
Pear

Dinner
Calories –716   Fat –6.3   Saturated Fat –3.7   Dietary Fiber –26.1

1 serving Macaroni and Spinach Casserole*
1 serving Garlic and Fava beans*
1 serving Pineapple Slaw*
Berry Surprise Fruit Smoothie*

Day 6

Calories	**1527**
Fat	**13.1**
Saturated Fat	**3.2**
Dietary Fiber	**36.4**

Breakfast
Calories –265   Fat –1.3   Saturated Fat –0.4   Dietary Fiber –6.4

1 cup shredded whole grain cereal
¾ cup skim milk or equivalent
½ cup blueberries

Lunch
Calories –544   Fat –7.5   Saturated Fat –2.2   Dietary Fiber –9.1

1 Frozen Entrée (no more than 6 grams fat and at least 5 grams of fiber)
2 cups mixed baby greens salad
2 tablespoons fat-free Italian salad dressing
1½ cups watermelon
½ cup cantaloupe
10 thin twisted pretzels

Dinner
Calories –718   Fat –4.3   Saturated Fat –0.6   Dietary Fiber –20.9

1 serving Texas BBQ Pasta*
1 serving Apple Glazed Peas and Carrots*
1 serving Vegetarian South of the Border*
1 serving banana Bread*

Day 7

Calories	**1645**
Fat	**14.7**
Saturated Fat	**3.5**
Dietary Fiber	**50**

Breakfast
Calories –394   Fat –1.9   Saturated Fat –0.7   Dietary Fiber –7.4

1 serving Berry Surprise Smoothie*
1 serving Apple Streusel Muffins*
1 banana

Lunch
Calories –468   Fat –4.0   Saturated Fat –0.7   Dietary Fiber –21.2

1 serving Vegetarian South of the Border Chili*
Vegetables and dip
   ½ cup broccoli
   ½ cup cauliflower
   3 tablespoons fat-free ranch salad dressing
2 slices whole wheat bread
1 orange

Dinner
Calories –783   Fat –8.8   Saturated Fat –2.1   Dietary Fiber –21.4

2 servings Vegetable Fried Rice*
1 serving Garlic Greens*
8 oz. skim milk or equivalent

Day 8

Calories	1714
Fat	12.5
Saturated Fat	1.4
Dietary Fiber	39.3

Breakfast
Calories –486   Fat –3.4   Saturated Fat –0.3   Dietary Fiber –16.0

2 cups Raisin Bran cereal
8 oz skim milk or equivalent

Lunch
Calories –566   Fat –2.2   Saturated Fat –0.3   Dietary Fiber –7.5

4 oz Orange Roughy
½ cup spinach, steamed
1 cup long grain white rice
2 cups mixed baby greens salad
   2 tablespoons fat-free ranch salad dressing
1 serving Apple Streusel Muffins*

Dinner
Calories –662   Fat –6.9   Saturated Fat –0.8   Dietary Fiber –15.8

5 Morningstar Chik Nuggets
1 serving Coleslaw*
½ cup sweet corn
1 serving baked Potatoes with Herbed Cheese Topping*
2 tablespoons barbecue sauce

Day 9

Calories	1642
Fat	17.3
Saturated Fat	3.6
Dietary Fiber	30.5

Breakfast
Calories –452   *Fat –4.7*   *Saturated Fat –0.9*   *Dietary Fiber –9.3*

Breakfast Sandwich
   1 Morningstar Breakfast Pattie
   1 whole wheat English muffin
   1 slice fat-free cheese
8 oz orange juice with calcium
1 banana

Lunch
Calories –675   *Fat –7.0*   *Saturated Fat –1.7*   *Dietary Fiber –14.3*

1 serving Vegetable Fried Rice*
1 cup chopped broccoli
8 oz skim milk
10 pretzels

Dinner
Calories –515   *Fat –5.6*   *Saturated Fat –1.0*   *Dietary Fiber –6.9*

Portabella Sandwich
   1 whole wheat bun
   1 ½ oz portabella mushrooms
   2 slices fat-free Swiss cheese
   1 slice red onion
   1 tablespoon honey mustard barbecue sauce
1 serving Seasoned Red Potatoes*
1 cup fat-free ice cream

Day 10

Calories	1538
Fat	14.9
Saturated Fat	3.3
Dietary Fiber	35.9

Breakfast
Calories –475   *Fat –2.5*   *Saturated Fat –0.8*   *Dietary Fiber –9.1*

Pancakes
   ½ cup whole wheat pancakes mix
   4 oz skim milk
   1 egg white
1 cup strawberries
1 pkg sugar-free hot cocoa mix
8 oz skim milk

Lunch
Calories –451   *Fat –3.1*   *Saturated Fat –0.6*   *Dietary Fiber –11.9*

Vegetarian Reuben
   2 slices rye bread
   2 tablespoons fat-free 1000 Island dressing
   2 slices fat-free Swiss cheese
   1 serving Coleslaw*
1 orange
Fruit Fizzie
   4 oz apple juice
   3 oz club soda
   8 baby carrots

Dinner
Calories –612   *Fat –9.3*   *Saturated Fat –1.9*   *Dietary Fiber –14.9*

1 serving 3 Pepper Tofu Stir Fry*
1 ½ cup whole wheat spaghetti
1 serving Crimini Mushroom Chowder*

Day 11

Calories	**1651**
Fat	**17.6**
Saturated Fat	**4.1**
Dietary Fiber	**50.3**

Breakfast
Calories –306   *Fat –1.7*   *Saturated Fat –0.3*   *Dietary Fiber –11.9*

1½ cup wheat bran flakes
½ cup blueberries
8 oz skim milk

Lunch
Calories –739   *Fat –6.7*   *Saturated Fat –0.7*   *Dietary Fiber –25.3*

1 serving West Coast Pasta Salad*
1 serving Lentil Soup with Herbs and Lemon*
2 cups mixed baby greens salad
   2 tablespoons fat-free salad dressing
1 Hard roll

Dinner
Calories –606   *Fat –9.2*   *Saturated Fat –3.1*   *Dietary Fiber –13.1*

1 serving 3 Bean Chili with Rice*
1 serving Banana Split Supreme Smoothie*
12 low-fat Graham Crackers
1 apple

Day 12

Calories	1712
Fat	16.2
Saturated Fat	4.1
Dietary Fiber	36.5

Breakfast
Calories –405   *Fat –3.6*   *Saturated Fat –0.8*   *Dietary Fiber –4.3*

1 pkg instant Flavored oatmeal
4 oz skim milk
1 slice whole wheat bread
1½ teaspoons jelly
6 oz orange juice with calcium

Lunch
Calories –593   *Fat –7.4*   *Saturated Fat –1.7*   *Dietary Fiber –17.1*

Vegetarian a la king
  2 slices whole wheat bread
  1 serving Pea Delight*
Salad
  1 cup mixed baby greens salad
  1 cup spinach
  2 tablespoons fat-free ranch dressing
1 orange
6 Gingersnaps

Dinner
Calories –714   *Fat –5.2*   *Saturated Fat –1.6*   *Dietary Fiber –15.1*

1 serving Filet of Sole Florentine*
1 serving Creamy broccoli Salad with Dried Cherries
1 cup pearl barley
8 oz skim milk
1 serving Crimini Mushroom Chowder*

Day 13

Calories	1557
Fat	10.7
Saturated Fat	1.9
Dietary Fiber	31.7

Breakfast
Calories –338   *Fat –1.9*   *Saturated Fat –0.5*   *Dietary Fiber –6.3*

Banana Split Supreme Smoothie*
1 whole wheat English muffin
1 tablespoon jelly

Lunch
Calories –535   *Fat –3.0*   *Saturated Fat –0.6*   *Dietary Fiber –11.7*

1 serving West Coast Pasta Salad*
1 cup non-fat low calorie fruit yogurt
1 peach
10 baby carrots

Dinner
Calories –684 *Fat –5.8* *Saturated Fat –0.8* *Dietary Fiber –13.7*

1 serving Portabella Fajitas*
1 serving Mexican Layered Bean Dip*
2 oz baked tortilla chips
8 oz orange juice with calcium

Day 14

Breakfast
Calories –329 *Fat –4.6* *Saturated Fat –1.0* *Dietary Fiber –6.4*

Calories	1529
Fat	18.0
Saturated Fat	3.3
Dietary Fiber	45.6

Breakfast Sandwich
  1 Morningstar Breakfast Pattie
  1 whole wheat English muffin
  1 egg white
  1 slice cheese single
8 oz skim milk

Lunch
Calories –582 *Fat –6.2* *Saturated Fat –0.9* *Dietary Fiber –24.1*

¾ cup fat-free cottage cheese
1 serving Lentil Soup with Herbs and Lemon*
½ cup broccoli
½ cup cauliflower
8 reduced-fat crackers, whole grain
1 cup grapes

Dinner
Calories –618 *Fat –7.2* *Saturated Fat –1.4* *Dietary Fiber –15.1*

1 serving Chicken Marsala*
1 serving Indian Pumpkin Soup*
1 cup steamed spinach
½ cup steamed mushrooms

Day 15

Breakfast
Calories –483 *Fat –6.1* *Saturated Fat –1.1* *Dietary Fiber –7.4*

Calories	1850
Fat	17.1
Saturated Fat	3.3
Dietary Fiber	37.8

2 slices whole grain bread
2 tablespoons Peanut Wonder
1 banana
1 pkg sugar-Free Hot cocoa
8 oz skim milk or equivalent

Lunch
Calories –521   *Fat –7.0*   *Saturated Fat –1.4*   *Dietary Fiber –19.6*

1 serving Warm Italian Sandwich*
1 serving Bean Salad with Dijon Marinade*
4 dried figs

Dinner
Calories –846   *Fat –4.0*   *Saturated Fat –0.8*   *Dietary Fiber–10.8*

Stir Fry
   1 serving Teriyaki Sauce*
   1 ½ cup long-grain brown rice
   6 oz Chinese cabbage
   ¼ cup water chestnuts
   ¼ cup mushrooms
   ½ cup sweet red peppers
   1 ½ cup long-grain white rice

Day 16

Calories	**1562**
Fat	**15.2**
Saturated Fat	**2.8**
Dietary Fiber	**33.7**

Breakfast
Calories –236   *Fat –1.5*   *Saturated Fat –0.4*   *Dietary Fiber –6.3*

1 cup shredded whole grain cereal
8 oz skim milk
1 cup strawberries

Lunch
Calories –700   *Fat –8.7*   *Saturated Fat –1.1*   *Dietary Fiber –12.6*

1 serving Indian Pumpkin Soup*
"Peanut Butter" Sandwich
   2 slices whole wheat bread
   2 tablespoons Peanut Wonder Spread
   1 tablespoon jelly
2 Dutch pretzels
1 orange
1 cup fat-free low calorie fruit yogurt

Dinner
Calories –626   *Fat –5.0*   *Saturated Fat –1.3*   *Dietary Fiber–14.8*

1 serving Jerked Veggie Burger*
1 whole wheat bun
1 serving Italian Fries*
1 serving Gingered Peach Smoothie*

Day 17

Breakfast
Calories –440   Fat –3.0   Saturated Fat –0.4   Dietary Fiber –13.4

1½ cup Raisin bran cereal
8 oz skim milk
1 banana

Calories	**1519**
Fat	**12.2**
Saturated Fat	**2.0**
Dietary Fiber	**40.6**

Lunch
Calories –497   Fat –6.8   Saturated Fat –1.2   Dietary Fiber –13.1

Salad
   3 cups mixed baby greens salad
   ½ tomato
   ¼ cucumber
   ½ cup chick peas
   4 tablespoons fat-free dressing
¼ cup 2% fat cottage cheese
1 hard roll
½ cup sliced peaches

Dinner
Calories –582   Fat –2.4   Saturated Fat –0.4   Dietary Fiber –14.1

1 serving whole wheat Pasta with Honey Mustard Dressing*
1 cup asparagus
2 fat-free Fig Newton cookies

Day 18

Calories	**1563**
Fat	**14.6**
Saturated Fat	**3.7**
Dietary Fiber	**30.8**

Breakfast
Calories –366   Fat –3.9   Saturated Fat –1.0   Dietary Fiber –4.3

1 pkg flavored instant oatmeal
1 slice whole grain bread
1½ teaspoons jelly
8 oz skim milk or equivalent

Lunch
Calories –701   Fat –6.8   Saturated Fat –1.7   Dietary Fiber –14.9

1 serving Jerked Veggie Burger*
2 slices whole grain bun
1 cup grapes
2 Oatmeal Cookies with a Touch of Chocolate*
8 oz skim milk or equivalent
10 baby carrots

Dinner
Calories –496   *Fat –3.9*   *Saturated Fat –1.0*   *Dietary Fiber –11.6*

1 serving Sweet and Sour Chicken on Rice*
½ cup mixed vegetables
Salad
    1 cup mixed baby greens salad
    1 cup spinach
    2 tablespoons fat-free 1000 Island dressing

Day 19

Calories	**1666**
Fat	**15.8**
Saturated Fat	**2.3**
Dietary Fiber	**50.8**

Breakfast
Calories –433   *Fat –2.8*   *Saturated Fat –0.7*   *Dietary Fiber –16.9*

2 cups wheat bran cereal
½ cup blueberries
8 oz skim milk

Lunch
Calories –644   *Fat –6.6*   *Saturated Fat –1.1*   *Dietary Fiber –18.1*

Seafood Sandwich
    1 ½ serving King Crab Spread*
    2 slices whole grain bread
    ½ cup spinach
    ⅓ tomato
1½ apple
Salad
    1 cup mixed baby greens salad
    1 cup spinach
    ¼ cup chick peas
    2 tablespoons fat-free Italian salad dressing
2 Oatmeal Cookies with a Touch of Chocolate*

Dinner
Calories –589   *Fat –6.4*   *Saturated Fat –0.5*   *Dietary Fiber –15.8*

1 serving Mediterranean Barley*
1 serving Lite Hummus*
1 piece pita bread
¾ cup cantaloupe
½ cup watermelon

Day 20

Breakfast
Calories –453   *Fat –2.4*   *Saturated Fat –0.7*   *Dietary Fiber –9.1*

Pancakes
     4 whole wheat pancakes (replace oil with applesauce in equal amounts, and use only egg whites)
1 cup strawberries
1 pkg sugar-Free Hot cocoa mix
8 oz skim milk

Calories	**1648**
Fat	**18.9**
Saturated Fat	**5.4**
Dietary Fiber	**44**

Lunch
Calories –561   *Fat –10.5*   *Saturated Fat –3.7*   *Dietary Fiber –14.7*

Grilled Chicken Caesar Salad
     4 oz boneless skinless chicken breast
     2 cup mixed baby greens salad
     1 cup spinach
     ¼ cup croutons
     2 tablespoons parmesan cheese
     ⅓ tomato
     4 tablespoons fat-free Italian salad dressing
2 slices whole wheat bread
1 cup mixed Fruit

Dinner
Calories –634   *Fat –6.0*   *Saturated Fat –1.0*   *Dietary Fiber –20.2*

1 serving Couscous Casserole*
1 serving Herbed Lima Beans*
1 cup green beans
1 hard roll

Day 21

Breakfast
Calories –462   *Fat –4.7*   *Saturated Fat –0.9*   *Dietary Fiber –9.2*

Breakfast Sandwich
     1 Morningstar Breakfast Pattie
     1 whole grain English muffin
     1 egg white
     1 slice fat-free sharp cheese, single
1 banana
8 oz orange juice with calcium

Calories	**1778**
Fat	**16.3**
Saturated Fat	**2.6**
Dietary Fiber	**53.6**

Lunch
Calories –622   Fat –5.8   Saturated Fat –0.1   Dietary Fiber –22.5

1 serving Carrot Soup*
1 Frozen Entrée (no more than 6 grams of fat and at least 5 grams of fiber)
15 fat-free twisted pretzels
1 pear

Dinner
Calories –694   Fat –5.8   Saturated Fat –1.6   Dietary Fiber –21.9

1 serving Cassoulet*
1 serving Marinated Mushrooms*
Salad
    2 cups mixed baby greens salad
    2 tablespoons fat-free ranch salad Dressing
1 serving Apple Glazed Peas and Carrots*
1 cup pearl barley, cooked

Day 22

Calories	**1752**
Fat	**14.3**
Saturated Fat	**2.7**
Dietary Fiber	**37.5**

Breakfast
Calories –483   Fat –6.1   Saturated Fat –1.1   Dietary Fiber –7.4

Peanut Butter Sandwich
    2 slices whole grain bread
    2 tablespoons Peanut Wonder Spread
1 banana
1 pkg sugar-free hot cocoa mix
8 oz skim milk

Lunch
Calories –639   Fat –4.6   Saturated Fat –1.1   Dietary Fiber –12.3

1 serving Sweet and Sour Chicken on Rice*
2 fat-free Fig Newton cookies
1 cup broccoli
1 apple

Dinner
Calories –630   Fat –3.6   Saturated Fat –0.5   Dietary Fiber –17.8

1 ½ oz Portabella Mushrooms, Grilled
1 serving Strawberry Soup in Melon Bowl*
1 serving Baked Potato with Herbed Cheese Topping*
Spinach Salad
    2 cups spinach
    2 tablespoons fat-free Catalina salad Dressing, warmed
    ¾ cup salad vegetables
1 hard roll

Day 23

Breakfast
Calories –422   *Fat –3.1*   *Saturated Fat –0.3*   *Dietary Fiber –13.0*

1½ cup Raisin Bran cereal
8 oz skim milk
1 plum

Calories	**1793**
Fat	**16.4**
Saturated Fat	**4.1**
Dietary Fiber	**33.3**

Lunch
Calories –456   *Fat –2.5*   *Saturated Fat –0.6*   *Dietary Fiber –9.4*

1 serving Asian Chicken Salad*
1 serving Granny's Apple Cake*
1 cup sliced cucumber

Dinner
Calories –915   *Fat –10.8*   *Saturated Fat –3.2*   *Dietary Fiber –10.9*

1 serving Asparagus Potato Soup*
1 serving Quick Italian Scallops*
1 serving Chocolate Eclair Dessert*
Salad
　2 cups mixed baby greens salad
　2 tablespoons fat-free ranch salad dressing

Day 24

Calories	**1662**
Fat	**10.3**
Saturated Fat	**1.4**
Dietary Fiber	**38.5**

Breakfast
Calories –359   *Fat –1.5*   *Saturated Fat –0.2*   *Dietary Fiber –7.6*

½ grapefruit
1 cup fat-free low calorie fruit yogurt
½ cup Grape Nuts cereal

Lunch
Calories –604   *Fat –5.5*   *Saturated Fat –0.9*   *Dietary Fiber –9.3*

"Peanut Butter" Sandwich
　2 slice whole wheat bread
　2 tablespoons Peanut Wonder Spread
　1 tablespoon jelly
12 oz skim milk
Vegetables with Dip
　1 serving Creamy Pesto Sauce Dip*
　5 baby carrots
　½ cup sliced cucumbers
　½ cup broccoli
1 peach
1 Oatmeal Cookie with a Touch of Chocolate*

Dinner
Calories –699   Fat –3.3   Saturated Fat –0.3   Dietary Fiber –21.6

  1 serving Black Beans with Rice*
  2 servings Guacomole Gone Skinny*
  2 oz baked tortilla chips
  1 cup mixed Fruit

Day 25

Calories	**1638**
Fat	**10.6**
Saturated Fat	**2.5**
Dietary Fiber	**46.8**

Breakfast
Calories –436   Fat –3.0   Saturated Fat –0.7   Dietary Fiber –15.9

  2 cups wheat bran cereal
  1 cup strawberries
  8 oz skim milk

Lunch
Calories –551   Fat –2.4   Saturated Fat –0.5   Dietary Fiber –15.9

  1 serving Black Beans and Rice*
  1 serving Pineapple Slaw*
  8 baby carrots
  1 Oatmeal Cookie with a Touch of Chocolate*

Dinner
Calories –651   Fat –5.2   Saturated Fat –1.3   Dietary Fiber –15.0

  2 appetizer servings of Tasty Tangy Sweet and Sour Meatballs*
  1 ½ cup long grain brown rice
  1 serving Garlicky Fava Beans*
  1 cup green beans
  8 oz skim milk

Day 26

Calories	**1581**
Fat	**10.5**
Saturated Fat	**2.7**
Dietary Fiber	**35.9**

Breakfast
Calories –313   Fat –2.5   Saturated Fat –0.8   Dietary Fiber –3.2

  1 pkg of Flavored instant oatmeal
  4 oz skim milk
  1 pkg sugar-Free Hot cocoa
  8 oz skim milk

Lunch
Calories –538   Fat –3.8   Saturated Fat –1.2   Dietary Fiber –13.3

1 pkg Frozen Entrée (no more than 6 grams of fat, at least 5 grams of fiber)
1 serving Granny's Apple Cake*
2 plums

Dinner
Calories –730   Fat –4.2   Saturated Fat –0.7   Dietary Fiber –19.4

1 serving Spinach and Artichoke Stuffed Pasta Shells*
1 serving Broiled Cheese Bread*
1 serving Red Bean and Rice Salad*
¾ cup zucchini
1 serving Lemon Torte with Raspberries*

Day 27

Calories	1619
Fat	15.4
Saturated Fat	4.9
Dietary Fiber	42.5

Breakfast
Calories –354   Fat –4.2   Saturated Fat –0.7   Dietary Fiber –6.4

Breakfast Sandwich
   1 Morningstar Breakfast Pattie
   1 whole grain English muffin
   1 egg white
   1 slice fat-free sharp cheese, single
8 oz orange juice with calcium

Lunch
Calories –648   Fat –4.0   Saturated Fat –0.8   Dietary Fiber –17.1

2 servings Quick Kasha Pilaf*
1 serving Zesty Cucumber Salad*
1 apple
2 fat-free Fig Newton cookies
15 fat-free pretzels

Dinner
Calories –617   Fat –7.2   Saturated Fat –3.4   Dietary Fiber –19.0

1 serving Roasted Red Pepper and Feta Cheese Sauce*
2 cups whole wheat spaghetti
Greek salad
   1 cup romaine lettuce
   1 cup spinach
   1 oz reduced-fat feta (3 grams of fat/ 1 oz)
   ¼ cup sliced red onions
   ½ cup sliced beets
   ¼ cup plain croutons
   2 tablespoons fat-free Italian salad Dressing

Day 28

Calories	**1679**
Fat	**10.8**
Saturated Fat	**1.9**
Dietary Fiber	**43.1**

Breakfast
Calories –327   Fat –1.7   Saturated Fat –0.5   Dietary Fiber –8.3

1½ cup shredded whole grain cereal
1 cup blueberries
8 oz skim milk

Lunch
Calories –690   Fat –4.9   Saturated Fat –1.0   Dietary Fiber –17.2

1 serving Spinach and Artichoke Stuffed Pasta Shells*
2 slices French bread
Salad
  1 cups mixed baby greens salad
  1 cup spinach
  ¼ tomato
  2 tablespoons fat-free salad Dressing
  2 tablespoons fat-free ranch salad Dressing
2 Oatmeal Cookies with a Touch of Chocolate*

Dinner
Calories –662   Fat –4.2   Saturated Fat –0.4   Dietary Fiber –17.6

1 serving Sun-Dried Tomatoes and Shitake Mushroom Orzo*
1 serving Black-eyed Peas with Garlic and Kale*
1 cup okra, topped with 4 tablespoons fat-free Italian salad dressing
1 serving Lemon Torte with Raspberries*

Fat and Fiber Counter

The following chart was put together so you would have a reference on fat and fiber. In addition you will find that the foods have been rated on a scale from 0-10. Like the continuum diet 0 is least desirable and 10 is the most desirable. The foods have been rated based on their nutritional value; this includes fat, saturated fat, fiber, calories, vitamins, minerals, portion and processing of the food. Glycemic Index was not considered in these values due to the likelihood of the foods being consumed in a meal versus by themselves. For food products which are not identified by brand, the data shown are average values reported by the FDA.

Grains and Breads

Food	Portion	Calories	Fat	Sat Fat	Fiber	Rating
GRAINS						
Barley, pearled, light, cooked	1 cup	193	1	0	9	10
Buckwheat groats,						
roasted, cooked	1 cup	182	1	na	4	8
Bulgur, cooked	1 cup	152	0	0	7	10
Cornmeal, whole grain, dry	1 cup	442	4	na	19	10
Granola, Kellogg's, low fat	½ cup	210	3	1	3	5
Granola, Nature Valley,						
100% Natural Oat	¾ cup	240	8	1	3	3
Cinnamon & Raisin						
100% Natural Oat, Fruit & Nut	⅔ cup	250	11	2	3	3
Granola, Uncle Roy's						
Fat Free Apple	½ cup	175	1	0	3	6
Cinnamon & Raisin						
Low Fat Crispy	½ cup	160	3	1	3	6
Organic Golden Honey	½ cup	190	6	1	3	7
Grits, hominy, cooked	1 cup	123	0	0	0	5
Millet, cooked	1 cup	286	2	na	11	10
Millet, raw	1 cup	756	9	na	29	10
Oat bran, raw	1 cup	231	7	na	13	10
Oats, whole grain, uncooked	1 cup	607	11	na	21	10
Rye, whole, dry	1 cup	566	4	na	9	10
Wheat, durum	1 cup	651	5	na	10	10
Wheat, hard red spring	1 cup	632	4	na	10	10
Wheat, hard red, winter	1 cup	628	3	na	10	10
Wheat, hard white	1 cup	657	3	na	7	10
Wheat, soft white	1 cup	571	3	na	6	9
Wheat, soft red winter	1 cup	556	3	na	9	10
Wheat, sprouted	1 cup	214	1	na	3	7
Wheat bran, crude	1 cup	130	3	na	8	10
FLOUR						
Amaranth	1 cup	729	13	3	30	
Pastry	⅓ cup	100	1	0	3	10
Potato	1 cup	628	1	0	na	5
Rice, white	1 cup	578	2	0	2	5
Rye, dark	1 cup	415	3	0	na	
Rye, light	1 cup	374	1	0	7	10
Rye, medium	1 cup	361	2	0	7	10
White, all-purpose	1 cup	455	1	0	2	5

Food	Portion	Calories	Fat	Sat Fat	Fiber	Rating
White, bread	1 cup	495	2	0	3	6
Whole wheat	1 cup	407	2	0	8	10
ARROWHEAD						
Kamut	¼ cup	110	1	0	4	10
Spelt	¼ cup	100	1	0	5	10
Teff	1 slice	140	1	0	5	10
Oat Blend, Gold Medal	1 cup	390	3	na	na	na

PASTA

Food	Portion	Calories	Fat	Sat Fat	Fiber	Rating
Cellophane noodles, rice	1 cup	491	0.1	0	0	4
Chow mein, canned, La Choy	1 cup	300	16	na	1.7	5
Corn, cooked	1 cup	176	1	0	7	10
Elbows, cooked	1 cup	197	1	0	2	7
Soba noodles, buckwheat	1 cup	190	0.6	0	1	4
Somen noodles, wheat	1 cup	202	0.4	0	1	4
Spaghetti, cooked	1 cup	197	1	0	2	7
Spelt, cooked, VitaSpelt	1 cup	190	1.5	na	5	10
Whole wheat spaghetti, cooked	1 cup	174	1	0	6	10
EDEN						
Elbows, whole wheat organic	2 oz	210	2	0	6	10
Ribbons, whole wheat spinach organic	2 oz	200	2	0	7	10
Spaghetti, Kamut, organic	2 oz	210	2	0	6	10
HEALTH VALLEY						
Lasagna, whole wheat	2 oz	170	1	na	7	10
Spaghetti, amaranth	2 oz	170	1	na	9	10
Spaghetti, oat bran	2 oz	120	1	na	4	8
Spaghetti, whole wheat	2 oz	170	1	na	7	10
SAN GIORGIO						
Bowties, egg	2 oz	210	3	na	na	7
Capellini	2 oz	210	1	na	2	7

RICE

Food	Portion	Calories	Fat	Sat Fat	Fiber	Rating
Brown, medium grain, cooked	½ cup	109	0	0	na	8
White, medium grain, cooked	½ cup	132	0	0	na	7
ARROWHEAD						
Basmati, brown	¼ cup	150	1	0	2	10
Basmati, white	¼ cup	150	0	0	0	6

Food	Portion	Calories	Fat	Sat Fat	Fiber	Rating
RICE COMBINATIONS						
GREEN GIANT						
Rice & Broccoli	1 package	320	12	4	2	3
Rice Medley	1 package	240	3	2	2	6
Rice Pilaf	1 package	230	3	2	3	6
White & Wild	1 package	250	5	1	3	6
LIPTON						
Golden Saute						
Onion Mushroom	½ cup	240	4	2	2	4
Rice & Sauce Alfredo Broccoli,						
as prepared	1 cup	320	12	5	1	2
Rice & Sauce Chicken Broccoli,						
as prepared	1 cup	280	9	2	2	4
MINUTE RICE						
Boil-in-Bag White as prep	1 cup	190	0	0	0	6
Instant Brown as prepared	1 cup	170	2	0	2	7
Instant White as prepared	1 cup	160	0	0	0	6
NEAR EAST						
Barley Pilaf as prepared	1 cup	220	4	1	5	5
Long Grain & Wild as prep	1 cup	220	5	1	2	4
BAGELS						
BRUEGGER'S						
Blueberry	1 (3.5 oz)	300	2	0	2	6
Egg	1 (3.5 oz)	280	1	1	3	7
Honey grain	1 (3.6 oz)	300	3	1	3	7
Plain	1 (3.5 oz)	280	2	0	2	6
Wheat bran	1 (3.5 oz)	280	2	0	5	10
DUNKIN' DONUTS						
Garlic	1 (4.4 oz)	330	1	0	3	7
Onion	1 (4.4 oz)	320	1	0	3	7
Plain	1 (4.4 oz)	330	1	0	3	7
Salt	1 (4.4 oz)	320	1	0	3	7
EINSTEIN BROS.						
Chopped garlic	1 (4.2 oz)	377	4	1	5	8
Cinnamon raisin	1 (4 oz)	360	1	0	2	6
Dark pumpernickel	1 (3.8 oz)	330	1	0	5	10
Honey 8 grain	1 (4 oz)	320	1	0	4	9
Plain	1 (3.7 oz)	330	1	0	2	6

Food	Portion	Calories	Fat	Sat Fat	Fiber	Rating
SARA LEE						
Plain	1 (2.8 oz)	210	1	0	2	6
Blueberry	1 (2.8 oz)	210	1	1	3	7
Oat Bran	1 slice	71	1	0	1	6
Pita	1 regular	165	1	0	1	6
Pita, whole wheat	1 regular	170	2	0	5	10
Sourdough	1 slice	78	1	0	1	6
White	1 slice	67	1	0	1	6
Whole Wheat	1 slice	70	1	0	2	10

BREAD

Food	Portion	Calories	Fat	Sat Fat	Fiber	Rating
ARNOLD						
12 Grain Natural	1 slice	60	0	0	1	6
Pumpernickel	1 slice	70	1	0	1	6
Rye Bakery Soft-Seeded	1 slice	70	1	0	1	6
BEEFSTEAK						
Rye Hearty	1 slice	70	1	0	1	6
Rye Light	2 slice	70	1	0	5	10
BREAD DU JOUR						
Italian	1 slice	130	2	0	1	4
Sourdough	1 slice	130	1	0	1	4
BROWNBERRY						
Bran'nola Country Oat	1 slice	90	2	na	3	10
Bran'nola Hearty Wheat	1 slice	88	2	na	3	10
Wheat, Soft	1 slice	74	2	na	1	7
HOME PRIDE						
Seven Grain	1 slice	60	1	0	1	7
Wheat	1 slice	70	1	0	1	7
White	1 slice	70	1	0	0	4
NATURAL OVENS						
Cracked Wheat	2 slice	140	1	0	4	10
Honey 'n Flax	2 slice	140	1	0	4	10
Nutty Natural Wheat Bread	2 slice	140	2	0	6	10
PEPPERIDGE FARM						
7 Grain Hearty Slice	2 slice	180	2	0	2	7
Cracked Wheat	1 slice	70	1	na	1	7
French Fully Baked	2 oz	150	2	na	1	7
White Sandwich	2 slice	130	2	na	0	4
ROMAN MEAL						
Brown & Serve Soft	1 slice	181	3	0	3	9

Food	Portion	Calories	Fat	Sat Fat	Fiber	Rating
Seven-Grain	1 slice	67	1	0	1	7
Twelve-Grain	1 slice	70	2	0	1	7
Whole Wheat 100%	1 slice	64	1	0	2	10
Whole Wheat 100%, Light	1 slice	42	0	0	2	10
WONDER						
Calcium-Enriched	1 slice	70	1	0	0	4
Granola	1 slice	100	2	0	2	10
Italian	1 slice	80	1	0	0	4
Nine Grain Light	2 slice	80	1	0	6	10
Wheat, Family	1 slice	70	1	0	0	4
Wheat, Light	2 slice	80	1	0	6	10
Whole Wheat, 100% Stoneground	1 slice	80	2	0	2	10

BISCUITS

Food	Portion	Calories	Fat	Sat Fat	Fiber	Rating
Buttermilk, home recipe	1	212	10	3	na	2
Buttermilk, mix	1	191	7	2	1	2
Plain, home recipe	1	212	10	3	na	2
Plain, mix	1	191	7	2	1	2
JIFFY						
Biscuit	¼ cup mix	130	5	1	1	2
Buttermilk as prepared	1	170	4	2	0	1

BREAD STICKS

Food	Portion	Calories	Fat	Sat Fat	Fiber	Rating
Plain	1	41	1	0	na	4
KEEBLER						
Garlic	2	30	0	0	na	4
Onion	2	30	0	0	na	4
Plain	2	30	0	0	na	4
Sesame	2	30	0	0	na	4

CRACKERS

Food	Portion	Calories	Fat	Sat Fat	Fiber	Rating
KEEBLER						
Club	2	30	2	0	na	4
Oyster, large	26	80	2	0	na	4
Oyster, small	50	80	2	0	na	4
KRISPY						
Mild Cheddar	5	60	2	1	0	4
Original	5	60	2	0	0	4
Soup & Oyster	17	60	2	0	0	4
Whole Wheat	5	60	2	0	0	4

Food	Portion	Calories	Fat	Sat Fat	Fiber	Rating
Melba toast, plain, Lance	2	20	0	0	na	3
NABISCO						
Wheat Thins, original	16	140	6	1	2	4
Wheat Thins, reduced fat	18	120	4	1	2	4
SNACKWELL'S						
Cracked Pepper	7	60	0	0	0	4
Fat Free Wheat	5	60	0	0	1	4
TRISCUIT						
Crackers	7	140	5	1	4	6
Garden Herb	6	130	5	1	3	6
Reduced Fat	8	130	3	1	4	10
Wheat 'n Bran	7	140	5	1	4	6

CROISSANTS

Food	Portion	Calories	Fat	Sat Fat	Fiber	Rating
Almond	1	360	21	5	2	1
Cheese	1	236	12	5	2	1
Plain	1	232	12	7	2	1

ENGLISH MUFFINS

Food	Portion	Calories	Fat	Sat Fat	Fiber	Rating
PEPPERIDGE FARMS						
Cinnamon Raisin	1	150	2	na	na	6
Plain	1	140	1	na	na	5
Sourdough	1	135	1	na	na	5
THOMAS						
Oat Bran	1	116	1	na	3	9
Regular	1	130	1	na	na	5
Sandwich size	1 (92g)	210	2	1	2	6
WONDER						
English Muffin	1 (2 oz)	120	1	0	1	5
Raisin Rounds	1 (2.1 oz)	150	2	0	2	6

FRENCH TOAST

Food	Portion	Calories	Fat	Sat Fat	Fiber	Rating
Frozen, Campbell's	1 slice	94	5	0	2	2
Home Recipe	1 slice	153	7	0	2	2
Sourdough, Krusteaz frozen	1 slice	140	2	0	0	4

MUFFINS

Food	Portion	Calories	Fat	Sat Fat	Fiber	Rating
HOME RECIPES						
Blueberry, as prepared with 2% milk	1	163	6	1	na	3

Food	Portion	Calories	Fat	Sat Fat	Fiber	Rating
Corn, as prepared with 2% milk	1	180	7	1	na	3
JIFFY						
Apple cinnamon as prep	1	190	7	3	1	3
Bran with dates as prep	1	170	6	3	3	5
HOSTESS						
Mini Chocolate Chip	5	260	15	5	1	2
Oat Bran	1	160	8	1	0	2
WEIGHT WATCHERS						
Fat Free, Banana	1	170	0	0	3	8
Fat Free, Blueberry	1	160	0	0	2	8

PANCAKES

Food	Portion	Calories	Fat	Sat Fat	Fiber	Rating
FROZEN						
Buttermilk	1 (4-inch diameter)	83	1	0	na	4
Plain	1 (4-inch diameter)	83	1	0	na	4
AUNT JEMIMA						
Blueberry	3	210	4	1	2	3
Lowfat	3	130	2	0	8	10
QUAKER						
Lite Pancakes & Lite Syrup	1 package (6 oz)	260	3	na	na	5
ARROWHEAD						
Multigrain, Pancake & Waffle mix	¼ cup (1.2 oz)	120	1	0	3	6
AUNT JEMIMA						
Original Pancake & Waffle mix	⅓ cup	150	1	0	1	4
BISQUICK						
Apple Cinnamon, Shake n' Pour	3 (4-inch diameter)	240	3			

POPOVERS

Food	Portion	Calories	Fat	Sat Fat	Fiber	Rating
Home recipe as prepared with 2% milk	1	87	3	1	na	4

ROLLS

Food	Portion	Calories	Fat	Sat Fat	Fiber	Rating
Brown & Serve	1	85	2	0	na	6
Dinner	1	85	2	0	na	6
Egg	1	107	2	1	1	6
Hamburger	1	123	2	1	na	6
Hamburger, multigrain	1	113	2	1	2	10

Food	Portion	Calories	Fat	Sat Fat	Fiber	Rating
Hamburger reduced calorie	1	84	1	0	3	10
Hot dog	1	123	2	1	na	6
Hot dog, multigrain	1	113	2	1	2	10
Hot dog, reduced calorie	1	84	1	0	3	10
Kaiser	1	167	2	0	na	6

SCONES

Food	Portion	Calories	Fat	Sat Fat	Fiber	Rating
Raisin	1	270	6	4	2	3
Orange Poppy	1	260	6	4	2	3

STUFFING/DRESSING

Food	Portion	Calories	Fat	Sat Fat	Fiber	Rating
Bread, dry as prepared	½ cup	178	9	2	3	4
Cornbread, as prepared	½ cup	178	9	2	na	

STOVE TOP

Food	Portion	Calories	Fat	Sat Fat	Fiber	Rating
Chicken, prepared with margarine	½ cup	170	9	2	0	2
Cornbread, prepared with margarine	½ cup	170	8	2	1	2
Beef, prepared with margarine	½ cup	180	9	2	1	2

WAFFLES

FROZEN

Food	Portion	Calories	Fat	Sat Fat	Fiber	Rating
Buttermilk	1 4-in square	88	3	0	1	4
Plain	1 4-in square	88	3	0	1	4

AUNT JEMIMA

Food	Portion	Calories	Fat	Sat Fat	Fiber	Rating
Blueberry	2	190	7	2	1	3
Buttermilk	2	170	6	2	1	3
Oatmeal	2	170	7	1	3	3
Whole Grain	2	170	7	1	2	3

EGGO

Food	Portion	Calories	Fat	Sat Fat	Fiber	Rating
Blueberry	2	220	8	2	0	2
Buttermilk	2	220	8	2	0	2
Common Sense	2	200	7	2	3	3

OAT BRAN

Food	Portion	Calories	Fat	Sat Fat	Fiber	Rating
Homestyle	2	220	8	2	0	2
Nutri-Grain	2	190	6	1	4	3
Nutri-Grain Multi-	2	180	6	1	6	5

BRAN

Food	Portion	Calories	Fat	Sat Fat	Fiber	Rating
Special K	2	140	0	0	0	4

Food	Portion	Calories	Fat	Sat Fat	Fiber	Rating
VANS						
7 Grain Belgian	2	152	4	0	8	7
Belgian Original	2	145	4	0	2	2

Vegetables

Food	Portion	Calories	Fat	Sat Fat	Fiber	Rating
Amaranth, raw	1 cup	729	13	3.2	30	4
Artichoke, edible portion, medium sized	1 serving	25	0	0	3	8
Artichoke hearts, marinated, quartered, S&W	2 pieces	20	2	na	1	6
Artichoke hearts, boiled	1 cup	84	0.6	0	8.3	9
Asparagus spears, canned, drained	1 cup	46	1.6	0	3.9	8
Asparagus, frozen, boiled, drained, tips	1 cup	50	0.8	0	2.2	6
Asparagus	5 spears	20	0	0	2	8
Bamboo shoots, fresh	1 cup	41	0.5	0	3.9	8
Bamboo shoots, canned, La Choy	1 cup	25	0.5	0	2	6

BEANS

Food	Portion	Calories	Fat	Sat Fat	Fiber	Rating
Adzuki, boiled	1 cup	294	0.2	0	14.3	10
Adzuki, sweetened	1 cup	702	0.1	0	13.7	10
Baked beans, home recipe	1 cup	382	13	na	19.5	6
Baked beans, canned	1 cup	236	1.1	1.5	19.6	10
Baked beans with pork	1 cup	268	3.9	0	13.9	8
Black, canned, Sun-Vista	1 cup	140	2	0	14	10
Black, canned, S&W	1 cup	140	0	0	12	10
Black-eyed, Canned, Sun-Vista	1 cup	140	0	0	8	10
Boston baked, fat free, canned, Health Valley	1 oz	25	0.1	0	0.7	10
Brick oven baked, canned, S&W	1 cup	320	1	0	14	10
Butter, canned, S&W	1 cup	140	0	0	10	10
Chili, canned, Sun-Vista	1 cup	220	2	na	14	10
Cranberry, boiled	1 cup	240	0.8	0	9.8	10
French, cooked, boiled	1 cup	228	1.3	na	14.9	10
Garbanzo, canned, S&W	1 cup	160	3	0.3	14	10
Great northern, canned, Sun-Vista	1 cup	140	0	0	12	6
Green, dietary, low sodium, canned	1 cup	26	0.1	0	2.6	6

Food	Portion	Calories	Fat	Sat Fat	Fiber	Rating
Green, frozen, boiled, Health Valley	1 cup	50	2	0	2	8
Green, snap, fresh	1 cup	19	0	0	4	7
Homestyle, Campbell's, canned	1 oz	28	0.5	0	1.6	10
Honey baked, fat free, canned, Health Valley	1 cup	110	0	0	7	10
Hot chipolte chili, canned, S&W	1 cup	180	0	0	12	6
Hot chili, canned, Campbell's	1 oz	23	0.5	0	0.4	6
Italian/green/yellow, boiled	1 cup	44	0.4	0	3	6
Italian/green/yellow, frozen, boiled	1 cup	35	0.2	0	3.4	6
Italian/green/yellow, canned	1 cup	27	0.1	0	2.9	10
Kidney, all types, canned	1 cup	207	0.8	0	13.3	10
Kidney, light red's, canned, Luck's	1 cup	240	0	0	10	10
Lima, canned, solids & liquids	1 cup	186	0.7	0	10.4	10
Mung, boiled	1 cup	213	1	0	11	10
Mung, sprouted, boiled	1 cup	26	0	0	3	7
Mung, sprouted, raw	1 cup	32	0	0	2	6
Pink, boiled	1 cup	252	1	0	8	10
Pinquitos, canned, S&W	1 cup	160	1	0	12	10
Pinto, Texas style barbecue, canned, S&W	1 cup	200	3	1	16	10
Pinto, canned	1 cup	160	1	0	6	8
Pinto, Smoky Ranch Beans, canned, S&W	1 cup	220	5	na	12	9
Red, Cajun Style, canned, S&W	1 cup	160	4	na	16	9
Red kidney, canned, solids and liquids	1 cup	230	1	0	13	10
Refried, sausage, canned, Old El Paso	1 cup	388	26	10	16	3
Refried, vegetarian	1 cup	200	4	2	12	8
Snap, green, drained, cut, canned	1 cup	27	0	0	2	6
Snap with liquids, canned	1 cup	36	0	0	3	6
Snap, yellow/wax, canned	1 cup	27	0	0	2	7
Vegetarian	1 cup	260	2	0	14	8
White, boiled	1 cup	249	0	0	9	10
White, small, maple sugar, canned, S&W	1 cup	300	1	0	12	10
Winged, boiled	1 cup	252	10	1	3	5
Yellow, boiled	1 cup	254	2	0	2	6
Yellow, wax, fresh	1 cup	19	0	0	4	8

Food	Portion	Calories	Fat	Sat Fat	Fiber	Rating
Bean salad, deli style, canned, S&W	1 cup	160	0	0	8	10
Bean salad, marinated, canned, S&W	1 cup	140	0	0	6	8
Bean sprouts, canned	1 cup	11	0	0	0	6
Beets, boiled, drained	1 cup	77	0	0	2	9
Beets, fresh	1 medium	50	0	0	1	9
Beet greens, boiled, drained	1 cup	39	0	0	4	10
Beets, pickled with liquid, canned	1 cup	149	0	0	3	8
Beets, sliced, drained, canned	1 cup	53	0	0	3	8
Beets, sliced, canned	1 cup	60	0	0	2	7
Beets, canned, solids& liquids	1 cup	84	0	0	1	6
Beets, whole, canned	1 cup	7	0	0	3	6
Broccoli, fresh, boiled, drained	1 cup	43	0	0	4	10
Broccoli, fresh, medium sized	1 stalk	50	0	0	4	10
Broccoli, frozen, boiled	1 cup	50	0	0	4	10
Brussels sprouts, fresh	4 pieces	40	1	0	4	10
Brussels sprouts, fresh, boiled	1 cup	61	1	0	6	10
Brussels sprouts, frozen, boiled	1 cup	65	0	0	6	10
Cabbage, Chinese, fresh	1 cup	6	0	0	0	6
Cabbage, green, boiled, drained	1 cup	31	0	0	4	10
Cabbage, green, fresh	$^1/_{12}$ medium	25	0	0	1	7
Cabbage, red, fresh, shredded	1 cup	19	0	0	1	7
Carrots, boiled, drained, sliced	1 cup	70	0	0	3	10
Carrots, fresh, scraped	1 medium	40	0	0	1	6
Carrots, fresh, scraped, shredded	1 cup	47	0	0	2	10
Carrots, sliced, drained, canned	1 cup	34	0	0	2	10
Carrots, sliced, canned	1 cup	50	1	0	4	10
Cauliflower, fresh, medium head	$^1/_6$ head	25	0	0	2	10
Cauliflower, frozen, boiled	1 cup	34	0	0	3	10
Celery, boiled	1 cup	42	0	0	4	8
Celery, fresh	1 stalk	13	0	0	1	6
Celery, fresh, diced	1 cup	19	0	0	2	7
Chard, Swiss, boiled, drained	1 cup	35	0	0	4	10
Chard, Swiss, fresh	1 cup	7	0	0	1	8
Chayote, fruit, raw	½ fruit	28	0	0	1	6
Chestnuts, water, canned	1 cup	75	0	0	3	6
Chicory greens, fresh, chopped	1 cup	41	0	0	4	9
Chives, fresh or freeze dried	1 tablespoon	3	0	0	0	7
Chop suey vegetables, canned, La Choy	1 cup	17	0	0	0	5
Collards, fresh, boiled, drained	1 cup	35	0	0	2	8
Collards, frozen, cooked	1 cup	60	0	0	2	8

Food	Portion	Calories	Fat	Sat Fat	Fiber	Rating
Corn, frozen, boiled	1 cup	160	2	0	4	8
Corn, sweet, fresh, medium size	1 ear	75	1	0	3	7
Corn, cream style, canned	1 cup	184	1	0	3	7
Corn, drained, canned	1 cup	134	2	0	3	7
Corn, frozen, boiled, drained	1 cup	134	1	0	4	8
Corn, vacuum pack, Niblets	1 cup	166	1	0	4	8
Corn, whole kernel, canned	1 cup	180	2	0	4	8
Cowpeas, common, canned with pork	1 cup	199	4	1	15	8
Cowpeas, common, pods and seeds, cooked	1 cup	54	1	0	3	6
Cress, garden, boiled	1 cup	31	1	0	1	6
Cress, garden, fresh	1 cup	16	0	0	1	6
Cucumber, fresh	1 cup	29	0	0	2	6
Cucumber, fresh, medium size	1/3	15	0	0	1	6
Dandelion greens, boiled	1 cup	35	1	0	4	8
Dandelion greens, fresh	1 cup	25	0	0	2	7
Eggplant, boiled, drained	1 cup	27	0	0	2	6
Eggplant, fresh, medium size	1/5	25	0	0	2	6
Eggplant, fresh, medium size	1 cup	22	0	0	2	6
Endive, fresh, chopped	1 cup	13	0	0	1	6
Fennel, leaves	1 cup	17	0	0	3	6
Garden salad, dill, S&W	1 cup	100	0	0	6	7
Garden salad, marinated, S&W	1 cup	100	0	0	6	7
Garlic, fresh, clove	1 clove	5	0	0	0	6
Ginger root, fresh, sliced	1 cup	66	1	0	1	6
Gourd, white flowered, boiled	1 cup	22	0	0	2	6
Hominy, white or golden, canned, Van Camp's	1 cup	160	2	0	2	6
Horseradish, fresh	1 cup	206	1	0	5	5
Horseradish, raw	1 tablespoon	13	0	0	0	5
Hyacinth beans, fresh pods	1 cup	32	0	0	2	5
Jerusalem artichokes, fresh	1 cup	114	0	0	2	6
Kale, fresh, boiled, drained	1 cup	42	1	0	4	10
Kale, frozen, boiled, drained	1 cup	39	1	0	4	10
Kohlrabi, boiled, drained	1 cup	48	0	0	3	9
Kohlrabi, fresh	1 cup	38	0	0	3	9
Leeks, boiled, drained	1	38	0	0	4	8
Leeks, fresh	1	76	0	0	3	7
Lentils, sprouted, fresh	1 cup	82	0	0	6	10
Lentils, whole, cooked	1 cup	231	1	0	10	10
Lettuce, butterhead, head	1	21	0	0	2	6
Lettuce, butterhead, leaves	1 slice	2	0	0	0	6
Lettuce, iceberg, fresh, medium head	1/6	20	0	0	1	6
Lettuce, leaf, fresh, shredded	1 cup	13	0	0	1	8
Lettuce, looseleaf, fresh	1 cup	10	0	0	1	8

Food	Portion	Calories	Fat	Sat Fat	Fiber	Rating
Lettuce, romaine, fresh, shredded	1 cup	9	0	0	1	8
Miso, fermented soybeans	1 cup	567	16	na	10	7
Mixed Chinese vegetables, canned, La Choy	1 cup	17	0	0	0	5
Mixed vegetables, canned	1 cup	70	0	0	4	8
Mixed vegetables, frozen, boiled	1 cup	140	2	0	4	10
Mushrooms, drained, canned	1	3	0	0	0	7
Mushrooms, drained, solids, canned	1 cup	61	1	0	6	7
Mushrooms, fresh	5 medium	20	0	0	0	7
Mushrooms, shiitake, cooked	1 cup	80	0	0	3	7
Mushrooms, shiitake, dried	1	11	0	0	0	7
Mustard greens, boiled, drained	1 cup	21	0	0	3	10
Mustard greens, fresh	1 cup	10	0	0	0	10
Mustard greens, frozen, boiled	1 cup	28	0	0	3	10
Okra, fresh	6 pods	30	0	0	1	9
Okra, fresh, boiled, drained	1 cup	51	0	0	2	9
Onions, boiled	1 cup	98	0	0	3	8
Onions, fresh, medium. size	1	60	0	0	3	8
Onions, green, chopped	1 cup	40	0	0	3	8
Onions, mature, fresh, chopped	1 cup	61	0	0	3	8
Onions, canned, solids & liquids	1 cup	22	0	0	3	8
Parsley, fresh, chopped	1 cup	22	0	0	2	8
Parsnips, fresh	1 large	132	1	0	4	8
Parsnips, sliced, boiled, drained	1 cup	126	0	0	4	9
Peas, green, canned	1 cup	117	1	0	8	9
Peas, green, fresh	1 cup	117	1	0	5	9
Peas, green, fresh, boiled	1 cup	134	1	0	5	9
Peas, green, frozen, boiled	1 cup	160	1	0	6	9
Peas, green, canned	1 cup	140	1	0	8	9
Peas, black-eyed/cowpeas, boiled, drained	1 cup	179	1	0	15	10
Peas, black-eyed/cowpeas, fresh, boiled	1 cup	160	1	0	11	10
Peas, black-eyed/cowpeas, frozen, boiled	1 cup	224	1	0	10	10
Peas, podded, boiled	1 cup	67	0	0	4	9
Peas, podded, fresh	1 cup	61	0	0	4	9
Peas, split, boiled	1 cup	231	0	0	8	10
Peas, split, dry, cooked	1 cup	230	1	0	10	10
Peas, split, fresh	1 cup	671	2	0	8	10
Peas & carrots, canned	1 cup	97	1	0	9	10
Peas & carrots, frozen, boiled	1 cup	77	1	0	7	10
Peas & onions, canned	1 cup	61	1	0	4	9
Peas & onions, frozen, boiled	1 cup	81	0	0	5	9

Food	Portion	Calories	Fat	Sat Fat	Fiber	Rating
Peppers, bell, green, red, yellow, fresh	1 medium	30	0	0	2	8
Peppers, hot, red, dried	1 tablespoon	5	0	0	1	7
Peppers, hot chili, canned	1 cup	34	0	0	2	7
Peppers, hot chili, fresh	1 cup	60	0	0	4	7
Peppers, jalapeno, chopped, canned	1 cup	33	1	0	2	7
Peppers, jalapeno	1	7	0	0	0	7
Peppers, Mexican, hot, tiny-Vlasic	1 oz	6	0	0	0	7
Pickle, cucumber, dill, medium.	1	5	0	0	1	6
Pickle, cucumber, dill, whole, 3¾	1	12	0	0	1	6
Pickle, sweet/gherkin, small, whole	1	20	0	0	0	6
Potato, canned, solids & liquids	1 cup	110	0	0	2	6
Potato, canned, new	1 cup	120	0	0	2	7
Potato, fresh, flesh	1 cup	190	0	0	4	9
Potato, fresh, whole	1 medium	120	0	0	4	9
Potato, baked, flesh only	1 cup	237	0	0	6	9
Potato, baked, flesh and skin	1 cup	257	0	0	6	9
Potato, french fried, restaurant cooked	1 cup	180	6	na	2	5
Potato, frozen, fried in oil	1 cup	180	9	na	2	5
Potato, hash brown, prepared from fresh	1 cup	326	22	8	3	4
Potato, hash brown, prepared from frozen	1 cup	340	18	7	2	4
Potato, mashed, from dehydrated, with milk	1 cup	260	12	7	1	2
Potato, mashed, from fresh, with milk, butter	1 cup	222	9	6	1	4
Potato puffs, frozen, heated	½ cup	130	7	3	na	na
Prickly pear, fresh, average size	1	39	0	10	1	7
Prickly pear, fresh, with seeds, average size	1	39	1	0	4	9
Pumpkin, boiled, drained	1 cup	49	0	0	7	10
Pumpkin, canned	1 cup	83	1	0	7	10
Pumpkin, canned, Libby's	1 cup	80	1	0	10	10
Pumpkin, fresh, cubed	1 cup	30	0	0	2	7
Pumpkin pie mix, canned, Libby's	1 cup	200	0	0	4	8
Purslane, leaves & stems, raw	1 cup	13	0	0	1	6
Radish, daikon, sliced, boiled, drained	1 cup	25	0	0	3	8
Radish, oriental, fresh	1 cup	18	0	0	1	6
Radish, red, fresh	1	2	0	0	0	6
Rutabaga, boiled, drained, cubes	1 cup	70	0	0	2	8
Rutabaga, (swede), boiled	1 cup	83	1	0	5	8

Food	Portion	Calories	Fat	Sat Fat	Fiber	Rating
Rutabaga, (swede), fresh	1 oz	10	0	0	1	6
Sauerkraut, solids & liquids	1 cup	27	0	0	1	6
Seaweed, dried, (hai-tai)	1 oz	71	0	0	2	9
Seaweed, kelp (kombu), fresh	1 oz	12	0	0	1	7
Shallots, fresh	3 tablespoons	20	0	0	0	6
Soybeans, boiled	1 cup	298	15	2	8	6
Soybeans, dry roasted	1 cup	775	37.5	6	8	4
Soybeans, roasted	1 cup	811	43.7	7	8	4
Soybeans, sprouted, boiled and drained	1 cup	48	2	na	1	6
Soybeans, sprouted, fresh	1cup	48	2	na	1	6
Spinach, canned, drained	1 cup	50	1	0	7	10
Spinach, canned, solids & liquids	1 cup	45	1	0	5	10
Spinach, canned	1 cup	60	0	0	4	10
Spinach, fresh, boiled, drained	1 cup	41	1	0	4	10
Spinach, frozen, boiled	1 cup	50	1	0	4	10
Spinach, raw	1 cup	27	0	0	3	10
Squash, acorn, baked	1 cup	113	0	0	4	10
Squash, butternut, baked	1 cup	139	0	0	4	10
Squash, crookneck, fresh	1 cup	20	0	0	2	8
Squash, Hubbard, baked	1 cup	103	1	0	4	8
Squash, spaghetti, fresh	1 cup	50	0	0	2	7
Squash, zucchini, boiled	1 cup	38	0	0	3	7
Squash, zucchini, canned, Italian style	1 cup	60	0	0	2	6
Squash flowers	1 large	3	0	0	0	6
Succotash, canned	1 cup	200	2	na	4	6
Succotash (corn & lima beans)	1 cup	150	1	na	1.4	6
Sweet potato, canned in syrup, drained	1 cup	213	1	0	3.3	9
Sweet potato, canned, mashed	1 cup	258	1	0	4.6	10
Sweet potato, canned, vacuum pack	1 cup	182	0	0	4.8	10
Sweet potato, fresh	1 medium	140	0	0	3	10
Sweet potato, baked, peeled	1	117	0	0	3	10
Taro root (poi)	1 cup	269	0	0	4.8	8
Tofu, Lite firm	3 oz	35	1	0	na	7
Tofu, extra firm, Nasoya	3.2 oz	92	5	1	0	6
Tofu, firm, Nasoya	3.2 oz	76	4	1	0	7
Tofu silken, extra firm, Mori Nu	1-inch slice	55	2	0	0	7
Tofu silken, firm, Mori Nu	1-inch slice	56	3	0	0	7
Tofu silken, soft, Mori Nu	1-inch slice	45	3	0	0	7
Tomatillo, fresh, chopped	1 cup	42	1	0	3	6
Tomato, canned, ripe, stewed	1 cup	66	0	0	3	8
Tomato, canned, ripe, whole	1 cup	48	1	0	3	8
Tomato, cooked, stewed	1 cup	60	0	0	4	7

Food	Portion	Calories	Fat	Sat Fat	Fiber	Rating
Tomato, diced	1 cup	47	0	0	2	8
Tomato, fresh	1 medium	35	0	0	2	7
Tomato, green, fresh	1 small	24	0	0	1	7
Tomato paste, canned	1 cup	204	1	0	2	5
Tomato paste, canned	2 tablespoons	30	0	0	2	9
Tomato puree, canned	1 serving	52	0	0	2	9
Tomato, red, fresh, boiled	1 cup	65	1	0	2	9
Turnips, boiled, drained	1 cup	35	0	0	1	8
Turnips, fresh	1 cup	40	0	0	1	8
Turnip greens, boiled	1 cup	29	0	0	5	10
Turnip greens, fresh	1 cup	56	0	0	2	8
Water chestnuts, canned	1 cup	70	0	0	1	7
Water chestnuts, fresh	1 cup	57	0	0	1	6
Water chestnuts, leaves and stems, fresh	1 cup	7	0	0	0	5
Yams, canned, old-fashioned candied, S&W	1 cup	340	0	0	8	7

Fruits

Food	Portion	Calories	Fat	Sat Fat	Fiber	Rating
Apple, unpeeled	1 medium	140	1	0	3	9
Apple, rings, dried	10	155	0	0	5	8
Apple, spiced rings, canned, S&W	2	25	0	0	1	4
Applesauce, sweetened, canned	½ cup	97	0	0	2	8
Applesauce, unsweetened, canned	½ cup	53	0	0	2	8
Apricots, dried, cooked, sugar added	1 cup	305	0	0	8	7
Apricots, dried sulfured	10 halves	83	0	0	3	9
Apricots, frozen, sweetened	1 cup	237	0	0	4	7
Apricots, in light syrup, canned	1 cup	159	0	0	5	8
Apricots, packed in water, canned	1 cup	66	0	0	4	9
Banana, fresh	1	110	1	0	4	10
Banana flakes, dehydrated or powdered	1 tablespoon	22	0	0	1	7
Blackberries, fresh	1 cup	75	1	0	7	10
Blackberries, frozen, unsweetened	1 cup	97	1	0	7	10
Blackberries, in heavy syrup, canned	1 cup	236	1	0	6	7
Blueberries, dried, Trader Joe's	½ cup	320	0	0	10	7
Blueberries, fresh	1 cup	81	1	0	3	10
Blueberries, frozen, unsweetened	1 cup	79	1	0	3	10

Food	Portion	Calories	Fat	Sat Fat	Fiber	Rating
Blueberries, in heavy syrup, canned	1 cup	255	1	1	2	7
Boysenberries, frozen, unsweetened	1 cup	66	0	0	5	9
Boysenberries, in heavy syrup, canned	1 cup	225	0	0	6	7
Breadfruit, fresh, medium size	¼	99	0	0	11	10
Cantaloupe, medium size	¼	50	0	0	1	8
Carambola (Star Fruit), fresh	1	42	0	0	1	7
Casaba melon, fresh	1 cup	44	0	0	2	8
Cherimoya, fresh	1	514	2	na	13	7
Cherries, dried	½ cup	240	1	0	3	7
Cherries, sour, fresh	1 cup	77	0	0	2	6
Cherries, sour, red, in light syrup, canned	1 cup	189	0	0	2	6
Cherries, sour, red, in water, canned	1 cup	88	0	0	2	6
Cherries, sweet	21	90	1	0	3	8
Cherries, sweet, in light syrup, canned	1 cup	170	0	0	2	6
Cherries, sweet, in water, canned	1 slice	114	0	0	1	6
Cherries, sweet, frozen, sweetened	1 cup	231	0	0	2	6
Coconut, dried, shredded	1 oz	187	18	16	2	3
Cranberry sauce, sweetened, canned	½ cup	209	0	0	3	6
Cranberries, dried	½ cup	180	1	0	5	7
Cranberries, fresh	1 cup	54	0	0	5	9
Currants, black, fresh	½ cup	36	0	0	2	8
Currants, zante, dried	½ cup	204	0	0	4	7
Date	1	26	0	0	1	8
Elderberries, fresh	1 cup	106	1	0	12	10
Figs, dried, uncooked	1 cup	507	2	0	19	7
Figs, fresh	1	37	0	0	3	10
Figs, in heavy syrup	1 cup	228	0	0	9	7
Figs, in water	1 cup	131	0	0	5	10
Fruit cocktail, in light syrup	1 cup	145	0	0	3	8
Fruit cocktail, in heavy syrup	1 cup	184	1	0	7	7
Gooseberries, fresh	1 cup	66	1	0	4	8
Gooseberries, in heavy syrup	1 cup	184	1	0	7	7
Grapefruit, medium size	½	70	1	0	5	10
Grapefruit, in juice, canned	1 cup	92	0	0	2	8
Grapes	1½ cups	90	1	0	1	6
Guava, common, fresh	1 medium	46	1	0	5	10
Guava, strawberry, fresh	1 medium	65	1	0	6	10
Honeydew melon	1/10 medium	50	0	0	1	6
Kiwifruit	2 medium	100	1	0	4	10

Food	Portion	Calories	Fat	Sat Fat	Fiber	Rating
Kumquat, fresh	2 medium	12	0	0	1	7
Lemon, fresh, w/o peel	1	17	0	0	1	6
Lime, fresh	1 medium	20	0	0	3	6
Litchi, canned, drained	1 oz	21	0	0	0	6
Litchi, dried	1	6	0	0	0	6
Loganberries, frozen	1 cup	81	1	0	7	9
Mango, fresh	1	135	1	0	5	10
Mixed fruit, frozen/sweet	1 cup	245	1	0	3	8
Mulberries, fresh	1 cup	60	1	0	2	7
Nectarine, fresh	1	67	1	0	2	7
Olive, canned, large	1	5	1	0	0	4
Orange	1 medium	80	0	0	5	10
Oranges, mandarin, light	1 cup	133	0	0	1	7
Papaya, fresh	1 medium	247	1	0	8	8
Passion fruit, fresh	1	18	0	0	2	10
Peach	1 medium	40	0	0	2	8
Peaches, dried	1 cup	382	1	0	14	7
Peaches, frozen, sweet	1 cup	235	0	0	6	7
Peaches, in juice, canned	1 cup	160	0	0	2	8
Peaches, in light syrup, canned	1 cup	136	0	0	3	8
Pear	1 medium	100	1	0	4	9
Pears, dried	1 cup	472	1	0	14	7
Pears, fresh, Asian	1 medium	57	0	0	4	9
Pears, fresh, Bartlett	1 medium	98	1	0	5	9
Pears in juice, canned	1 cup	160	0	0	4	9
Pears, in syrup, canned	1 cup	116	0	0	4	7
Persimmons, dried	1	93	0	0	1	7
Persimmons, fresh	1	32	0	0	0	7
Pineapple, fresh	1 cup	76	1	0	2	7
Pineapple, frozen, sweet	1 cup	208	0	0	5	7
Pineapple, in juice, canned	1 cup	150	0	0	2	7
Pineapple, in water, canned	1 cup	79	0	0	2	7
Plaintains, cooked	1 cup	179	0	0	4	7
Plaintains, fresh	1	218	1	0	4	8
Plum, fresh	1	20	0	0	1	7
Plum, Japanese	1	36	0	0	1	7
Plum, in light syrup, canned	1 cup	158	0	0	3	6
Plum, whole, canned	1 cup	260	0	0	4	6
Pomegranates, fresh	1	105	1	0	1	6
Prickly pears, fresh	1	42	1	0	6	10
Prunes, dried	1 cup	385	1	0	11	7
Prunes, cooked w/o sugar	1 cup	227	1	0	8	8
Prunes, heavy syrup	1 cup	246	1	0	9	7
Quince, fresh	1	52	0	0	2	7
Raisins, seeded	1 cup	488	1	0	9	7
Raisins, seedless	1 cup	435	1	0	6	7

Food	Portion	Calories	Fat	Sat Fat	Fiber	Rating
Raspberries, fresh	1 cup	261	1	0	9	10
Raspberries, frozen, sweet	1 cup	258	0	0	11	8
Raspberries, heavy syrup	1 cup	234	0	0	7	7
Rhubarb, fresh	1 cup	26	0	0	2	8
Rhubarb, frozen w/ sugar	1 cup	278	0	0	5	7
Rhubarb, raw w/ sugar	1 cup	380	0	0	5	7
Star fruit, see carambola						
Strawberries, fresh	8 medium	70	1	0	3	10
Strawberries, frozen, sweet	1 cup	199	0	0	6	7
Tangerines	1 medium	80	1	0	3	9
Watermelon	$1/18$ medium	90	0	0	1	7

Dairy

CHEESE

Food	Portion	Calories	Fat	Sat Fat	Fiber	Rating
American	1 oz	93	7	4	0	1
American Cheese Food	1 slice	110	8	6	0	0
Brie	1 oz	95	8	4	0	1
Cheddar	1 oz	114	9	6	0	1
Colby	1 oz	112	9	6	0	1
Feta	1 oz	75	6	4	0	1
Mozzarella	1 oz	80	6	4	0	1
Parmesan, grated	1 tablespoon	23	2	1	0	1
Ricotta, part skim	½ cup	171	10	6	0	1
Ricotta, whole milk	½ cup	216	16	10	0	1
Swiss	1 oz	107	8	5	0	1
Alpine Lace						
American	1 slice	50	3	2	0	5
American Fat Free	1 piece	45	0	0	0	5
Feta Reduced Fat	1 oz	60	4	3	0	5
Frigo						
Asiago	1 oz	110	9	0	0	1
Healthy Choice						
Cheddar Fancy Shreds	¼ cup	45	0	0	0	5
Mozzarella	¼ cup	45	0	0	0	5
Mozzarella Fancy Shreds	¼ cup	45	0	0	0	5
Kraft						
Cheddar, Medium	1 oz	110	9	6	0	1
Deluxe Singles, American	1 slice	70	6	4	0	1
Free Shredded Cheddar	¼ cup	40	0	0	0	5
Free Shredded Mozzarella	¼ cup	45	0	0	0	5

Food	Portion	Calories	Fat	Sat Fat	Fiber	Rating
Grated Parm Plus!,						
Garlic Herb	2 teaspoon	15	0	0	0	4
Pizza Shredded						
Mozzarella & Cheddar	⅓ cup	120	9	6	0	1
Reduced Fat, Cheddar Sharp	1 oz	90	6	4	0	1
Shredded Lower Fat Cheddar,						
Sharp	¼ cup	80	6	4	0	1
Shredded Lower Fat,						
Mozzarella	⅓ cup	80	5	3	0	1
Singles, American	1 slice	60	5	3	0	1
Singles, Swiss	1 slice	70	5	4	0	1
Singles, Nonfat American	1 slice	30	0	0	0	5
Sargento						
Blue Crumbled	¼ cup	100	8	5	0	1
Cheddar, Mild Shredded						
Fancy Supreme	¼ cup	110	9	6	0	1
Cheddar, Mild Shredded						
Preferred Light	¼ cup	70	5	3	0	1
MooTown Snackers String	1 piece	70	5	3	0	1
MooTown Snackers						
String Light	1 piece	60	3	2	0	5

COTTAGE CHEESE

Food	Portion	Calories	Fat	Sat Fat	Fiber	Rating
Knudsen						
2% Fat Small Curd	½ cup	100	3	2	0	5
4% Fat Small Curd	½ cup	120	5	4	0	1
Light N' Lively						
1% Fat	½ cup	80	1	1	0	5
Fat Free	½ cup	80	0	0	0	5

MILK

Food	Portion	Calories	Fat	Sat Fat	Fiber	Rating
Evaporated, canned	½ cup	169	10	6	0	2
Evaporated, canned, skim	½ cup	99	0	0	0	5
Sweetened, condensed, Eagle	⅓ cup	320	9	0	0	2
1%	1 cup	102	3	2	0	5
2%	1 cup	121	5	3	0	1
Buttermilk	1 cup	99	2	1	0	5
Goat	1 cup	168	10	7	0	0
Nonfat	1 cup	86	0	0	0	4
Sheep	1 cup	264	17	11	0	0
Whole	1 cup	150	8	5	0	1
1%, Bordon, Acidophlius	8 fl oz	100	2	0	0	5

Food	Portion	Calories	Fat	Sat Fat	Fiber	Rating
MILK DRINKS						
Chocolate milk	1 cup	208	8	5	0	1
Chocolate milk, 1%	1 cup	158	3	2	0	5
Chocolate milk, 2%	1 cup	179	5	3	0	1
Cocoa mix, regular, Swiss Miss	1 serving	110	1	0	1	4
Cocoa mix, sugar free	1 serving	67	0	0	1	6
MILK SUBSTITUTES						
Better Than Milk, Carob	8 fl oz	130	5	0	0	1
Better Than Milk, Chocolate	8 fl oz	125	5	0	0	1
Better Than Milk, Light	8 fl oz	80	0	0	0	5
Better Than Milk, Natural	8 fl oz	90	5	0	0	1
Edensoy, Carob	8 fl oz	150	4	1	0	1
Edensoy, Extra Original	8 fl oz	130	4	1	0	1
Edensoy, Vanilla	8 fl oz	150	3	0	0	5
Soy Milk	1 cup	79	5	1	0	1
YOGURT						
Plain	8 oz	139	7	5	0	1
Plain lowfat	8 oz	144	4	2	0	4
Plain no-fat	8 oz	127	0	0	0	5
Dannon						
Chunky Fruit Nonfat						
Apple Cinnamon	6 oz	160	0	0	0	5
Danimals Lowfat Blueberry	4.4 oz	130	1	1	na	5
Double Delights						
Cheesecake Strawberry	6 oz	170	1	1	0	5
Fruit on the Bottom						
Lowfat Apple Cinnamon	8 oz	240	3	2	1	5
Light 'N Crunchy Nonfat						
Raspberry with Granola	8 oz	140	0	0	2	6
Light Duets Cherry Cheesecake	6 oz	90	0	0	0	5
Light Nonfat						
Strawberry Banana	8 oz	100	0	0	0	5
Light N' Lively						
Free Peach	4.4 oz	70	0	0	0	5
Lowfat Blueberry	4.4 oz	130	1	1	0	5
Weight Watchers						
Ultimate 90						
Blueberries & Cream	1 cup	90	0	0	3	7
Yoplait						
Custard Style Banana	6 oz	190	4	0	na	3

Food	Portion	Calories	Fat	Sat Fat	Fiber	Rating
Fat Free Blueberry	6 oz	150	0	0	na	4
Light Blueberry	6 oz	80	0	0	na	4
Original Peach	6 oz	190	3	0	na	4

SOUR CREAM

Breakstones

Free	2 tablespoons	35	0	0	0	4
Reduced Fat	2 tablespoons	45	4	3	0	0
Sour Cream	2 tablespoons	60	5	4	0	0

SOUR CREAM SUBSTITUTES

Tofutti, Better Than

Sour Cream Supreme	1 oz	50	5	2	0	0

Meats

BEEF

Flank steak	3 oz	220	13.2	5.6	0	1
Top round	3 oz	164	5.3	1.9	0	2
Round	3 oz	184	8	3	0	2
Sirloin	3 oz	219	13	5	0	0
Chuck	3 oz	293	22	9	0	0
Steak, eye of the round, trimmed	3 oz	145	5	2	0	3
Steak, top sirloin, trimmed	3 oz	162	6	2	0	3
Porterhouse, trimmed	3 oz	278	22	8	0	0
T-bone, trimmed	3 oz	202	15	6	0	0
Tenderloin, trimmed	3 oz	207	12	5	0	0
Corned beef	3 oz	213	16	5	0	0
Brisket	3 oz	185	9	3	0	1
Liver	3 oz	137	4	2	0	2
Veal, stew	3 oz	200	10.9	5.2	0	1
Veal, round	3 oz	141	9.4	4.5	0	1

PORK

Bacon	3 oz	489	42	15	0	0
Ham	3 oz	151	8	3	0	2
Ribs	3 oz	306	24	9	0	1
Chop, center loin	3 oz	196	8.9	3.1	0	1
Tenderloin	3 oz	141	4.1	1.4	0	5
Shoulder	3 oz	196	12	4	0	0

Food	Portion	Calories	Fat	Sat Fat	Fiber	Rating
FISH						
Bass, freshwater	3 oz	97	3.1	0.7	0	6
Bluefish	3 oz	105	3.6	0.8	0	6
Catfish, channel	3 oz	99	3.6	0.8	0	6
Cod, Atlantic	3 oz	70	0.6	0.1	0	7
Haddock	3 oz	74	0.6	0.1	0	7
Flounder/sole	3 oz	58	0.4	na	0	7
Mackerel, Atlantic	3 oz	174	11.8	2.8	0	1
Monkfish	3 oz	64	1.3	na	0	7
Perch, freshwater	3 oz	77	0.8	0.2	0	7
Perch, ocean	3 oz	81	1.3	0.2	0	7
Pike, pickerel	3 oz	72	0.5	na	0	7
Pike, walleye	3 oz	79	1	0.2	0	7
Orange roughy	3 oz	55	0.3	0.1	0	7
Salmon, chinook	3 oz	153	8.9	2.1	0	2
Salmon, chum	3 oz	102	3.2	0.7	0	6
Salmon, coho	3 oz	124	5.1	0.9	0	3
Salmon, pink	3 oz	99	2.9	0.5	0	6
Salmon, sockeye	3 oz	143	7.3	1.3	0	3
Sardine (2 canned)	3 oz	50	2.8	0.4	0	6
Trout, rainbow	3 oz	167	10	0.6	0	1
Tuna, albacore	3 oz	87	2.6	na	0	6
FISH EGGS						
Caviar, black & red	3 oz (1 tablespoon)	40	2.9	na	0	6
Roe (mixed species)	3 oz	39	1.8	0.4	0	7
SHELLFISH						
Clams (4 large, 9 small)	3 oz	63	0.8	0.1	0	7
Crab, Alaska king	3 oz	71	0.5	na	0	7
Crab, blue	3 oz	74	0.9	0.2	0	7
Crab, Dungeness	3 oz	73	0.8	0.1	0	7
Lobster	3 oz	77	0.8	na	0	7
Oysters ckd (6 medium)	3 oz	117	4.2	1.1	0	5
Scallops (6 large, 14 small)	3 oz	75	0.6	0.1	0	7
Shrimp (12 large)	3 oz	90	1.5	0.3	0	7
GAME						
Rabbit	3 oz	183	8.6	na	0	2
Venison, lean	3 oz	107	3.4	2.1	0	5
Beaver	3 oz	211	11.6	na	0	1
Opossum	3 oz	189	8.7	na	0	2
Raccoon	3 oz	255	12.4	na	0	1
Reindeer	3 oz	108	3.3	na	0	6
Turtle	3 oz	91	0.6	na	0	7

Food	Portion	Calories	Fat	Sat Fat	Fiber	Rating
POULTRY						
Chicken, breast (no skin)	3 oz	140	3	0.8	0	6
Chicken, breast (skin)	3 oz	167	6.6	1.9	0	2
Chicken, leg (no skin)	3 oz	163	7	1.9	0	2
Chicken, leg (skin)	3 oz	198	11.4	3.1	0	1
Duck (no skin)	3 oz	171	9.5	3.5	0	2
Duck (skin)	3 oz	287	24.1	8.2	0	0
Goose (no skin)	3 oz	202	10.7	3.9	0	1
Goose (skin)	3 oz	260	18.6	5.8	0	0
Pheasant (no skin)	3 oz	114	3	1	0	6
Pheasant (skin)	3 oz	130	4.4	na	0	5
Quail (no skin)	3 oz	115	3.8	1	0	5
Quail (with skin)	3 oz	198	12	3	0	1
Turkey, light (no skin)	3 oz	133	2.7	0.8	0	6
Turkey, light (skin)	3 oz	169	7.1	2	0	2
Turkey, dark (no skin)	3 oz	159	6.1	2	0	2
Turkey, dark (skin)	3 oz	189	9.8	3	0	2
Turkey, ground, Louis Rich	3 oz	183	10.5	3.6	0	2
Turkey, ground, extra lean, Mr. Turkey	3 oz	90	1.1	0.4	0	6

Nuts and Seeds

Food	Portion	Calories	Fat	Sat Fat	Fiber	Rating
Almond butter, plain	1 tablespoon	101	9.5	1.0	2.5	3
Almonds, assorted. varieties, 25 nuts, blue diamond	¼ cup	150	14	1.0	2.5	3
Almonds, unsalted	1 cup	910	76.5	7	4.3	
Beechnuts, dried	¼ cup	164	14.2	1.6	2.6	3
Brazil, dried, shelled	¼ cup	186	18.8	5.6	2.2	3
Butternuts, dried	¼ cup	174	16.2	0.4	2.4	3
Cashew butter, salt added, Marantha	1 tablespoon	105	8	1.6	3	2
Cashews, roasted/salted, 18 nuts, planters	¼ cup	170	14	3.1	1	1
Chestnuts, Chinese, dried	¼ cup	103	0.5	0	2.2	8
Chestnuts, Chinese, fresh	¼ cup	64	0.3	0	2.2	8
Chestnuts, roasted	¼ cup	68	0.3	0	2.2	8
Filberts/hazelnuts, roasted, salted	½ cup	477	45.8	3.2	6.1	3
Flax seed, linseed	1 oz	101	9.8	1.0	1.3	2
Hazelnuts, Oregon	1 oz	166	17	1.0	3.9	3
Hickory, dried	1 oz	187	18.3	2.1	2.4	3
Macadamia, oil roasted, 12 nuts, Mauna Loa	1 oz	200	21	na	3	2

Food	Portion	Calories	Fat	Sat Fat	Fiber	Rating
Mixed, roasted/salted, 20 nuts, Planters	1 oz	200	18	2.4	2	2
Peanuts, honey roasted, 35 nuts, Eagle	1 oz	180	14	2.5	2	2
Peanuts, roasted, 35 nuts	1 oz	166	14	2.5	2	2
Peanuts, roasted/salted, 53 nuts, planters	1 oz	180	14	2.5	2	2
Pecans, roasted	1 oz	195	20.2	1.7	2.2	2
Pistachios, natural/red, 22 nuts, Trader Joe's	1 oz	170	12	2.0	3	2
Pumpkin/squash seeds, roasted and salted	1 oz	148	12	1.0	3.9	3
Sesame butter (tahini), Westbrae organic	2 tablespoons	200	17	na	3	2
Sesame seed, roasted, whole	1 oz	161	13.6	2.0	5.3	4
Soybean kernels, roasted	1 cup	489	25.9	2.7	9.2	5
Sunflower kernels, roasted	½ cup	385	33.5	3.7	4.6	2
Walnuts, black/Persian/English	½ cup	380	35.3	3.7	2.4	2

NUT SPREADS

Food	Portion	Calories	Fat	Sat Fat	Fiber	Rating
Peanut butter, creamy	2 tablespoons	190	16	3	2	2
Peanut butter, crunchy	2 tablespoons	190	16	3	2	2
Peanut butter, reduced fat, Jiffy	2 tablespoons	190	12	3	2	2
Peanut wonder, Tree of Life	2 tablespoons	100	3	0.5	1	4

Fats and Oils

Food	Portion	Calories	Fat	Sat Fat	Fiber	Rating
Beef tallow	1 tablespoon	126	14	6.8	0	0
Butter	1 pat	36	4	2.5	0	0
Butter	1 tablespoon	100	11	7	0	0
Cooking spray, olive oil	1 serving	0	0	0	0	10
Flax seed, oil, unfiltered	1 tablespoon	115	14	1	1	0
Ghee (clarified butter of India)	1 oz	250	28	na	0	0
Margarine, corn oil, tub	1 tablespoon	102	12	3	0	0
Molly McButter	1 serving	8	0	0	0	10

OILS

Food	Portion	Calories	Fat	Sat Fat	Fiber	Rating
Canola	1 tablespoon	120	14	1	0	0
Corn	1 tablespoon	120	14	2	0	0
Olive oil	1 tablespoon	119	14	1	0	0
Palm kernel	1 tablespoon	106	12	3.1	0	0
Shortening	1 tablespoon	120	14	7	0	0

Beverages

Food	Portion	Calories	Fat	Sat Fat	Fiber	Rating
ALCOHOL						
Beer, light	12 fl oz	100	0	0	0	3
Beer, non-alcoholic	12 fl oz	60	0	0	0	4
Beer, regular	12 fl oz	146	0	0	0	3
Gin	1½ oz	110	0	0	0	3
Rum	1½ oz	97	0	0	0	3
Vodka	1½ oz	97	0	0	0	3
Whiskey	1½ oz	105	0	0	0	3
Wine Cooler, original Bartles & Jaymes	12 fl oz	190	0	0	0	3
Wine, dessert	2 fl oz	90	0	0	0	3
Wine, red	3½ fl oz	74	0	0	0	3
Wine, white	3½ fl oz	70	0	0	0	3
BREAKFAST DRINKS						
Carnation						
Instant Breakfast Café Mocha, as prepared	1 package	220	1	0	1	4
Instant Breakfast Café Mocha	1 can	220	3	1	0	4
Instant Breakfast, French Vanilla	1 package	130	0	0	0	4
COFFEE						
Cappuccino, Grande, Lowfat Milk, Starbucks	1 serving	110	4	3	0	0
Coffee	6 fl oz	4	0	0	0	3
Coffee, decaffeinated	6 fl oz	4	0	0	0	4
Espresso, Solo, Starbucks	1 serving	5	0	0	0	3
Latte, short w/ skim milk	1 serving	60	0	0	0	4
Latte, short w/ whole milk	1 serving	100	5	3	0	0
JUICE						
Apple juice, frozen, prepared	8 fl oz	111	0	0	0	6
Apple, Mott's natural	8 fl oz	120	0	0	0	6
Apple cider	8 fl oz	124	0	0	0	6
Apricot nectar	8 fl oz	141	0	0	2	9
Carrot juice, Hollywood	6 fl oz	80	0	0	2	9
Cranapple, Ocean Spray	8 fl oz	160	0	0	0	4

Food	Portion	Calories	Fat	Sat Fat	Fiber	Rating
Cranberry Cocktail, Ocean Spray	8 fl oz	140	0	0	0	4
Cranberry Cocktail, reduced calorie, Ocean Spray	8 fl oz	50	0	0	0	4
Cranberry Juice, Apple & Eve	6 fl oz	100	0	0	0	4
Grapefruit juice, fresh	8 fl oz	96	0	0	0	6
Orange juice, fresh	8 fl oz	111	0	0	0	6
Orange juice, frozen conc., diluted	8 fl oz	120	0	0	0	6
Papaya nectar	8 fl oz	142	0	0	0	5
Pineapple juice, canned	8 fl oz	139	0	0	0	6
Prune juice, Del Monte	8 fl oz	170	0	0	1	8
Tomato juice, Campbell's	6 fl oz	40	0	0	0	5
Tomato juice, Hunt's	8 fl oz	50	0	0	1	7
Vegetable Juice, V8	6 fl oz	35	0	0	0	9

MILK

Food	Portion	Calories	Fat	Sat Fat	Fiber	Rating
Milk—see Dairy				0	0	4

DIET SUPPLEMENT

Food	Portion	Calories	Fat	Sat Fat	Fiber	Rating
Slim Fast, Ultra Chocolate Coyote	11 fl oz	230	3	0	5	8

SOFT DRINKS, CARBONATED

Food	Portion	Calories	Fat	Sat Fat	Fiber	Rating
Soda, diet	12 fl oz	2	0	0	0	3
Soda, regular	12 fl oz	151	0	0	0	4

SOFT DRINKS, NON-CARBONATED

Food	Portion	Calories	Fat	Sat Fat	Fiber	Rating
Juicy Juice, Apple Grape	8.45 oz	120	0	0	0	6
Hi-C, Koolaid, Wyler's	8 fl oz	130	0	0	0	4
Minute Maid, Juices To Go Citrus Punch	11.5 oz	180	0	0	0	4
Lemonade, Minute Maid	8 fl oz	110	0	0	0	4
Crystal Light	12 fl oz	2	0	0	0	3

TEA

Food	Portion	Calories	Fat	Sat Fat	Fiber	Rating
Brewed, Lipton	6 fl oz	2	0	0	0	3

Soups

Food	Portion	Calories	Fat	Sat Fat	Fiber	Rating
Asparagus	1 cup	173	8.2	0	0.6	2
Bean, black	1 cup	235	3.4	0	4.6	8
Bean, Spicy with Couscous, Dry, Health Valley	⅓ cup	130	0	0	5	9
Bean, turtle	1 cup	218	0.7	0	4.3	9
Bean, turtle, boiled	1 cup	241	0.6	0	3.3	9
Bean, Vegetable, Fat Free, Health Valley	1 cup	110	0	0	12	10
Bean, Zesty with Rice, Health Valley	⅓ cup	100	0	0	4	8
Bean, Five Vegetable, Chunky, Health Valley	1 cup	140	0	0	13	10
Bean, Navy, Dry, Knorr	1 package	140	0	0	5	9
Bean with bacon	1 cup	347	11.9	0	9.2	4
Beef, Country Vegetable, Chunky, Single Serve, Campbell's	1 can	200	5	0	4	4
Beef, Oriental Ramen, Maruchan	½ package	190	8	0	1	2
Beef, Sirloin/Country Vegetable, Chunky, Campbell's	1 cup	190	9	0	4	4
Beef noodle	1 cup	84	3.1	0	1.5	4
Broccoli, Cream of, Healthy Request, Campbell's	1 cup	140	4	0	2	4
Broccoli Carotene Soup, Super, Health Valley	1 cup	70	0	0	7	10
Broth, chicken	1 cup	39	1	0	na	4
Broth, beef	1 cup	16	1	0	na	4
Broth, vegetable	9.25 fluid oz	20	1	0	na	4
Broth, Beef, Swanson's	7.25 fl oz	18	1	0	0	4
Broth, Chicken, Swanson's	7.25 fl oz	30	2	0	0	4
Broth, Vegetable, Swanson's	7.25 fl oz	20	1	0	0	6
Celery, Cream of, Campbell's	1 cup	220	14	0	2	2
Cheese	1 cup	155	10.5	0	2	2
Cheese, prepared with milk	1 cup	230	14.6	0	2	2
Chicken, Country Vegetable, Campbell's	1 cup	150	4	0	1.6	3
Chicken, Cream of, Campbell's	1 cup	260	16	0	2	2
Chicken, Cream	1 cup	233	14.7	0	0.5	2
Chicken Alphabet, Campbell's	1 cup	160	2	0	2	4
Chicken Chunky, Ready to Eat	1 cup	178	6.6	0	0.8	2
Chicken Corn Chowder, Chunky Soup, Campbell's	1 cup	250	15	0	3	2

Food	Portion	Calories	Fat	Sat Fat	Fiber	Rating
Chicken & Dumplings, with Milk	1 cup	96	5.5	0	0.7	2
Chicken Gumbo, Campbell's	1 cup	120	3	0	2	4
Chicken Minestrone, Tuscany, Home Style, Campbell's	1 cup	160	7	0	5	6
Chicken Noodle	1 cup	150	4.6	0	1.5	2
Chicken Noodle, Chunky Soup, Campbell's	1 cup	130	4	0	2	4
Chicken Noodle, Healthy Request, Campbell's	1 cup	160	3	0	2	4
Chicken Oriental Ramen, Maruchan	½ package	190	8	0	1	2
Chicken Pasta, Pritikin	1 slice	100	1	0	1	4
Chicken Pasta & Beans, Dry, Lipton	1 cup	110	1.5	0	3	6
Chicken Rice, Chunky Soup, Campbell's	1 cup	10	4	0	2	4
Chicken Rice, Healthy Choice	1 cup	100	3	0	3	6
Chicken Rice, Health Cookin', Campbell's	1 cup	120	4	0	1	4
Chicken Rice, Pritikin	1 cup	80	1	0	2	4
Chicken Vegetable	1 cup	149	5.7	0	1.5	3
Chili, Three Bean, Pritikin	1 cup	180	1	0	10	10
Chili Beef	1 cup	339	13.2	0	10	5
Clam Chowder, Manhattan, Progresso	1 cup	110	2	0	3	4
Clam Chowder, New England, Healthy Choice	1 cup	140	1	0	7	8
Corn Chowder	1 cup	153	2.7	0	1.8	4
Corn Chowder with Tomatoes, Healthy Valley	½ cup	90	0	0	3	6
Corn & Vegetable, Country, Fat Free, Health Valley	1 cup	70	0	0	7	8
Fiesta Nacho Cheese, Campbell's	1 cup	280	16	0	4	3
French Onion, Campbell's	1 cup	140	5	0	2	3
Garlic & Pasta, Healthy Classics, Progresso	1 cup	100	1.5	0	3	4
Lentil, Nile Spice	1 package	180	1.5	0	3	4
Lentil, Pritikin	1 cup	130	<1	0	8	10
Lentil & Carrot, Fat Free, Health Valley	1 cup	90	0	0	14	10
Lentil with Couscous, Health Valley	⅓ cup	130	0	0	5	9
Minestrone, Lipton	1 cup	110	2	0	4	8
Minestrone, Fat Free, Health Valley	1 cup	80	0	0	11	10
Minestrone, Pritikin	1 cup	90	1	0	3	9
Mushroom with Beef Stock	1 cup	171	8.1	0	0.6	2

Food	Portion	Calories	Fat	Sat Fat	Fiber	Rating
Mushroom, Cream of	1 cup	220	14	0	2	2
Noodle, Chicken Flavored with Vegetables, Health Valley	⅓ cup	100	0	0	4	8
Onion, dehydrated	1 cup	27	0.6	0	0.7	4
Pasta Italiano, Health Valley	½ cup	140	0	0	3	8
Pea, green	1 cup	165	2.9	0	4.8	8
Pork, Oriental Ramen, Maruchan	½ package	190	8	0	1	2
Potato, cream of, with milk	1 cup	148	6.5	0	0.5	3
Potato, creamy with broccoli, Health Valley	⅓ cup	70	0	0	2	4
Red Beans & Rice, Nile Spice	1 package	190	1.5	0	3	4
Shrimp, cream of	1 cup	180	10.4	0	0.3	2
Split Pea, Garden, with Carrots, Health Valley	½ cup	130	0	0	2	4
Split Pea, Healthy Classics Progresso	1 cup	180	2.5	0	5	9
Split Pea, Pritikin	1 cup	140	<1	0	10	10
Split Pea, Yellow	1 cup	379	8.8	0	8.6	7
Split Pea & Carrot, Fat Free, Health Valley	1 cup	110	0	0	4	4
Split Pea with Ham, Chunky Soup	1 cup	185	4	0	6	6
Steak & Potato, Chunky Soup, Campbell's	1 cup	160	4	0	3	4
Tomato Vegetable, Fat Free, Health Valley	1 cup	80	0	0	5	9
Turkey, Chunky, Ready to Serve	1 cup	135	4.4	0	2.5	4
Vegetable, 14 Garden, Fat Free, Health Valley	1 cup	80	0	0	4	4
Vegetable, Campbell's	1 cup	180	2	0	4	4
Vegetable, Hearty, Pritikin	1 cup	90	0.5	0	3	4
Vegetable, Homestyle, Dry, Mrs. Grass	½ package	70	0	0	2	4
Vegetable, Vegetarian, Pritikin	1 cup	100	0	0	3	4
Vegetable Barley, Fat Free, Health Valley	1 cup	90	0	0	4	4
Vegetable Beef, Campbell's	1 cup	160	4	0	4	4
Vegetable Power Carotene, Health Valley	1 cup	70	0	0	6	8
Vegetable with Pasta, Chunky Soup, Campbell's	1 cup	130	3	0	3	6
Vegetarian	1 cup	144	3.9	0	2.4	5

Prepared Foods

Food	Portion	Calories	Fat	Sat Fat	Fiber	Rating
BREAKFAST						
ROMAN MEAL						
Breakfast Sandwich						
with cheese & sausage	1	394	24	10	na	2
with egg, cheese & bacon	1	487	31	12	na	2
with egg, cheese &						
Canadian bacon	1	383	20	9	na	2
MORNINGSTAR FARMS						
Bagel Scramblers,						
pattie & cheese	1 (5.9 oz)	320	5	1	4	7
English muffin,						
Scrambler & pattie	1 (5.1 oz)	240	3	1	5	10
English muffin,						
Scrambler, pattie & cheese	1 (6 oz)	280	3	1	5	10
Breakfast patties	1	70	3	1	2	8
Breakfast Sandwich Muffin:						
pattie, cheese, Scramblers	1	280	3	1	5	8

Frozen Foods

Food	Portion	Calories	Fat	Sat Fat	Fiber	Rating
VEGETARIAN ENTREES						
Gnocchi (potato dumplings)						
raw, Bernardi	1 oz	60	0	na	0.3	4
Fettucini Alfredo,						
Linda McCartney's	1 package	520	18	na	5	4
Pasta & Garden Vegetable,						
Light Balance	1	190	1	na	5.4	8
Pasta Primavera, Ultra Slim Fast	1	340	9	na	4.2	2
Rigatoni Pomodoro Italiano,						
Michelina's	1 package	290	8	na	4	2
Sizzle Burger, Loma Linda	1 pattie	200	12	na	6	4
Vegetable, 3 Cheese, Kraft	1 cup	360	16	na	3.7	4
Vegetable Lasagna, Le Menu						
Frozen Dinner	1	400	24	na	5.1	2
ADVANTAGE 10						
Caribbean Sweet and Sour	10 oz	280	3	2	12	10

Food	Portion	Calories	Fat	Sat Fat	Fiber	Rating
Mediterranean pasta	10 oz	230	2	0	11	10
Mushroom burger	1 pattie	130	2	1	5	10
Pasta Santa Fe	10 oz	230	2	1	11	10
Roasted Vegetable Pizza	1 slice	210	3	0	6	10
Southwestern Style Burger	1 pattie	140	1	0	3	8
Vegetarian Pepperoni Pizza	1 slice	250	3	1	7	10
Vegetable Szechwan	10 0z	250	3	1	8	10
AMY'S KITCHEN						
Asian Noodle Stir Fry	10 oz	240	5	1	6	10
Black Bean and						
Vegetable Enchilada	9.5 oz	130	4	0	2	5
Canneloni with Vegetables	9.5 oz	330	12	8	6	5
Chili and Cornbread	10.5 oz	320	6	2	8	10
Mexican Tamale Pie	8 oz	220	3	0	11	10
Ravioli with cheese	8 oz	320	12	7	3	3
Bean, rice and cheese burrito	6 oz	280	8	3	6	6
Shepherd's Pie	8 oz	160	4	0	5	10
Tofu vegetable lasagna	9.5 oz	300	10	1	6	5
Vegetarian Pizza Pocket Sandwich	4 ½ oz	260	6	3	4	5
Whole Meals Country Dinner	1 package	380	12	4	9	5
HEALTHY CHOICE						
Cheese Ravioli Parmigiana	1 package	250	4	2	6	10
Macaroni & cheese	1 package	290	5	2	4	6
Three cheese manicotti	1 package	310	9	5	7	5
Vegetable Pasta Italiano	1 package	220	1	0	6	10
Zucchini lasagna	1 package	330	2	1	11	10
LEAN CUISINE						
Angel hair pasta	1 package	220	3	1	6	10
Bow Tie Pasta & Creamy						
Tomato Sauce	1 package	260	6	2	6	10
Cheddar Bake w/ Pasta	1 package	220	6	3	3	10
Fettucini Primavera	1 package	270	7	3	2	0
Five cheese lasagna	8 oz	210	4	2	4	7
Penne pasta w/ tomato basil sauce	1package	270	4	1	5	10
MORNINGSTAR/WORTHINGTON						
Better 'n Burgers, meatless	1 pattie	70	0	0	3	10
Better 'n Eggs, meatless	¼ cup	20	0	0	0	5
Bolono (meatless bologna)	3 slices	80	4	na	2	5
Breakfast links, meatless	2 links	90	5	na	2	4
Breakfast Strips, meatless	2 strips	60	5	na	1	2
Chik Nuggets	4 nuggets	160	4	1	5	6
Chik Patties	1	150	6	1	2	4
Deli Franks, Meatless	1 link	110	7	na	2	4

Food	Portion	Calories	Fat	Sat Fat	Fiber	Rating
Ground Meatless Crumbles	½ cup	60	0	0	2	8
Ground Meatless Vegetarian Beef	½ cup	80	3	na	3	8
Garden Veggie Patties	1 pattie	100	3	1	4	10
Prime Patties	1 pattie	130	5	na	3	5
Spicy Black Bean Burger	1 pattie	110	1	0	5	9
Smoked turkey slices, meatless	3 slice	140	10	na	2	4
Stripples, meatless	2 strips	60	5	na	3	4
Vegetarian beef pie	1 pie	410	24	na	6	4
Vegetarian chicken pie	1 pie	450	27	na	8	4
Vegetarian egg rolls	1 roll	180	8	na	2	4
STOUFFER'S						
Enchiladas, cheese, Stouffer's	1 serving	590	40	na	8	4
Fiesta Lasagna, Stouffer's	1 serving	430	22	na	4	0
Five cheese lasagna	1 package	360	13	7	6	2
Macaroni & cheese	1 cup	320	16	7	3	0
Vegetable lasagna, Stouffer's	1 serving	440	20	8	5	0
WEIGHT WATCHERS						
Angel hair marinara	1 package	170	2	0	4	8
Fettucini Alfredo w/Broccoli	1 package	230	6	3	3	4
Garden Lasagna, Weight Watchers	1 package	230	7	na	6	6
Pasta Penne with Sun Dried Tomatoes, Weight Watchers	1 package	290	9	3	4	0

FROZEN PIZZA

CHEESE

Food	Portion	Calories	Fat	Sat Fat	Fiber	Rating
Crisp & Tasty, Jeno's	1 serving	270	11	3.6	2.1	4
Microwave, Pillsbury	1 serving	240	10	na	2	4
Party, Totino's	1 serving	320	14	5.0	2.7	4

COMBINATION

Food	Portion	Calories	Fat	Sat Fat	Fiber	Rating
Microwave, Pillsbury	1 serving	310	15	na	2.3	4
Party, Totino's	1 serving	380	21	4.5	2.7	4

FRENCH BREAD

Food	Portion	Calories	Fat	Sat Fat	Fiber	Rating
Cheese, Lean Cuisine	1 serving	300	5	3	4	4
Cheese, Stouffer's	1 serving	370	16	6	3	0
Deluxe, Lean Cuisine	1 serving	300	6	3	4	4
Hamburger, Stouffer's	1 serving	410	19	na	1	0
Pepperoni, Lean Cuisine	1 serving	310	7	3	3	0
Pepperoni/Mushroom, Stouffer's	1 serving	440	20	7	5	0
Vegetable Deluxe, Stouffer's	1 serving	380	16	6	4	0
Golden Topping, Fox Deluxe	1 serving	240	11	na	2	0
Hamburger, Party, Totino's	1 serving	370	19	na	1	0
Party Pizza, Totino's	½ pie	380	21	na	2	0

Food	Portion	Calories	Fat	Sat Fat	Fiber	Rating
Pepperoni, Red Baron	⅕ pie	360	19	na	2	0
Sausage, Stouffer's	1 serving	420	18	7	3	0
Sausage, Party, Totino's	1 serving	390	21	na	3	0
Sausage & Pepperoni, Tombstone	⅕ pie	320	16	7	2	0
Spicy Chicken, Wolfgang Puck	½ pie	360	16	na	5	0
Supreme, Light, Tombstone	⅕ pie	270	9	4	3	0
Supreme Thin, Tombstone	¼ pie	380	22	10	2	0
Supreme, Tombstone	⅕ pie	320	16	7	2	0
Vegetable, Light, Tombstone	⅕ pie	240	7	3	3	0
Vegetable, Party, Totino's	1 serving	300	13	na	3.1	0
Pizza Rolls, Jeno's	1 serving	250	13	na	1.6	0

FROZEN DINNERS WITH MEAT

ARMOUR

Food	Portion	Calories	Fat	Sat Fat	Fiber	Rating
Classics Chicken Parmigiana	1 meal	360	18	6	7	4
Classics Chicken & Noodles	1 meal	280	9	5	6	4
Classics Chicken Mesquite	1 meal	280	13	4	5	3
Classics Meatloaf	1 meal	300	10	5	7	4
Classics Salisbury Steak	1 meal	330	18	8	4	2
Classics Lite Beef Pepper	1 meal	210	4	2	5	6
Classics Lite Chicken Burgundy	1 meal	210	5	2	4	6
Classics Lite Salisbury Steak	1 meal	260	7	4	6	4
Classics Lite Shrimp Creole	1 meal	220	1	0	16	
Classics Lite Sweet & Sour Chicken	1 meal	220	1	0	4	6

BANQUET

Food	Portion	Calories	Fat	Sat Fat	Fiber	Rating
Chicken & Dumplings	1 meal	260	8	3	16	
Extra Helping Fried Chicken	1 meal	790	39	9	8	4
Extra Helping Turkey Dinner	1 meal	560	20	5	7	4
Family Entrée Beef Stew	1 serving	160	4	2	4	4
Family Entrée Gravy and Sliced Turkey	1 serving	100	5	2	0	0
Family Entrée Veal Parmigiana	1 serving	230	14	4	2	4
Family Entrée Gravy & Sliced Beef	1 serving	100	3	2	0	4
Hot Sandwich Toppers Sloppy Joe	1 meal	140	7	3	1	0
Mexican Style Meal	1 package	340	13	5	10	5

BIRDS EYE

Food	Portion	Calories	Fat	Sat Fat	Fiber	Rating
Easy Recipe Meal Starter Orange Glaze Chicken, as prepared	1 serving	280	8	2	2	4
Easy Recipe Meal Starter, Southwestern	1 serving	280	8	2	2	4

BUDGET GOURMET

Food	Portion	Calories	Fat	Sat Fat	Fiber	Rating
Beef Stroganoff	1 meal	260	10	5	na	
Chicken Marsala	1 meal	260	8	na	na	na

Food	Portion	Calories	Fat	Sat Fat	Fiber	Rating
Chinese Style Vegetables and Chicken	1 meal	220	9	4	na	na
Glazed Turkey	1 meal	260	5	2	na	na
Oriental Beef	1 meal	290	8	3	na	na
Pot Roast Beef	1 meal	230	7	3	na	na
Swedish Meatballs with Noodles	1 meal	590	38	na	na	na
Teriyaki Chicken Breast	1 meal	300	8	1	na	na
HEALTHY CHOICE						
Beef Tips Francais	1 meal	280	5	2	4	6
Chicken Cantonese	1 meal	210	1	0	5	7
Chicken Dijon	1 meal	280	4	2	9	8
Chicken Picante	1 meal	220	2	2	6	8
Classics Mesquite Beef Barbecue	1 meal	310	4	2	6	8
Classics Salisbury Steak	1 meal	260	6	3	5	6
Country Roast Turkey with Mushrooms	1 meal	220	4	1	3	6
Country Turkey & Pasta	1 meal	300	4	2	6	8
Lemon Pepper Fish	1 meal	290	5	1	7	8
LE MENU						
Beef Stroganoff	10 oz	430	24	na	na	na
Chicken Cordon Bleu	11 oz	460	20	na	na	na
Entrée LightStyle Chicken Dijon	8 oz	240	7	na	na	na
Entrée LightStyle Traditional Turkey	8 oz	200	5	na	na	na
Pepper Steak	11½ oz	370	13	na	na	na
Salisbury Steak	10½ oz	370	20	na	na	na
Sweet & Sour Chicken	11¼ oz	400	18	na	na	na
LEAN CUISINE						
American Favorite Baked Chicken	1 package	230	4	2	5	6
American Favorite Baked Fish	1 package	270	6	2	3	6
American Favorite Beef Pot Roast	1 package	210	6	2	6	8
American Favorite Beef Tips Barbecue	1 package	290	6	2	7	8
Café Classics Chicken Carbonara	1 package	280	8	2	2	3
Café Classics Chicken Piccata	1 package	270	6	2	2	5
Café Classics Glazed Turkey	1 package	240	5	1	5	6
Café Classics Sirloin Beef Peppercorn	1 package	220	7	2	2	3
Mandarin Chicken	1 package	250	4	1	3	6
Stuffed cabbage with whipped potatoes	1 package	170	5	2	5	6

Food	Portion	Calories	Fat	Sat Fat	Fiber	Rating
STOUFFER'S						
Baked chicken breast with mashed potatoes	1 serving	330	14	5	3	2
Chicken a la king	1 package	350	13	4	2	2
Creamed chipped beef	½ cup	160	11	3	1	0
Escalloped chicken & noodles	1 package	430	27	5	3	1
Glazed chicken with rice	1 serving	290	6	1	2	5
Homestyle Fish Filet with Macaroni & Cheese	1 package	430	21	5	2	1
Homestyle Fried Chicken and Whipped Potatoes	1 package	310	12	4	5	3
Homestyle Meatloaf and Whipped Potatoes	1 package	330	16	6	3	2
SWANSON'S						
Beef in Barbecue Sauce	11 oz	460	17	na	na	na
Fish 'n' Chips	10 oz	500	21	na	na	na
Fried Chicken White Meat	10 ¼ oz	550	25	na	na	na
Homestyle Chicken Cacciatore	10.95 oz	260	8	na	na	na
Homestyle Seafood Creole with Rice	9 oz	240	6	na	na	na
Hungry Man Boneless Chicken	17 ¾ oz	700	28	na	na	na
Hungry Man Salisbury Steak	16 ½ oz	680	41	na	na	na
Hungry Man Sliced Beef	15 ¼ oz	450	12	na	na	na
Macaroni & Beef Meatloaf	12 oz	370	15	na	na	na
Meat Loaf	10 ¾oz	360	15	na	na	na
TYSON						
Chicken Picante	1 package	250	4	na	na	na
Grilled Chicken	1 package	220	3	na	na	na
Healthy Portions BBQ Chicken	1 package	400	8	na	na	na
Health Portions Italian Style Chicken	1 package	310	4	na	na	na
Honey Roasted Chicken	1 package	220	4	na	na	na
WEIGHT WATCHERS						
Smart One Grilled Salisbury Steak	1 package	260	10	5	3	2
Smart Ones Lemon Herb Chicken Piccata	1 package	200	2	1	3	6
Smart Ones Risotto with Cheese and Mushrooms	1 package	290	8	4	4	3
Smart Ones Shrimp Marinara	1 package	290	2	1	4	6
Smart Ones Stuffed Turkey Breast	1 package	260	7	2	5	4

Non-Frozen Entrees and Meals

Food	Portion	Calories	Fat	Sat Fat	Fiber	Rating
ABCs & 123s, Mini Meatballs, Chef Boyardee	7.5 oz	260	11	4	2	3
Beans & Weiners, Beanee Weenee, Van Camp's	1 cup	405	18	na	11	5
Beef Chow Mein/Chop Suey	1 cup	465	25	na	4	4
Beef potpie, Home Recipe, ⅓ of pie	1 slice	515	30	na	4	4
Beef ravioli, Chef Boyardee	7.5 oz	190	4	2	2	6
Beef stew, Dinty Moore	1 cup	230	14	na	2	2
Beef stew with vegetables	1 cup	220	11	na	3	4
Beefaroni, Chef Boyardee	1 cup	280	7	na	5	4
Cheese ravioli/in meat sauce, Chef Boyardee	7.5 oz	200	3	1	na	na
Chicken a la king, cooked home recipe	1 cup	470	34	na	1	1
Chicken & Cashew Take Out Cuisine	1 serving	440	17	na	2	1
Chicken & Dumplings, Luck's	1 serving	260	12	na	4	3
Chicken & Dumplings, Microwave, Luck's	1 serving	170	2	na	2	1
Chicken & Potatoes, Microwave, Luck's	1 serving	190	4	na	3	6
Chicken & Rice, Microwave, Luck's	1 serving	150	2	na	2	5
Chicken chow mein, canned	1 cup	95	1	0	3	8
Chicken chow mein, home recipe	1 cup	255	10	4	1	1
Chicken, fried, & potatoes	1 cup	431	21	na	3	2
Chicken potpie, baked, home recipe	1 slice	545	31	na	4	2
Chili, Beef & Beans, Hormel	1 cup	340	17	na	9	4
Chili with beans	1 cup	330	15	na	14	4
Chili con carne with beans	1 cup	290	9	na	13	4
Chili, No Beans, Hormel	1 cup	410	30	na	3	2
Chili Mac, Macaroni with Beef in Chili, Chef Boyardee	1 cup	260	11	na	8	4
Chimichanga, beef	1	425	20	na	4	3
Corn dog, plain	1	460	19	na	3	2
Corn beef hash, Libby's	1 cup	490	36	na	9	4
Enchirito, Cheese/Beef/Bean	1	344	16	na	3	2
Fajita, beef	1 serving	244	10	na	2	2
Fajita, chicken	1 serving	170	3	na	2	6

Food	Portion	Calories	Fat	Sat Fat	Fiber	Rating
Fettucine, Hearty Meat Sauce, Chef Boyardee	1 cup	230	6	na	4	6
Haddock, breaded/fried	1 slice	140	5	na	0	0
Fish cakes, fried	1 cup	361	17	na	3	1
Hot dog, plain with bun	1	242	15	na	1	0
Lasagna, Chef Boyardee	7.5 oz	230	9	na	0	0
Meatloaf with celery & onions	1 serving	213	14	na	0	0
Pork & beans, baked, canned	1 cup	268	4	na	14	8
Pork & beans with frankfurters, canned	1 cup	365	17	na	13	5
Pork & beans in tomato sauce, canned Van Camp's	1 cup	220	3	na	12	8
Pork chow mein/chop suey with noodles	1 oz	56	3	na	0	2
Ravioli, Beef & Garlic, Fresh, Contadina	1 cup	280	11	na	2	2
Rigatoni, Chef Boyardee	7.5 oz	210	6	na	4	2
Salmon rice loaf	1 cup	256	10	na	1	0
Shrimp, french fried	1 serving	206	10	na	0	0
Spaghetti/tomato/meat, home recipe	1 cup	330	12	na	3	2
Spaghetti/tomato/meat, canned	1 cup	260	10	na	3	2
Spaghetti & meatballs, Chef Boyardee	7.5 oz	230	7	na	3	2
Spaghettio's/meatballs, Franco-American	1 cup	260	11	na	5	3
Spaghettio's/sliced franks, Franco-American	1 cup	260	11	na	4	3
Sportyo's pasta/meatballs/sauce, Franco-American	1 oz	29	1	na	0	2
Stew, Brunswick, microwave, Luck's	1 serving	150	1	na	3	6
Sweet & sour chicken, Take Out Cuisine	1 serving	410	8	na	2	2
Tamales, beef, Hormel	1	93	7	na	1	1
Tamales, chicken & cheese, Trader Joe's	1	270	13	na	3	2
Tortellini, chicken & vegetable, Contadina	1 cup	347	9	na	3	2
Tortellini, chicken & prosciutto, Contadina	1 cup	360	13	na	3	2
Tortellini in meat sauce, Chef Boyardee	1 cup	260	3	na	8	4
Tortellini, sweet Italian sausage, Contadina	1 cup	330	10	na	3	2
Turkey chili, Hormel	1 cup	190	3	na	3	6

Food	Portion	Calories	Fat	Sat Fat	Fiber	Rating
Turkey pot pie, baked, home prepared	1 cup	569	32	na	3	2
Turkey pot pie, frozen	1 cup	473	25	na	3	2
Turnip greens & diced turnips, seasoned, pork, Luck's	1 cup	180	10	na	8	4

HELPER COMBINATIONS
(Serving size reflects portion of prepared dish)

Food	Portion	Calories	Fat	Sat Fat	Fiber	Rating
Chicken Helper, Stir-fried Chicken, Skillet	1 cup	14	1	0	1	6
Hamburger Helper, Cheeseburger Macaroni	1 cup	170	4	na	1	3
Hamburger Helper, Hamburger Stew	1 cup	100	1	0	3	8
Hamburger Helper, Pizza Pasta with Cheese Topping	1 cup	150	2	na	1	5
Hamburger Helper, Three Cheese	1 cup	190	6	na	1	2
Hamburger Helper, Zesty Italian	1 cup	160	1	0	1	6
Tuna Helper, Creamy Noodle	1 cup	190	6	na	1	2
Tuna Helper, Fettucine Alfredo	1 cup	180	4	na	1	2
Tuna Helper Tetrazzini	1 cup	180	3	na	1	5
Tuna Helper, Tuna Pot Pie	1 pie	340	20	na	1	2
Tuna Helper, Tuna Salad	1 cup	165	1	0	2	5

PASTA COMBINATIONS

Food	Portion	Calories	Fat	Sat Fat	Fiber	Rating
ABCs & 123s in Sauce, Chef Boyardee	1 serving	160	1	0	3	8
Cheese Ravioli in Sauce, Chef Boyardee	1 cup	210	0	0	4	8
Lasagna, Chef Boyardee	1 serving	240	8	na	3	2
Macaroni & cheese, Chef Boyardee	1 cup	210	3	na	2	5
Macaroni & cheese, home recipe	1 cup	430	22	na	1	2
Macaroni & cheese, Kraft	1 cup	260	3	na	1	5
Macaroni shells, Chef Boyardee	1 serving	150	1	0	2	6
Mini Bites, Chef Boyardee	1 serving	260	12	na	1	2
Mini Canneloni, Chef Boyardee	1 serving	230	7	na	5	4
Noodles, Alfredo & Sauce, Farmhouse	1 cup	260	4	na	2	2
Noodles, Creamy Chicken/Sauce, Farmhouse	1 cup	240	2	0	2	6
Noodles, Herb/Butter & Sauce, Farmhouse	1 cup	240	2	na	1	5
Noodles, Parmesano & Sauce, Farmhouse	1 cup	260	3	na	2	6

Food	Portion	Calories	Fat	Sat Fat	Fiber	Rating
Noodles, Stroganoff & Sauce, Farmhouse	1 cup	240	3	na	2	6
Pasta in Pizza Sauce, PizzaO's, Franco-American	1 cup	210	3	na	2	6
Roller Coaster, Chef Boyardee	1 serving	230	10	na	3	2
Sir Chompsalot Ravioli, Tomato/ Cheese Sauce, Chef Boyardee	1 cup	210	0	0	5	7
Smurf Ravioli, Pasta/Sauce, Chef Boyardee	1 serving	230	5	na	6	5
Spaghetti, tomato sauce, cheese, canned	1 cup	190	2	na	8	8
Spaghetti, tomato sauce, cheese, home recipe	1 cup	260	9	na	3	2
Teddyo's in Cheese Sauce, Franco-American	1 cup	190	2	na	2	6
Tic Tac Toes, pasta-tomato/cheese flavored sauce, Chef Boyardee	1 cup	190	0	0	3	6
Tortellini, cheese in tomato sauce, Chef Boyardee	1 cup	230	1	0	5	6
Tortellini, cheese, fresh, Contadina	1 cup	347	8	na	3	3

RICE COMBINATIONS

Food	Portion	Calories	Fat	Sat Fat	Fiber	Rating
Beef, Farmhouse	1 cup	200	1	0	2	5
Broccoli au Gratin, Farmhouse	1 cup	210	2	0	2	5
Broccoli au Gratin, Dry, Rice-a-Roni	⅓ cup	270	6	na	2	5
Chicken Pilaf, Farmhouse	1 cup	190	2	0	3	6
Chicken, Farmhouse	1 cup	180	2	0	4	7
Chicken & Broccoli, Dry, Rice-a-Roni	⅓ cup	240	2	0	2	5
Fried Rice, Dry, Rice-a-Roni	⅓ cup	240	2	0	2	5
Herb & Butter, Farmhouse	1 cup	210	2	na	2	5
Mexican, Farmhouse	1 cup	180	1	0	3	6
Oriental, Fried, Farmhouse	1 cup	200	2	na	2	5
Oriental & Vegetable, Quick Meal, Spice Island	1 package	180	3	na	13	8
Pilaf, Farmhouse	1 cup	200	1	0	2	5
Saffron Yellow, Farmhouse	1 cup	190	1	0	4	6
Spanish Rice, Rice-a-Roni	⅓ cup	190	1	0	4	6
Spicy Black Bean Quick Meal, Spice Island	1 package	190	1	0	7	7
Traditional Long Grain & Wild, Farmhouse	1 cup	190	2	na	3	6
Whole Grain Quick Brown, Farmhouse	1 cup	160	2	na	3	6

Food	Portion	Calories	Fat	Sat Fat	Fiber	Rating
SALADS						
Caesar, Suddenly Salad	¾ cup	220	9	2	1	5
Carrot Raisin, Home Recipe	1 cup	306	12	0	17	5
Chef with Ham & Cheese	1 serving	196	13	na	2	2
Chicken	1 cup	502	36	na	2	2
Classic Pasta, Suddenly Salad	1 cup	227	1	0	1	5
Coleslaw	1 tablespoon	6	0	0	0	4
Crab	1 serving	145	9	na	0	2
Creamy Macaroni, Suddenly Salad	1 cup	227	1	0	1	5
Elbow Macaroni	3.5 oz	160	5	2	na	2
Fruit, Canned, Water Pack	1 cup	74	0	0	5	8
Gelatin, Mandarin Orange	1 serving	23	0	0	1	4
Green salad, tossed	1 serving	32	0	0	2	5
Lobster with tomato & egg	1 cup	211	13	na	2	2
Macaroni	1 serving	51	3	na	0	4
Pasta, Creamy Dill, Kraft	1 cup	400	22	na	1	1
Pasta, Garden Primavera, Kraft	1 cup	340	14	na	1	2
Pasta, Herb/Garlic, Kraft	¾ cup	280	14	2	2	2
Pasta, Homestyle, Kraft	1 cup	480	32	na	2	1
Pasta, Rancher's Choice, Kraft	1 cup	480	32	na	1	1
Ranch & Bacon, Suddenly Salad	1 cup	200	1	0	1	5
Taco	1 serving	279	15	na	3	3
Three Bean, canned, Green Giant	1 cup	140	0	0	6	8
Tuna/celery/mayonnaise/ pickle/egg	1 cup	350	22	na	1	1

Dining Out

Food	Portion	Calories	Fat	Sat Fat	Fiber	Rating
BREAKFAST						
ARBY'S						
Danish, Cinnamon Nut	1	360	11	1	1	0
Egg Portion	1 serving	95	8	2	0	0
Toastix	6 pieces	430	21	5	3	1
BURGER KING						
Biscuit	1 (3.3 oz)	330	18	4	1	0
Biscuit with bacon, egg & cheese	1 (6 oz)	510	31	10	1	0
Biscuit with egg	1 (5.3 oz)	420	24	6	1	0
Biscuit with sausage	1 (4.8 oz)	530	36	11	1	0
Croissan'wich sausage egg & cheese	1 (5.7 oz)	550	42	14	1	0

Food	Portion	Calories	Fat	Sat Fat	Fiber	Rating
Croissan'wich with						
sausage & cheese	1 (3.7 oz)	450	35	12	1	0
French Toast Sticks	1 (4.9 oz)	500	27	7	1	0
Hash browns	1 (2.6 oz)	240	15	6	2	0
CARL'S JR.						
Burrito, Breakfast	1 (5.3 oz)	430	26	12	0	0
Burrito, Breakfast,						
Quesadilla Cheese	1 (5.2 oz)	300	14	6	1	0
Eggs, scrambled 1 (3.5 oz)	160	11	4	0	0	
English Muffin with margarine	1 (2.6 oz)	230	10	2	2	0
French Toast Dips						
without syrup	1 (3.7 oz)	410	25	6	3	0
Hash brown nuggets	1 (3.3 oz)	270	17	4	2	0
Sausage	1 (1.8oz)	200	18	7	0	0
Sunrise Sandwich	1 (4.6 oz)	370	21	6	2	0
DENNY'S						
All American Slam	1 (15 oz)	1028	87	21	2	0
Bacon, Canadian	1 (3oz)	110	5	2	0	3
Biscuit with Sausage gravy	1 (7oz)	570	38	10	0	0
Country Scramble	1 (16 oz)	795	50	11	2	0
Egg Beaters	1 (2 oz)	134	12	3	0	0
Hash browns	1 (4 oz)	218	14	2	2	0
Hash browns, covered	1 (6 oz)	318	23	7	2	0
Hash browns, covered						
and smothered	1 (8 oz)	359	26	7	2	0
Oatmeal	1 (4 oz)	100	2	0	3	10
Omelette, cheddar cheese	1 (13 oz)	770	62	20	2	0
Omelette, Farmer's	1 (18 oz)	912	69	19	3	0
Omelette, Ham 'n' Cheddar	1 (14 oz)	743	55	10	2	0
Omelette, sausage cheddar	1 (16 oz)	1036	86	29	2	0
Omelette, Senior	1 (12 oz)	623	47	10	3	0
Omelette, Veggie Cheese	1 (16 oz)	714	53	10	4	0
Original Grand Slam	1 (10 oz)	795	50	14	2	0
Pancakes	3 (5 oz)	491	7	1	3	6
Senior Starter	1 (7 oz)	336	24	5	2	0
Slim Slam	1 (14 oz)	638	12	3	1	3
Southern Slam	1 (13 oz)	1065	84	23	0	0
Steak & eggs, Chicken Fried	1 (14 oz)	723	56	18	8	0
Steak & eggs, sirloin	1 (13 oz)	808	64	18	2	0
Steak, Porterhouse	1 (18 oz)	1223	95	32	2	0
Waffle	1 (6 oz)	304	21	3	0	0
HARDEE'S						
Biscuits						
Bacon egg & cheese	1	610	37	13	na	0

Food	Portion	Calories	Fat	Sat Fat	Fiber	Rating
Bacon & egg	1	570	33	11	na	0
Ham	1	400	20	6	na	0
Ham Egg & Cheese	1	540	30	11	na	0
IHOP						
Pancake, Buckwheat	1	134	5	1	1	2
Pancake, Buttermilk	1	108	3	1	0	4
Pancake, Harvest Grain & Nut	1	160	8	1	1	1
Waffle, Belgian	1	408	20	11	1	0
MCDONALD'S						
Biscuit, Bacon Egg & Cheese	1 (5.5 oz)	470	25	8	1	0
Biscuit, Sausage	1 (4.5 oz)	470	31	9	1	0
Biscuit, Sausage with egg	1 (6.2 oz)	550	37	10	1	0
Breakfast Burrito	1 (4.1 oz)	320	19	7	1	0
Egg McMuffin	1 (4.8 oz)	290	14	5	1	3
Hash Browns	1 (1.9 oz)	130	8	2	1	0
Hotcakes, Margarine & Syrup	2 (7.8 oz)	570	16	3	2	0
McMuffin, sausage with egg	1 (5.7 oz)	440	28	10	1	0
Scambled Eggs	2 (3.6 oz)	160	11	4	0	2
SHONEY'S						
Bun, cinnamon honey	1	344	12	na	0	0
Bun, honey	1	265	14	na	0	0
Cake, brunch sour cream	1 square	160	8	na	0	3
Croissant	1	260	16	na	0	0
Egg, fried	1	159	15	na	0	0
Egg, scrambled	¼ cup	95	7	na	0	3
Hash browns	¼ cup	43	2	na	0	4
Muffin, blueberry	1	107	4	na	1	5
Toast, buttered	2 slices	163	5	na	1	4

LUNCH, DINNER & DESSERT

Food	Portion	Calories	Fat	Sat Fat	Fiber	Rating
ARBY'S						
Beef, Roast Deluxe, Light	1	296	10	3	6	4
Beef 'n' Cheddar, Roast	1	487	28	9	2	0
Beef, Regular Roast	1	388	19	7	2	0
Chicken Deluxe, Light	1	276	6	2	4	6
Chicken Salad, Light Roast	1 serving	149	2	1	5	6
Ham 'n' Swiss, Sub Roll Hot	1	500	23	7	2	0
Turkey Sub	1	550	27	7	2	0
Potato, Baked Deluxe	1	736	36	16	7	4
Potato, Baked Plain	1	355	0	0	7	8
Chowder, Boston Clam	1 serving	190	9	3	1	
Fries, Curly	1 serving (3.5 oz)	300	15	3	0	0
Fries, French	1 serving (2.5 oz)	246	13	3	0	0

Food	Portion	Calories	Fat	Sat Fat	Fiber	Rating
Soup, Lumberjack Mixed Vegetable	1 serving (8 oz)	90	4	2	1	3
Soup, Wisconsin Cheese	1 serving	280	18	7	2	0
Salad, Garden	1	61	1	0	5	6
Apple Turnover	1	330	14	7	0	0
Polar Swirl Heath	1	543	22	5	0	0
Polar Swirl Oreo	1	329	22	10	0	0
Arby's Sauce	1 serving	15	0	0	0	4
Italian Reduced Calorie	1 serving	20	1	0	0	4
Thousand Island	1 serving	260	26	4	0	0
BLIMPIE (6-inch subs)						
5 Meatball	1	500	22	8	2	0
Beef, Roast	1	340	5	1	2	5
Blimpie Best	1	410	13	5	4	1
Chicken, Grilled	1	400	9	2	2	2
Ham Salami	1	590	28	11	3	0
Tuna	1	570	32	5	2	0
Turkey	1	320	5	1	3	5
Grilled Chicken Salad	1 serving	350	12	0	0	1
BOSTON MARKET						
½ chicken with skin	1 serving	630	37	19	0	0
¼ dark meat chicken, no skin	1 serving	210	10	3	0	0
¼ dark meat chicken with skin	1 serving	330	22	6	0	0
¼ white meat chicken, no skin or wing	1 serving	160	4	1	0	4
¼ white meat chicken with skin	1 serving	330	18	5	0	0
Salad, Caesar	1 serving	520	43	12	3	2
Sandwich, ham & turkey club with cheese & sauce	1	890	44	20	4	0
Sandwich, ham & turkey club w/o cheese & sauce	1	430	6	2	4	6
Beans, BBQ Baked	¾ cup	330	9	3	9	4
Casserole, green bean	¾ cup	170	5	2	2	4
Cornbread	1	200	6	2	1	1
Macaroni & cheese	¾ cup	280	10	6	1	2
Potatoes, homestyle mashed with gravy	¾ cup	200	9	5	2	4
Potatoes, mashed	⅔ cup	180	8	5	2	4
Squash, butternut lowfat	¾ cup	160	6	4	3	4
Stuffing	¾ cup	310	12	2	3	2
Vegetables, steamed lowfat	⅔ cup	35	1	0	3	10

Food	Portion	Calories	Fat	Sat Fat	Fiber	Rating
BURGER KING						
BK Big Fish Sandwich	1	720	43	9	3	0
BK Broiler Chicken Sandwich	1	530	16	5	2	0
Cheeseburger	1	380	19	9	1	0
Chicken Tenders	8 pieces	350	22	7	1	0
Hamburger	1	330	15	6	1	0
Whopper	1	640	39	11	3	0
Whopper with Cheese	1	730	46	16	3	0
Whopper Jr	1	420	24	8	2	0
Whopper Jr with Cheese	1	460	28	10	2	0
Fries	1 medium	370	20	5	3	0
Fries, coated	1 medium	400	21	8	4	0
Salad w/o dressing	1	60	3	2	2	8
DENNY'S						
Burger, Classic	1	673	40	15	3	0
Cod, battered with tartar sauce	1 serving	732	47	7	3	2
Chicken Quesadilla	1 serving	827	55	23	2	1
Chicken, fried	1 serving	327	18	4	1	1
Gardenburger Patty Only	1	160	3	0	3	8
Pork chop with gravy	1 serving	386	24	8	0	0
Pork chop, senior	1 serving	193	12	4	0	0
Sandwich, club	1	485	35	6	na	0
Sandwich, fish, fried	1	905	56	8	3	0
Sandwich, patty melt	1	695	44	13	2	0
DOMINO'S PIZZA						
(14-inch Large Pizzas)						
Deep Dish Cheese	2 slices	455	20	8	3	2
Hand Tossed Cheese	2 slices	317	10	5	3	3
Thin Crust Cheese	⅙ of a pie	253	11	5	2	1
with extra cheese	1 topping serving	45	4	2	0	0
with fresh mushrooms	1 topping serving	3	0	0	0	4
with Italian sausage	1 topping serving	44	3	1	0	1
with pepperoni	1 topping serving	55	5	2	0	0
Buffalo Wings	1 piece	50	2	1	0	1
Cheesy Bread	1 piece	103	5	2	0	0
HARDEE'S						
Cheeseburger	1	310	14	6	na	0
Cheeseburger, Mesquite Bacon	1	370	18	7	na	0
Cheeseburger, Quarter Pound Double	1	470	27	11	na	0
Chicken breast, fried	1	370	15	4	na	0
Chicken leg, fried	1	170	7	2	na	0
Chicken sandwich, grilled	1	350	11	2	na	0
Hamburger	1	270	11	3	na	0

Food	Portion	Calories	Fat	Sat Fat	Fiber	Rating
Roast Beef, regular	1	320	16	6	na	0
The Works Burger	1	530	30	12	na	0
Fries	1 large	430	18	5	na	0
Salad, garden	1	220	13	9	na	0
Salad, grilled chicken	1	150	3	1	na	6
Salad, side	1	25	0	0	na	6
Big Cookie	1	280	12	4	na	0
Vanilla, cone	1	170	2	1	na	4
Strawberry Sundae	1	210	2	1	na	4
KENTUCKY FRIED CHICKEN						
Extra Tasty Crispy Breast	1	470	28	7	1	0
Extra Tasty Crispy Thigh	1	370	25	6	2	0
Original Recipe Breast	1	400	24	6	1	0
Original Recipe Thigh	1	250	18	5	1	0
Tender Roast Breast with Skin	1	251	11	3	0	0
Tender Roast Breast w/o Skin	1	169	4	1	0	4
Tender Roast Thigh with Skin	1	207	12	4	0	0
Tender Roast Thigh w/o Skin	1	106	6	2	0	4
Biscuit	1	180	10	3	0	0
Coleslaw	1 serving (5oz)	180	9	2	3	4
Corn on the Cob	1 ear	150	2	0	2	10
Macaroni & cheese	1 serving (5.4 oz)	180	8	3	2	4
Mashed potatoes with gravy	1 serving (4.8oz)	120	6	1	2	4
LITTLE CAESAR'S						
Crazy Bread	1 piece	106	3	1	1	4
Crazy Sauce	1 serving (6 oz)	170	0	0	1	4
Sandwich, Deli-Style Italian	1	740	37	12	3	0
Sandwich, Deli-Style Veggie	1	647	29	9	4	0
Sandwich, Hot Oven Baked Meatsa	1	1036	56	24	5	0
Pan!Pan! Cheese	1 medium slice	181	6	3	1	4
Pan!Pan! Pepperoni	1 medium slice	199	8	4	1	0
Pizza!Pizza! Cheese	1 medium slice	201	7	4	1	0
Pizza!Pizza! Pepperoni	1 medium slice	220	9	4	1	0
MAX & IRMA'S						
Black Bean Roll Up	1 serving	401	8	3	na	na
Garden Grill	1 serving	467	7	3	na	na
Gourmet Garden Grill	1 serving	484	8	3	na	na
Pasta, Grilled Zucchini and Mushroom	1 serving	448	10	4	na	na
Pasta, Grilled Zucchini and Mushroom, with Chicken	1 serving	621	18	6	na	na

Food	Portion	Calories	Fat	Sat Fat	Fiber	Rating
MCDONALD'S						
Big Mac	1	560	31	10	3	0
Cheeseburger	1	320	13	6	2	1
Chicken McNuggets	6	290	17	4	0	0
Chicken, Grilled Deluxe	1	440	20	3	3	0
Chicken, Grilled Deluxe Plain without Mayonnaise	1	300	5	1	3	6
Fish Filet Deluxe	1	560	28	6	4	0
Hamburger	1	260	9	4	2	1
Quarter Pounder	1	420	21	8	2	0
Quarter Pounder with Cheese	1	530	30	13	2	0
Fries	1 large	450	22	4	5	0
Fries	1 super	540	26	5	6	0
Apple Pie, Baked	1	260	13	4	0	0
Danish, Apple	1	360	16	5	1	0
Cookies, McDonaldland	1 package	180	5	1	1	1
PIZZA HUT						
Cheese, Hand Tossed	1 slice	280	10	5	2	1
Cheese Pan	1 slice	300	14	6	2	1
Cheese Stuffed Crust	1 slice	380	11	5	4	1
Meat Lover's Hand Tossed	1 slice	290	11	5	3	1
Pepperoni Hand Tossed	1 slice	260	9	4	3	2
Pepperoni Lover's Hand Tossed	1 slice	320	13	6	4	1
Veggie Lover's Pan	1 slice	240	9	4	3	2
SUBWAY (6-inch sandwiches)						
B.L.T.	1	327	10	na	na	na
Club	1	297	5	na	na	5
Cold Cut Trio	1	344	13	na	na	1
Italian B.M.T.	1	430	22	na	na	0
Roast Beef	1	295	5	na	na	5
Tuna with light mayonnaise	1	376	15	na	na	0
Turkey breast	1	213	4	na	na	5
Turkey breast & ham	1	271	5	na	na	5
Veggie Delight	1	219	3	na	na	6
Hot Subway Melt	1	357	12	na	na	1
TACO BELL						
Burrito, 7 Layer	1	530	23	7	13	0
Burrito, bean	1	380	12	4	13	5
Nachos	1 serving	320	18	4	3	0
Nachos Bellgrande	1 serving	770	39	11	17	0
Rice, Mexican	1 serving	190	9	4	1	1
Salad, Taco with Salsa	1	850	52	15	16	0
Taco	1	180	10	4	3	2
Taco, Double Decker	1	340	15	5	9	3

Food	Portion	Calories	Fat	Sat Fat	Fiber	Rating
Taco, Grilled Chicken Soft	1	240	12	4	3	2
Taco, Soft	1	220	10	5	3	2
Taco, Soft Supreme	1	260	14	7	3	1
Taco, Supreme	1	220	14	7	3	1
Tostada	1	300	15	5	12	3
Wrap, Veggie Fajita	1	420	19	5	3	1
Wrap, Steak Fajita	1	470	21	6	3	0
WENDY'S						
Cheeseburger, Jr. Bacon	1	380	19	7	2	0
Cheeseburger, Jr.	1	320	13	6	2	0
Chicken, breaded	1	440	18	4	2	0
Chicken Club	1	470	20	4	2	0
Chicken, Spicy Sandwich	1	410	15	3	2	0
Hamburger, plain Single	1	360	16	6	2	0
Hamburger, Single with everything	1	420	20	7	3	0
Pita, Chicken Caesar with Dressing	1	490	18	5	4	0
Pita, Garden Veggie with Dressing	1	400	17	4	5	1
Chicken Nuggets	5 pieces	230	16	3	0	0
Potato, baked, chili & cheese	1	630	24	9	9	0
Salad, Deluxe Garden without dressing	1	110	6	1	3	6
Salad, grilled chicken without dressing	1	200	8	2	3	2
Salad, side without dressing	1	60	3	0	2	6
Fries	1 Biggie	470	23	4	6	0
Potato, baked plain	1	310	0	0	7	10

Sauces and Dressings

DIPS

BREAKSTONE'S						
Bacon & Onion	2 tablespoons	60	5	3	0	0
Free French Onion	2 tablespoons	25	0	0	0	4
French Onion	2 tablespoons	50	5	3	0	0
CHEEZ WHIZ						
Medium Cheese & Salsa	2 tablespoons	100	8	5	0	0
CHI CHI'S						
Fiesta Bean	2 tablespoons	35	2	1	1	6

Food	Portion	Calories	Fat	Sat Fat	Fiber	Rating
Fiesta Cheese	2 tablespoons	40	3	1	0	4
GUILTLESS GOURMET						
Black Bean Mild	1 oz	25	0	0	1	6
Black Bean Spicy	1 oz	25	0	0	1	6
Pinto Bean	1 oz	25	0	0	1	6
KRAFT						
Avocado	2 tablespoons	60	4	3	0	0
Bacon & Horseradish	2 tablespoons	60	5	3	0	0
Free Ranch	2 tablespoons	25	0	0	0	4
French Onion	2 tablespoons	60	4	3	0	0
Premium Sour Cream						
French Onion	2 tablespoons	45	4	3	0	0
LAY'S						
Low Fat Sour Cream & Onion	2 tablespoons	40	1	0	0	4
LOUISE'S						
Fat Free Honey Mustard	1 oz	40	0	0	0	4
Fat Free White Cheese	1 oz	25	0	0	0	4
RUFFLES						
Low Fat French Onion	1 tablespoon	40	1	0	0	4
TACO BELL						
Fat Free Black Bean	2 tablespoons	30	0	0	2	6
Salsa Con Queso Medium	2 tablespoons	45	3	1	0	5
Salso Con Queso Mild	2 tablespoons	45	3	1	0	5
Salsa, Chile,						
Green Tomatillo, Rosarita	2 tablespoons	10	0	na	1	4
Salsa, Thick & Chunky, Pace	2 tablespoons	10	0	na	1	4

DRESSINGS

Food	Portion	Calories	Fat	Sat Fat	Fiber	Rating
Cheese, Cheddar,						
All Natural, Kraft	1 tablespoon	60	4		0	1
Horseradish, prepared	1 tablespoon	6	0	0	0	4
Jelly, assorted flavors	1 teaspoon	6	0	0	0	4
Mayonnaise	1 tablespoon	99	11	2	na	0
Mayonnaise, reduced calorie	1 tablespoon	34	3	1	0	4
Mayonnaise, fat-free, Kraft	1 tablespoon	10	0	0	0	10
Mayonnaise, light, Kraft	1 tablespoon	50	5	1	0	2
Mayonnaise, Kraft	1 tablespoon	100	11	2	0	0
Miracle Whip Free	1 tablespoon	15	0	0	0	10
Miracle Whip light	1 tablespoon	35	3	0	0	5
Miracle Whip	1 tablespoon	70	7	1	0	0
Mustard, Dijon, Grey Poupon	1 teaspoon	5	0	0	0	4

Food	Portion	Calories	Fat	Sat Fat	Fiber	Rating
Mustard, yellow, prepared	1 teaspoon	5	0	na	0	4
Pickle relish, dill, Vlasic	1 tablespoon	5	0	na	1	4
Gravy, chicken	¼ cup	25	1	na	na	

SALAD DRESSINGS

Food	Portion	Calories	Fat	Sat Fat	Fiber	Rating
Blue Cheese	2 tablespoons	130	13	3	trace	0
French	2 tablespoons	150	13	2	0	0
Italian	2 tablespoons	110	11	1	0	0
Ranch	2 tablespoons					
Sweet & Sour	2 tablespoons	160	13	2	0	0
Thousand Island	2 tablespoons	110	10	2	0	0
KRAFT						
⅓ Less Fat Italian	2 tablespoons	70	7	1	0	0
⅓ Less Fat Ranch	2 tablespoons	110	11	2	0	0
Free Italian	2 tablespoons	20	0	0	0	4
Free Ranch	2 tablespoons	50	0	0	1	4
Honey Mustard	2 tablespoons	110	10	2	0	0

GRAVY

Food	Portion	Calories	Fat	Sat Fat	Fiber	Rating
Au jus, dehydrated, prepared	1 cup	32	1		3	5
Mushroom, Franco-American	¼ cup	25	1	na	na	3
Turkey, Franco-American	¼ cup	30	2	na	na	3
PILLSBURY						
Brown	¼ cup	15	0	0	0	6
Chicken	¼ cup	25	1	0	0	6

SAUCES

Food	Portion	Calories	Fat	Sat Fat	Fiber	Rating
Barbecue, ready to serve	1 cup	188	5		2	4
Bernaise, dehydrated	1 serving	362	9		0	0
Catsup, tomato, regular	2 tablespoons	30	0	0	1	4
Chili, Hunt's	1 serving	117	0	0	6	5
Cocktail, Kraft	¼ cup	60	1	0	1	4
Curry, dry mix, made with milk	1 cup	269	15		1	0
Enchilada, Rosarita	1 oz	6	0	0	0	4
Marinare Ventian, Newman's Own	½ cup	60	2	0	3	8
Peanut, House of Tsang	1 tablespoon	45	3		1	3
Peppers, hot chili, red, canned, sauce	1 cup	51	2	0	5	4
Pizza, Ragu	1 cup	120	4		4	6
Plum, Canned, La Choy	1 tablespoon	20	0	0	0	4
Soy	1 tablespoon	10	0	0	0	4

Food	Portion	Calories	Fat	Sat Fat	Fiber	Rating
Spaghetti, Bombolina, Newman's Own	½ cup	100	5	2	5	5
Spaghetti, Chunky Garden, Ragu	½ cup	120	4	1	3	5
Spaghetti, Garlic-Herb & Ex Chunky Garden, Healthy Choice	1 cup	100	1	0	4	6
Spaghetti, Sun-dried Tomato, Classico	1 cup	160	9	na	4	4
Spaghetti, Sweet Peppers & Onions, Classico	4 oz	50	4	na	na	3
Spaghetti, Regular, Prego	4 oz	130	5	na	na	3
Sandwich Spread, Kraft	1 tablespoon	50	4	1	0	1
Stroganoff mix, prepared	1 cup	272	11		1	1
Sweet & Sour, Kraft	2 tablespoons	60	0	0	0	4
Taco, Green, LaVictoria	1 tablespoon	0	0	0	1	4
Taco, Red, Taco Bell	1 tablespoon	5	0	0	1	4
Tamari	1 tablespoon	10	1	0	0	4
Tartar	2 tablespoons	90	9	2	0	0
Teriyaki, Lawry's	2 tablespoons	72	0	0	0	4
Tomato, canned	1 cup	74	0	0	3	6
Tomato, Italian Recipe, S&W	1 cup	70	0	0	4	6
White	1 cup	241	13	6	0	0

Snack Foods

GRANOLA BARS

Quaker

Food	Portion	Calories	Fat	Sat Fat	Fiber	Rating
Chewy chocolate Coated chocolate Chip	1	132	7	4	1	3
Chewy raisin	1	191	8	4	2	3
Chocolate chip	1	124	5	3	1	3
Peanut butter, chewy	1	121	5	1	1	3
Plain chewy	1	126	5	2	1	3

CARNATION

Honey & Oats	1	130	4	2	1	3

GENERAL MILLS

Nature Valley, Cinnamon	1	120	5	1	1	3

KUDOS

Chocolate Chunk	1	90	3	1	1	4
Low Fat Blueberry	1	90	2	0	1	4

Food	Portion	Calories	Fat	Sat Fat	Fiber	Rating
Low Fat Strawberry	1	80	2	0	1	4
NATURE'S CHOICE						
Carob Chip	1	80	3	0	2	5
Oats 'n' Honey	1	80	2	0	2	5
POTATO CHIPS						
Barbecue	1 oz	139	9	2	0	0
Light	1 oz	134	6	1	0	0
Regular	1 oz	152	10	3	0	0
LAY'S						
Baked KC Masterpiece	1 oz	120	3	0	2	8
Baked Original	1 oz	110	2	0	2	8
Salt & Vinegar	1 oz	150	10	na	1	2
WOW Original	1 oz	75	0	0	1	5
LOUISE'S						
1g Mesquite BBQ	1 oz	110	1	na	2	8
70% Less Fat Original	1 oz	110	3	na	2	8
PRINGLES						
Fat Free	1 oz	75	0	0	2	8
Original	1 oz	160	11	3	1	2
Right Original	1 oz	140	7	2	1	2
RUFFLES						
Cheddar Cheese & Sour Cream	1 oz	160	10	3	1	2
French Onion	1 oz	150	10	3	1	2
Regular	1 oz	150	10	2.5	1	2
Reduced Fat	1 oz	140	7	1	1	2
TORTILLA CHIPS						
Nacho	1 oz	141	7	1	2	4
DORITOS						
Nacho Cheese	1 ozs	140	7		1	2
Reduced Fat Nacho	1 oz	130	5	1	1	2
Reduced Fat Cooler Ranch	1 oz	130	5	1	1	2
Wow Nacho Cheese	1 oz	90	1	na	1	6
TOSTITOS						
Baked Original	1 oz	110	0	0	2	8
Chips	1 oz	140	8	1	1	2
CORN CHIPS						
Plain	1 oz	153	10	1	1	2

Food	Portion	Calories	Fat	Sat Fat	Fiber	Rating
Puffs Cheese	1 oz	157	10	2	0	0
FRITOS						
Crisp 'N' Thin	1 oz	160	10	na	1	2
Dip Size, Fritos	1 oz	150	10	na	1	2
PLANTERS						
Corn Chips	1 oz	170	10	2	2	4

PRETZELS

Food	Portion	Calories	Fat	Sat Fat	Fiber	Rating
Chocolate covered	1 oz	130	5	2	na	na
Whole Wheat	1 oz	103	1	0	2	9
ROLD GOLD						
Bavarian	3 pieces	120	2	na	na	na
Fat Free Hard Sourdough	1	80	0	0	1	6
Fat Free Thins	1 oz	100	0	0	1	6
Sticks	1 oz	110	2	na	1	6
SNYDER'S						
Rods	1 oz	310	0	0	na	na
Sourdough Hard Honey Mustard & Onion	1 oz	130	5	1	0	2

RICE CAKES

Food	Portion	Calories	Fat	Sat Fat	Fiber	Rating
PRITIKIN						
Multigrain	1	35	0	0	na	na
Plain	1	35	0	0	na	na
QUAKER						
Apple Cinnamon	1	50	0	0	0	4
Mini Apple Cinnamon	5	50	0	0	0	4
Mini White Cheddar	6	50	0	0	0	4
Salted	1	35	0	0	0	4

POPCORN CAKES

Food	Portion	Calories	Fat	Sat Fat	Fiber	Rating
Popcorn cake	1	38	0	0	0	4
Popcorn Bars, Caramel, General Mills	1	70	1	1	0	4
Chocolate Peanut Crunch Mini, Orville Redenbacher's	6	60	1	0	1	6
QUAKER						
Butter Popped	1	35	0	0	2	9
Cheddar Cheese Mini	6	50	1	na	1	6

Food	Portion	Calories	Fat	Sat Fat	Fiber	Rating
POPCORN						
Air-popped	1 cup	31	0	0	2	8
Cheese	1 cup	58	4	1	1	2
Cracker Jack, Original	1 oz	120	3	na	na	
JIFFY POP						
Bag Butter	3 cups	90	5	1	2	4
Microwave Butter	4 cups	140	7	na	na	
LOUISE'S						
Fat Free Apple Cinnamon	1 oz	100	0	0	na	
Fat Free Caramel	1 oz	100	0	0	na	
NEWMAN'S OWN						
Microwave Butter	3½ cups	170	11	2	3	4
Microwave Butter Light	3½ cups	110	3	1	3	8
Microwave Light Natural	3½ cups	110	3	1	3	8
ORVILLE REDENBACHER'S						
Gourmet Hot Air	3 cups	40	0	na	3	8
Microwave Gourmet Butter	3 cups	100	6	1	3	4
Gourmet Cheddar Cheese	3 cups	130	8	2	3	4
Microwave Gourmet Light Butter	3 cups	70	3	1	3	8
POP SECRET						
Microwave 94% Fat Free Butter	6 cups	110	2	0	4	8
Microwave Light Butter	6 cups	120	5	1	4	5
WEIGHT WATCHERS						
Butter	1 package	90	3	0	3	8

Sweets, Candies and Desserts

Food	Portion	Calories	Fat	Sat Fat	Fiber	Rating
CANDY						
Butterscotch	1 piece	24	0	0	0	3
Candy corn	1 oz	105	0	0	na	3
Caramels	1 piece	31	1	1	na	3
Gumdrops	10 small	135	0	0	na	3
Hard Candy	1 oz	106	0	0	na	3
Jelly Beans	10 small	40	0	0	na	3
Lollipop	1	22	0	0	na	3
Circus Peanuts, Brock	11 pieces	260	0	0	na	3
Gummy Bears, Brock	5 pieces	130	0	0	na	3
Breath Mints, Certs	1 piece	6	0	0	na	3
Good 'N' Fruity Candy	1 box	140	1	na	2	3

Food	Portion	Calories	Fat	Sat Fat	Fiber	Rating
Jolly Rancher Candies	3 pieces	60	0	0	na	3
Lifesavers Roll Five Flavor	2 pieces	20	0	0	na	3
Lifesavers Roll Pep-O-Mint	3 pieces	20	0	0	na	3
Payday Candy Bar	1 bar	240	12	2	2	0
Skittles Original Flavors	1 package	250	3	1	0	2
Starburst Original Fruits	8 pieces	160	3	1	0	2
Switzer's Licorice Bites	12 pieces	46	0	0	na	3
Tootsie Roll Candy	1	110	2	0	na	3

CHOCOLATE CANDY

Food	Portion	Calories	Fat	Sat Fat	Fiber	Rating
Peanuts, chocolate covered	1.4 oz	210	14	5	2.5	0
Pretzels, chocolate covered	1 oz	130	5	2	na	0
100 Grand	1 bar	200	8	5	0	0
3 Musketeers	1 bar	260	8	4	1	0
Baby Ruth	1 bar	270	13	7	2	0
Butterfinger	1 bar	280	11	6	1	0
Chunky Bar	1 bar	200	11	6	2	0
Junior Mints Candies	1 package	190	4	3	na	0
M&M's, Almond	1.5 oz	220	12	4	2	0
M&M's, Mint	1.5 oz	200	9	5	1	0
M&M's, Peanut	1.5 oz	220	11	5	2	0
M&M's, Peanut Butter	1.6 oz	240	13	8	2	0
M&M's, Plain	1.5 oz	200	9	5	1	0
Milk Duds	1 box	230	8	6	0	0
Milky Way Bar	1 bar	280	11	5	1	0
Nestle Crunch	1 bar	230	12	7	1	0
Raisinets	1 package	200	8	4	2	0
Reese's Peanut Butter sticks	1	120	7	3	na	0
Snickers Bar	1 bar	280	14	5	1	0
Snickers, Peanut Butter bar	1 bar	310	20	7	1	0
Twix, Caramel	1 oz	140	7	3	0	0
Twix, Peanut Butter	1 bar	130	8	3	1	0
Whoppers Candy	1 package	230	10	8	1	0
York Peppermint Patty	1 snack size	57	1	1	na	3

CHOCOLATE

Food	Portion	Calories	Fat	Sat Fat	Fiber	Rating
Bitter, for baking	1 oz	145	15	9	4	0
Chips, Semi-Sweet Morsels, Nestle	30 chips	70	4	3	2	0
Chips, sweet, German	5 oz	60	4	2	0	0
Cocoa, Powder, Nestle	1 tablespoon	15	1	0	na	3
Cocoa, Mix, Nestle's Quick	2 tablespoons	75	1	0	na	3
Fudge, chocolate, plain	1 oz	115	3	na	0	0
Semisweet, Baker's	1 square	140	10	6	2	0
Unsweetened, Nestle	¼ bar	80	7	2	3	0
White, Baking, Nestle	¼ bar	80	5	3	0	0

Food	Portion	Calories	Fat	Sat Fat	Fiber	Rating
BROWNIES						
Brownie Bites, Hostess	5	260	14	na	2	na
Brownie Bites, Walnut, Hostess	5	270	15	na	2	na
German Chocolate Supreme, Betty Crocker	1/18 of package	160	7	2	1	na
Supreme Mix, Betty Crocker	1/18 of package	140	6	1	1	na
Supreme with Walnuts Mix, Betty Crocker	1/18 of package	140	7	1	1	na
CAKES						
Apple Spice Crumb, Fat Free, Entenmann's	⅛ of cake	130	0	na	2	3
Banana, Suzy Q's, Hostess	1 cake	220	10	na	1	2
Banana Crunch, Entenmann's	⅛ of cake	220	9	na	0	2
Banana Crunch, Fat Free, Entenmann's	⅛ of cake	140	0	na	2	3
Blueberry Crunch, Fat Free, Entenmann's	⅛ of cake	140	0	0	2	3
Boston Crème, Supreme, Pepperidge	⅛ of cake	260	9	na	1	2
Butter Chocolate, Supermoist, Betty Crocker	1/12 of package	190	4	na	1	3
Butter, Mix, Pillsbury Plus	1 serving	170	3	na	1	3
Cake, Banana Mix, Pillsbury Plus	1 serving	190	4	na	0	3
Carrot, Entenmann's	⅛ of cake	290	16	na	0	1
Carrot, Fat Free, Entenmann's	⅛ of cake	170	0	0	1	3
Carrot, Supermoist Mix	1 serving	180	3	na	1	2
Cheesecake, Frozen, Sara Lee	¼ of cake	330	12	na	2	1
Cheesecake, Frozen, Weight Watchers	1 slice	180	6	na	1	2
Cheesecake, New York Style, Jell-O	1 serving	175	3	na	0	3
Chocolate Free & Light, Sara Lee	1 slice	110	0	0	2.4	3
Chocolate Fudge, 3 Layer, Pepperidge	1/6 of cake	300	16	na	2	1
Chocolate Fudge, Entenmann's	1/6 of cake	320	15	na	2	1
Chocolate Fudge, Supermoist, Betty Crocker	1/12 of package	180	4	na	1	
Chocolate Fudge, Iced, Fat Free, Entenmann's	1/6 of cake	210	0	0	2	3
Chocolate Loaf, Fat Free, Entenmann's	⅛ of loaf	130	0	0	1	2
Chocolate Mousse, Light, Pepperidge	⅛ cake	190	9	na	0	1

Food	Portion	Calories	Fat	Sat Fat	Fiber	Rating
Cinnamon Apple Coffee, Fat Free, Entenmann's	⅛ of cake	130	0	0	2	3
Cinnamon Streusel Swirl Mix	1 serving	200	5	na	0	2
Coconut, 3 Layer, Pepperidge	⅙ of cake	300	14	na	1	1
Coffee Crumb, Sara Lee	⅛ of cake	220	9	na	1	1
Crème, Regular, Hostess	1 cake	190	5	na	0	2
Crumb, Hostess	1 cake	105	4	na	0	2
Crumb, Light, Hostess	1 cake	75	0.5	0	0	2
Cupcake, Chocolate, Hostess	1 cake	170	5	na	1	2
Cupcake, Chocolate, Light, Hostess	1 cake	120	1	0	0	2
Cupcake, devil's food with chocolate icing	1 cupcake	120	4	na	0	1
Devil's Food, Layer, Pepperidge	1 oz	111	5	na	0	1
Devil's Food, Light, Supermoist, Betty Crocker	1/10 of package	210	5	na	1	3
German Chocolate Mix, Supermoist	1 serving	180	4	na	1	1
German Chocolate, Entenmann's	⅙ of cake	320	16	na	1	1
Gingerbread Mix	1 slice	175	4	na	2	3
Golden, Fudge Iced, Fat Free, Entenmann's	⅙ of cake	220	0	na	2	3
Golden, Thick Fudge, Entenmann's	⅙ of cake	330	16	na	2	1
Golden, French Crumb, Fat Free, Entenmann's	⅛ of cake	140	0	na	2	3
Golden Pound, Classic Dessert Mix	1 serving	190	8	na	0	1
Lemon Mix, Supermoist	1 serving	180	4	na	0	2
Lemon Chiffon, Classic Dessert Mix	1 serving	190	4	na	0	2
Pound, All-Butter, Sara Lee	¼ of cake	320	16	na	0	1
Pound, Hostess	⅕ of cake	350	16	na	1	1
Sheet, no icing, home recipe	1 slice	315	12	na	1	1
Sno Balls, Hostess	1 cake	160	5	na	1	2
Sour Cream Chocolate, Supermoist, Betty Crocker	1/12 of package	190	5	na	1	1
Spice Mix, Supermoist	1 serving	180	4	na	0	2
Strawberry Mix, Pillsbury Plus	1 serving	180	4	0	1	2
Strawberry shortcake	1 serving	344	9	na	2	1
Streusel with icing, mix	1 slice	172	8	na	1	1
Suzy Q's, Hostess	1 cake	220	9	na	2	1
White, Pillsbury Plus	1 serving	180	4	na	1	2
White/chocolate icing, home recipe	1 slice	271	11	na	1	1
Yellow Mix, Pillsbury Plus	1 serving	180	5	na	1	2

Food	Portion	Calories	Fat	Sat Fat	Fiber	Rating
COOKIES						
Animal Crackers, Sunshine	14 pieces	140	4	1	0	2
Arrowroot, Nabisco	1	20	1	na	0	2
Chocolate Chip, Barbara's	1	85	1	na	2	2
Chocolate Chip, Fiber, Keebler	1	70	4	na	1	2
Chocolate Chip, Pillsbury	1	70	3	na	0	2
Chocolate Cinnamon, Teddy Grahams	1 serving	70	3	na	0	2
Chocolate Fudge Sandwich, Keebler	1	80	4	na	0	2
Chocolate Wafer, Nabisco	1	28	1	na	0	2
Fancy Peanut Chunk, Health Valley	1	45	2	na	1	2
Fiber Jumbo, Health Valley	1	100	3	na	3	3
Fig, Ultra Slim Fast	1	60	1	0	1	2
Fig Bar, Sunshine	2	110	3	1	1	2
Fig Bar, Whole Wheat, Fat Free, Mother's	1	70	0	0	1	2
Fig Newton, Nabisco	1	55	1	0	1	2
Fig Newton, Fat Free, Nabisco	1	50	0	0	1	3
Fortune, La Choy	1	15	0	0	0	1
French Vanilla Crème, Keebler	1	80	4	0	0	1
Fruit Centers, Fat Free, Assorted Flavors, Health Valley	1	25	0	0	1	2
Fruit Centers, Regular, Health Valley	1	70	1	0	4	2
Fruit Centers, Raspberry, Health Valley	1	70	0	0	2	2
Fruit Centers, Jumbo, Health Valley	1	70	1	0	4	3
Fruit, Golden, Apple, Sunshine	1	80	2	0	0	2
Fruit, Golden, Cranberry, Sunshine	1	70	1	0	0	2
Fruit & Nut, Barbara's	1	85	4	0	2	1
Fudge Royals, Mini	15	160	8	na	1	1
Ginger Snaps, Sunshine	7	130	5	na	0	1
Grahams, Fudge Dipped, Sunshine	4	170	9	1	1	2
Grammy Bears, Sunshine	10	140	5	6	1	1
Health Chip, Health Valley	1	100	0	1	4	3
Healthy Grahams, Health Valley	1	110	3	0	3	3
Honey Jumbo, Cinnamon, Health Valley	1	70	2	na	1	1
Honey Jumbo, Oat Bran, Health Valley	1	60	2	na	2	2
Honey Jumbo, Peanut, Health Valley	1	70	2	na	1	1
Macaroon	1	90	5	na	0	1
Molasses, Iced, Bakery Wagon	1	100	3	na	1	1
Oat Bran, Apple, Fiber, Keebler	1	70	3	1	1	1

Food	Portion	Calories	Fat	Sat Fat	Fiber	Rating
Oat Bran, Fruit Jumbos, Health Valley	1	60	2	na	2	2
Oat Bran Fruit/Nut, Health Valley	1	110	4	na	3	1
Oatmeal, Country Style, Sunshine	3	170	7	2	1	1
Oatmeal, Fiber Enriched, Keebler	1	70	3	na	1	1
Oatmeal, Iced, Sunshine	1	60	3	1	0	1
Oatmeal, Keebler	1	80	4	na	0	1
Oatmeal Chocolate Chip, Fat Free, Entenmann's	2	80	0	0	1	1
Oatmeal Raisin, Health Valley	1	100	0	0	3	3
Oatmeal Raisin, Pillsbury	1	60	2	na	0	1
Original Vanilla, Fiber Classic	1	210	8	na	0	1
Peanut Butter, Fiber Classic	1	220	9	na	7	2
Peanut Butter Mix	1	50	3	na	0	1
Peanut Butter, Pillsbury	1	70	3	na	0	1
Sandwich, Chocolate, Ultra Slim Fast	3	130	3	na	1	1
Sandwich, Choc/Cream, SnackWell's	1	50	1	0	0	1
Sandwich, Hydrox, Sunshine	1	50	2	0	0	1
Sandwich, Hydrox, Reduced Fat, Sunshine	1	43	1	na	0	1
Sandwich, Oreo, Nabisco	1	53	2	0	0	1
Sandwich, Peanut Butter, Nutter Butter Bites, Nabisco	10	150	7	2	1	1
Sandwich, Vanilla/Crème Filling, Snackwells	1	55	1	0	1	1
Sugar, Fiber Enriched, Keebler	1	70	3	na	1	1
Sugar, Old Fashioned, Keebler	1	80	3	na	1	1
Sugar, Pillsbury	1	70	3	na	0	1
Sugar Wafer/Crème Filling, Lady Lee	1	40	2	na	0	1
Tea Biscuit, Peek Freans	1	40	1	na	0	1
Vanilla, Dixie, Sunshine	2	120	5	na	1	1
Vanilla Wafer, Nabisco Nilla Wafers	7	150	7	2	0	1
Vienna Fingers, Sunshine	1	70	3	1	0	1
Vienna Fingers, Low Fat, Sunshine	1	65	1.8	na	0	1
Wheat-Free, The Great, Health Valley	1	40	1.5	na	2	1

PIES

Food	Portion	Calories	Fat	Sat Fat	Fiber	Rating
Apple, French, Hostess Fruit Pie	1 pie	410	19	na	2	1
Apple, Homestyle, Entenmann's	1/6 of pie	300	14	na	2	1
Apple, Hostess Fruit Pie	1 pie	410	19	na	2	1

Food	Portion	Calories	Fat	Sat Fat	Fiber	Rating
Apple, Mrs. Smith	1/6 of pie	270	11	2	1	1
Apple Beehive, Fat Free, Entenmann's	1/5 of pie	270	0	0	2	3
Banana Cream, Mrs. Smith's	1/4 of pie	250	9	3	1	1
Banana custard	1 cup	396	16	na	1	1
Blackberry, 2 crusts, baked	1 cup	467	21	na	6	2
Blackberry, Hostess Fruit Pie	1 pie	400	17	na	2	1
Blueberry	1/8 cup	360	18	4	3	1
Blueberry, Hostess Fruit Pie	1 pie	400	17	na	2	1
Butter Tarts, Baked	1 cup	534	15	na	2	1
Cherry, Hostess Fruit Pie	1 pie	430	19	na	1	3
Cherry Beehive, Fat Free, Entenmann's	1/5 of pie	270	0	0	1	3
Cherry Streusel, Free/Light, Sara Lee	1 slice	160	2	na	1	1
Chocolate meringue	1 cup	474	22	na	3	1
Coconut custard	1 cup	421	22	na	3	1
Custard	1/8 cup	262	11	4	1	1
Lemon, Hostess Fruit Pie	1 pie	420	20	na	1	1
Lemon chiffon	1 cup	454	18	na	1	2
Lemon meringue, Sara Lee	1/6 of pie	350	11	3	5	1
Mince, Mrs. Smith's	1/6 of pie	300	11	2	2	1
Peach, Hostess Fruit Pie	1 pie	400	18	na	2	1
Pecan	1/8 cup	502	27	5	4	1
Pineapple, Hostess Fruit Pie	1 pie	400	16	na	2	1
Pumpkin	1/8 cup	316	14	5	4	1
Pumpkin custard, Mrs. Smith's	1/5 of pie	270	8	2	1	1
Rhubarb, 2 crusts, baked	1 cup	486	21	na	3	1
Strawberry	1 cup	345	14	na	4	1
Strawberry, Hostess Fruit Pie	1 pie	390	18	na	2	1
Sweet potato	1 cup	381	20	na	2	1
Pie crust, baked, prepared from mix	1	743	47	na	4	1
Pie crust, graham, Keebler	1 slice	110	5	na	0	1
Pie filling, cherry, canned	1 serving	85	0	na	1	4
Pie filling, apple, canned	1 serving	74	0	na	0	4

PUDDINGS

Food	Portion	Calories	Fat	Sat Fat	Fiber	Rating
Chocolate, as prepared, Jell-O	1/2 cup	150	3	2	0	4
Chocolate, Ready-to-eat, Hunt's	1 serving	160	6	na	0	2
Chocolate, sugar free with skim milk, Jell-O	1/2 cup	80	0	0	0	4
Chocolate Fudge, Lite, Ready-to-eat, Jell-O	1 serving	101	1	na	0	1

Food	Portion	Calories	Fat	Sat Fat	Fiber	Rating
Chocolate/Caramel, Ready-to-eat, Jell-O	1 serving	175	6	na	1	2
Chocolate/Vanilla, Lite, Ready-to-eat, Jell-O	1 serving	104	2	na	1	3
Coconut, instant	1 serving	383	4	na	0	1
Coconut, cream	½ cup	157	3	na	na	1
Corn	1 cup	273	13	na	1	1
Custard, baked	1 cup	305	15	na	1	1
Double chocolate, Yoplait	1 serving	180	4	na	1	1
Flan, caramel custard, prepared, 2% Milk	1 cup	270	5	na	1	1
Fudge/milk chocolate, Ready-to-eat, Jell-O	1 serving	171	6	na	1	1
Gelatin, typical variety with or w/o sugar	1 oz	18	0	na	0	2
Lemon, dry mix, Jell-O	⅙ of package	50	0	na	0	2
Milk chocolate, Ready-to-eat, Jell-O	1 serving	173	6	na	0	1
Mousse, Chocolate, Instant, Prep, San Sucre	1 cup	150	3	na	0	2
Mousse, skim milk	1 cup	140	4	na	0	2
Rice with Raisins	1 cup	387	8	na	1	1
Tapioca Cream, Starch, Home Recipe	1 cup	220	8	na	1	1
Vanilla, Regular, Dry	1 serving	325	0.4	na	0	3
Vanilla/Chocolate, Ready-to-eat, Jell-O	1 serving	178	6	na	1	1

OTHER SWEETS & PASTRIES

Food	Portion	Calories	Fat	Sat Fat	Fiber	Rating
Apple Butter	1 tablespoon	37	0	0	0	3
Apple Crisp, Berkshire, Pepperidge	1 oz	53	2	1	1	3
Apple Crisp, Easy Delicious, Betty Crocker	⅕ of package	310	11	na	3	1
Apple Dumplings, Pepperidge	1 oz	87	4	na	0	2
Banana Chips	1 oz	147	10	na	2	1
Carob Powder	1 oz	51	0	0	2	4
Carob Chips	1 serving	151	9	na	2	1
Chutney, Mango	1 cup	632	0	0	7	6
Cobbler, Frozen, Weight Watchers	1 slice	160	6	na	1	1
Danish, Black Forest, Fat Free, Entenmann's	⅑ of package	130	0	0	2	2
Danish, Orange with Icing, Pillsbury	1	150	7	na	1	1
Danish, Plain	1	250	14	na	1	1
Éclair, Custard with Chocolate Icing	1	239	14	na	1	3

Food	Portion	Calories	Fat	Sat Fat	Fiber	Rating
Éclair, Weight Watchers	1	150	5	na	2	2
Honey, Strained/Extracted	1 tablespoon	65	0	0	0	2
Honey, Strained or Extracted	1 cup	1016	0	0	1	3
Jam/Preserves, Regular	1 tablespoon	55	0	0	0	4
Jam/Preserves, Strawberry, Low Calorie	1 teaspoon	8	0	0	0	3
Marmalade, Citrus	1 tablespoon	49	0	0	0	3
Marmalade	1 oz	67	0	0	1.0	3
Muffin, Apple Streusel, Hostess Breakfast	1	100	1	0	1	3
Muffin, Blueberry, Hostess Breakfast	1	100	1	0	1	3
Pastry Pockets, Pillsbury	1	240	13	na	1	2
Pears, Candied	1 cup	566	1	0	4	1
Pecan Danish Ring, Entenmann's	⅛ package	130	15	na	1	1
Pecan Spinners, Hostess	1 piece	110	5	na	1	2
Pineapple, Candied	1 cup	590	1	0	1	2
Raspberry Cheese, Fat Free, Entenmann's	⅑ package	140	0	0	1	1
Roll, Cinnamon with Icing, Pillsbury	1	110	5	na	0	1
Sugar, beet, maple or cane	1 cup	666	0	0	1	1
Swirls, Caramel Pecan, Hostess	1 swirl	250	15	na	1	1
Toaster pastries, Strawberry, Kellogg's Pop Tarts	1	210	6	2	1	1
Toaster pastries, Frosted Blueberry/ Cherry, Kellogg's Pops Tarts	1	200	5	na	1	1
Topping, strawberry or pineapple	1 cup	863	1	0	2	3
Turnover, Apple, Pepperidge	1	330	14	na	6	1
Turnover, Apple, Pillsbury	1	170	8	na	1	1
Turnover, Cherry, Pepperidge	1	320	13	na	6	1
Turnover, Cherry, Pillsbury	1	170	8	na	7	1
Turnover, Peach, Pepperidge	1	340	15	na	6	1
Twinkie, Hostess	2	280	9	na	1	1
Sugar, brown, packed	1 cup	828	0	0	na	1
Sugar, powdered	1 tablespoon	31	0	0	na	1
Sugar, white	1 tablespoon	45	0	0	na	1
Sugar substitute, Sweet 'N Low	1 package	4	0	0	na	4

DONUTS

Food	Portion	Calories	Fat	Sat Fat	Fiber	Rating
Plain	1	210	14	3	1	1
Chocolate glazed	1	250	14	3	1	1
Powdered	1	310	19	4	1	1
Coffee roll	1	280	13	3	2	1
Yeast donut, jelly filled	1	240	10	3	1	2

Food	Portion	Calories	Fat	Sat Fat	Fiber	Rating
FRUIT-FLAVORED PRODUCTS						
Health Valley Fruit Bars:						
Apple, fat free	1	140	1	0	4	7
Apricot, fat free	1	140	1	0	4	7
Date, fat free	1	140	2	na	4	7
Raisin, fat free	1	140	1	0	4	7
Oat Bran Jumbo	1	140	2	na	4	7
Rice Bran Jumbo	1	160	5	na	4	7
Real Fruit, Assorted, Barbara's	1 bar	50	0	0	0	3
Taz. Devil Snack, B.Crocker	1 pouch	90	1	0	0	3
X-Men Snacks, B. Crocker	1 pouch	90	1	0	0	3

Endnotes

Chapter 1

1. *The Journal of the American Medical Association (JAMA)*, Dec. 1, 1999, Vol. 282, No. 21, p. 2068
2. *JAMA*, June 4,1973, Vol. 224, No. 10, pp. 1418-1419
3. *Dr. Atkins' New Diet Revolution*, p. 173
4. *Natural Health*, June 1999, p. 103

Chapter 2

1. *Scientific American*; Gaining of Fat, Aug. 1996, Vol. 275(2), pp. 88-94
2. Sister Tribe Avoids Health Pitfalls, *The Arizona Republic*, Nov. 2, 1999
3. *Journal of Clinical Endocrinology and Metabolism*, July 1991, No. 73, pp.156-165
4. Fujimoto WY: *Nature, Nurture, and the Metabolic Epidemiology of Diabetes-The Saga of Japanese in America*; 59th Annual Scientific Sessions of ADA, San Diego, California, 1999
5. Golay et al., *American Journal of Clinical Nutrition*, 1996, 63:174-178
6. *Natural Health*, June 1999, p. 100
7. *International Journal of Obesity*, 1987, 11 Suppl 1:9-25

Chapter 3

1. Piatti PM et al., *Metabolism*, 1994, 43:1481-1487
2. *American Journal of Clinical Nutrition*, 1993, 58:398; *European Journal of Clinical Nutrition*, 1994, 48:591
3. Linkswiler HM et al., *Protein-Induced Hypercalciuria*, Fed Proc, 40:2429-2433, 1981
4. *American Journal of Epidemiology*, 1996, 143:472
5. *American Journal of Clinical Nutrition*, 1998, 48:880-883
6. www.healthwealthsolutions.com
7. *Journal of Gerontology*, 1976, 31:155; *New England Journal of Medicine*, 1982, 307:652

Chapter 4

1. *Dr. Atkins' New Diet Revolution*, p. 4

2. *Ibid.*, p. 338

3. *Natural Health,* June 1999, p. 100

4. *Ibid.,* June 1999, p. 100

5. *Public Health Nutrition,* Sept. 1999, 2(3A):363-368

6. *Journal of Clinical Endocrinology and Metabolism,* 1991, 73:156-165

7. *Natural Health,* June 1999, p. 100

8. *Diabetes Care,* June 1999, 22(6):889-895

9. *JAMA,* 1999, Oct. 27:282(16):1539-1546

10. *Natural Health,* June 1999, p. 101

11. *Ibid.,* June 1999, p. 103

12. McNamara, DJ, et al., *Journal of Clinical Investigation,* 1987, 79:1729-1739; Wood, PD, et al., *Dietary Regulation of Cholesterol Metabolism; Lancet,* 1966, 2:604-607; Keys A, ed., *Coronary Heart Disease in Seven Countries:* American Heart Association, Monograph 29, Circulation, 1970, 41(suppl 1): 1-211

13. *Natural Health,* June 1999, p. 141

14. *Ibid.,* June 1999, p. 141

15. *Dr. Atkins' New Diet Revolution,* p. xii

16. *Ibid.,* p. xii

17. *Ibid.,* p. 4

18. *JAMA,* June 4, 1973, Vol. 224, No. 10

19. *Dr. Atkins' New Diet Revolution,* p. 4

20. *Ibid.,* p. 6

21. *Journal of the American Dietetic Association,* April 1990, 90(4):534-540

22. *The American Journal of Clinical Nutrition,* Feb. 1996, 63(2):174-178.

23. *Dr. Atkins' New Diet Revolution,* p. 10

24. *Ibid.,* pp. 22-23

25. *Ibid.,* p. 59

26. *Ibid.,* pp. 63-64

27. *Journal of Clinical Investigation,* 1966; 45 1648

28. *Dr. Atkins' New Diet Revolution,* p. 65

29. *Ibid.,* pp. 144-145

30. *Ibid.,* p. 153

31. *Ibid.,* p. 153

32. *Ibid.,* p. 172

33. *Ibid.,* p. 184

34. www.americanheart.org

35. www.mayohealth.org/mayo/9706/htm/medical.htm

36. *Dr. Atkins' New Diet Revolution,* p. 48

37. *Nutrition Action Health Letter,* March 2000
38. *Dr. Atkins' New Diet Revolution,* p. 103
39. *Ibid.,* p. 195
40. *Nutrition Action Health Letter,* March 2000, Vol. 27, No. 2, p. 6
41. *Dr. Atkins' New Diet Revolution,* p. 197
42. *American Journal of Clinical Nutrition,* April 1995, 61(4 Suppl):960S-967S
43. *Dr. Atkins' New Diet Revolution,* p. 203
44. Nutrition Society Proceedings, U.K., May 1999, 58(2):243-248
45. Surgical Clinics of North America, October 1986, 66(5):917-929
46. *International Journal of Cancer,* Suppl 1998, 11:85-89
47. *Dr. Atkins' New Diet Revolution,* p. 205
48. *Ibid.,* p. 234
49. *Ibid.,* pp. 268, 276-277
50. *Ibid.,* p. 319
51. *Journal of Nutrition,* 1982, 112:338-349
52. *American Journal of Clinical Nutrition,* 1993, 58:398; *European Journal of Clinical Nutrition,* 1994; 48:591; *Calcified Tissue International,* 1992, 50:14

Chapter 5

1. *American Journal of Clinical Nutrition,* May 1994, 59 (5 Suppl):1153S-1161S
2. *JAMA,* Dec. 1, 1999, Vol. 282, No. 21
3. *Lancet,* 1966, 2:604-607; *Journal of Clinical Investigation,* 1987, 79; 1729-1739
4. *JAMA,* Dec. 1, 1999, Vol. 282, No. 21
5. *JAMA,* 1986, 256:2849-2858; *Archives of Internal Medicine,* 1991, 151:1181-1187; *Cardiology Clinics,* 1996, Feb:14(1):69-83
6. *JAMA,* 1991, 265:3285-3291
7. *JAMA,* Dec. 16, 1998, Vol. 280, No. 23
8. *Journal of the American Dietetic Association,* 1997, 97:151-156
9. *American Journal of Clinical Nutrition,* 1988, 48:830-832; *American Journal of Clinical Nutrition,* 1988, 48:833-836; *Public Health Nutrition:* 1(1), 33-41
10. *Archives of Family Medicine,* 1995, 4:551-554; *JAMA,* 1995, 274:894-901; *JAMA,* Dec. 16, 1998, Vol. 280, No. 23
11. *New England Journal of Medicine,* July 1, 1993, 329(1):21-26
12. *Canadian Journal of Cardiology,* Oct. 1995, 11 Suppl G:55G-62G

13. *JAMA*, Nov. 26, 1997, Vol. 278, No. 20
14. *Annals of Epidemiology*, Sept. 1993, 3(5):550-554
15. *New England Journal of Medicine*, 1997, 336:1117-1124
16. *JAMA*, March 24/31, 1999, Vol. 281, No. 12
17. *Public Health Report*, July-Aug. 1987, Suppl:22-5
18. *Diabetes Care*, Feb. 1988, 112:160-73

Chapter 7

1. The nutritional adequacy of a vegetarian diet is obtained from *Position of the American Dietetic Association: Vegetarian Diets* (1997)
2. *American Journal of Clinical Nutrition*, 1994, 59:1356-1361
3. *Ibid.*, 1994, 59(suppl):1238S-1241

Chapter 9

1. *New England Journal of Medicine*, 1976, 263:935
2. *Exercise Physiology* by McArdle, et al., 1986, 549
3. *Journal of Consulting and Clinical Psychology*, 1979, 47:898; *International Journal of Obesity*, 1981, 5:57

Chapter 12

1. www.detnews.com/2000/health/0003/19/A12-19027.htm

Chapter 13

1. *British Medical Journal*, Jan. 1, 2000, 320:53
2. *Mortality and Morbidity Weekly Review*, Jan. 28, 2000, 49(o3):49-53
3. *Newsletter of the University of California*, School of Public Health, August 1997

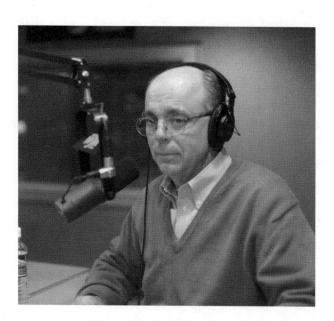

Fred W. Stransky, Ph.D.

Fred W. Stransky, Ph.D., is Director of the Meadow Brook Health Enhancement Institute at Oakland University in Rochester, Michigan. For nearly three decades, he has been a pioneer in advocating disease prevention and a healthy lifestyle in Michigan and nationwide.

Dr. Stransky received his Bachelor's and Master's degrees in Education from the University of Miami at Coral Gables, Florida. He earned his Ph.D. in Exercise Science from Florida State University, where he was an offensive lineman on the Hurricanes football team for two years. In 1999, he served as Adjunct Professor to the College of Osteopathic Medicine at Michigan State University. His first book, *Fitness and Fallacies,* with Rick DeLorme, was published in 1990.

He came to Oakland University in 1973 and established numerous programs emphasizing health promotion and disease prevention. These programs represented some of the earliest attempts in Michigan to emphasize the importance of disease prevention and the role of lifestyle in containing health care costs. Among the most celebrated have been the Institute's Primary Prevention Program; a Preventive Medicine Rotation in Internal Medicine and Family Practice, through which Dr. Stransky has trained more than 500 physicians; and the Cardiac Rehabilitation Program, the first Phase III program in the State of Michigan.

Dr. Stransky has presented to more than 20,000 people across the country including General Motors, ITT, DuPont, DaimlerChrysler and the United States Government, as well as hospitals, school districts, physician associations and other community and corporate groups.

He is host of the popular radio program, *The Secrets to Good Health*, on Detroit-based WJR-AM 760, one of the oldest and most-heard radio stations in the nation. He also serves as a health advisor to two of Michigan's professional sports teams —the Detroit Pistons and the Detroit Lions.

The Meadow Brook Health Enhancement Institute, designed and created by Dr. Stransky, offers unique preventive medicine programs that help patients assume more responsibility for their health. The Institute's programs address the lifestyle aspects of good health, nutrition, weight control, physical fitness, substance control and stress management. The goal is to give patients a greater feeling of well-being and to prevent chronic degenerative diseases, hypertension and obesity. The Institute also offers cardiac rehabilitation, corporate health promotion and special programs for women, older adults and diabetics and can be contacted at:

Meadow Brook Health Enhancement Institute
Oakland University
Rochester, Michigan 48309-4401
(248) 370-3198
fwstrans@oakland.edu

R. Todd Haight

Todd Haight is President of Todd Haight Communications in Rochester, Michigan. He has been writing professionally for more than 22 years, since joining a community newspaper as a reporter at the age of 15. After five years in the print and broadcast media, he worked in the field of health care marketing and public relations for 13 years, much of that in management, before opening his consulting firm.

Todd Haight Communications has provided media and publicity for the 1998 North American International Auto Show Charity Preview in Detroit; national presentations for insurance executives; executive media training and marketing consultation; and publicity for clients' celebrity appearances of Gen. Colin Powell, Penelope Leach, Dr. T. Barry Brazelton and U.S. Surgeon General Dr. David Satcher, among others.

Todd earned his Bachelor's degree in Journalism from Oakland University and his Master's degree in Advertising from Michigan State University. He has earned six professional awards for writing, communications, publications and photography.

Pamela Hardin

A native of San Diego, California, Pamela Hardin is an accomplished and diversified artist who, for the past 30 years, has worked in acrylic color, oil paint, water color and pencil.

Her subject matter includes portraits, wildlife, landscapes and still life. Pam's favorite theme is the southwestern United States, such as various historical and contemporary Indian tribal portraits, mountain men, cowboys, pony and "Buffalo" soldiers.

Pam was asked for input to the Smithsonian Institution Indian Museum, and has had commissioned work hang in offices at the U.S. Senate office building, the Pentagon and the White House. She currently lives and maintains her "Back In Time" Portrait and Fine Art studio in Tyrone, Georgia.

Yvonne Moses

Yvonne Moses, Dietician for the Meadow Brook Health Enhancement Institute for more than six years, received her bachelor's degree in Dietetics from Western Michigan University. A registered dietician, she directs the Institute's successful Weight Management Program and leads nutrition lectures for cardiac rehabilitation patients and participants in the 60+ and Just For Women programs at the MBHEI. She also lectures primary care physicians who rotate through the Institute.

Yvonne has worked for the Maternal Support Services and Infant Support Services programs offered by the Oakland County Health Department and Saginaw County Health Department, both in Michigan. For more than six years, she has also served as a nutrition consultant for the Detroit Public Schools' Head Start Program.